Key Concepts in
Mental Health

The SAGE Key Concepts series provides students with accessible and authoritative knowledge of the essential topics in a variety of disciplines. Cross-referenced throughout, the format encourages critical evaluation through understanding. Written by experienced and respected academics, the books are indispensable study aids and guides to comprehension.

Fifth Edition

Key Concepts in
Mental Health

DAVID PILGRIM

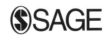

Los Angeles | London | New Delhi
Singapore | Washington DC | Melbourne

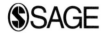

Los Angeles | London | New Delhi
Singapore | Washington DC | Melbourne

SAGE Publications Ltd
1 Oliver's Yard
55 City Road
London EC1Y 1SP

SAGE Publications Inc.
2455 Teller Road
Thousand Oaks, California 91320

SAGE Publications India Pvt Ltd
B 1/I 1 Mohan Cooperative Industrial Area
Mathura Road
New Delhi 110 044

SAGE Publications Asia-Pacific Pte Ltd
3 Church Street
#10-04 Samsung Hub
Singapore 049483

Editor: Alex Clabburn
Assistant Editor: Jade Grogan
Production Editor: Manmeet Kaur Tura
Copyeditor: Sarah Bury
Proofreader: Sharon Cawood
Indexer: Martin Hargreaves
Marketing Manager: George Kimble
Cover Design: Wendy Scott
Typeset by: C&M Digitals (P) Ltd, Chennai, India
Printed in the UK

Library of Congress Control Number: 2019943671

British Library Cataloguing in Publication data

A catalogue record for this book is available from
the British Library

ISBN 978-1-5264-9314-9 (HB)
ISBN 978-1-5264-9313-2 (PB)

At SAGE we take sustainability seriously. Most of our products are printed in the UK using responsibly sourced
papers and boards. When we print overseas we ensure sustainable papers are used as measured by the PREPS
grading system. We undertake an annual audit to monitor our sustainability.

Contents

contents

List of Figures and Tables

FIGURES

TABLES

About the Author

David Pilgrim is Honorary Professor of Health and Social Policy, University of Liverpool, and Visiting Professor of Clinical Psychology, University of Southampton. After training and working as a clinical psychologist, he completed a PhD examining psychotherapy in the organisational setting of the British NHS. He then went on to complete a Master's in sociology. He has worked at the boundary between clinical psychology and medical sociology for the past 30 years and has produced more than a hundred articles based upon his research into mental health policy and practice that were published in peer-reviewed journals. His years working in the British NHS provided him with extensive everyday experience of the theoretical and policy aspects of mental health expressed in practical settings. One of his books, *A Sociology of Mental Health and Illness* (3rd edn, Open University Press, 2005), co-authored with Anne Rogers, won the British Medical Association's Medical Book of the Year Award for 2006. The sixth edition is set to be published in 2020. His most recent sole-authored book, *Critical Realism for Psychologists*, will be published by Routledge in 2019.

Publisher's Acknowledgements

The publisher is grateful to the following academics for their feedback and insights provided for this fifth edition:

Peter Hall, University of Suffolk

Herbert Mwebe, Middlesex University

Carlos Pires, University of Coimbra

Robin Sen, University of Sheffield

Louise Ward, La Trobe University

publisher's
acknowledgements

xiii

Author's Acknowledgement

I want to repeat acknowledgements from earlier editions. I am particularly grateful to Anne Rogers for working with me since 1993 on editions of *A Sociology of Mental Health and Illness*, which has informed many entries here. I have also been helped in my editing task by conversations in recent years with Richard Bentall, Roy Bhaskar, Mary Boyle, Pat Bracken, Tim Carey, Jacqui Dillon, Chris Dowrick, Bill Fulford, John Hall, Dave Harper, Lucy Johnstone, Peter Kinderman, Eleanor Longden, Ann McCranie, Nick Manning, Joanna Moncrieff, Nimisha Patel, John Read, Helen Spandler, Nigel Thomas, Phil Thomas, Floris Tomasini and Ivo Vassilev. In the preface to the first edition of this book, I acknowledged an even longer list of helpers, who remain important here. As with the previous editions, any errors of omission or commission, which might be spotted in the coming pages by the reader, are my responsibility alone.

David Pilgrim

Introduction to the Fifth Edition

This new edition allows me to update the entries, re-order them a little, lose some with less utility and add a few new ones. This editing has been enabled by useful feedback about the previous edition. Where I have deleted some entries, the material involved has not been lost but incorporated elsewhere in the book. Where I have added entries, this is in response to some changes in practice and the challenges that current service organisation poses for practitioners on the ground. I would emphasise, though, that the book is not intended to guide specific forms of practice for particular practitioners. It primarily offers a generic resource from, and for, an interdisciplinary community of students and researchers.

The book is divided into four parts: Mental Health, Mental Abnormality, Mental Health Services and Mental Health and Society. However, sometimes an entry could have been placed in a different part than the one allocated. For example, I have put 'Secondary Prevention' in Part 3: Mental Health Services because it connects readily to its neighbour on 'Primary Care'. It could have gone easily in either the part on Mental Abnormality or even Mental Health and Society.

Not surprisingly, a recurring discussion about all of the editions to date has been about terminology. The dilemma, about which words to use reasonably but inoffensively, is always present when discussing mental health. This is hardly surprising, given that most of the discussion tends to arise when the latter 'breaks down'. When that happens, there are often negative personal and social connotations, such as stigma, and a range of other proven personal disadvantages for those who become identified as patients in a new role in society. This encourages an understandable reticence about mental health problems in any discussion by professionals, lay people or politicians. In past times, a similar reluctance could be found about TB, cancer and epilepsy.

Today, calling 'a mental disorder' or 'a mental illness' 'a mental health problem' is an example of this cautious and euphemistic feature. Journalists (and even some experts) can get into tangles, such as talking vaguely about 'mental health issues'. They might also use the oxymoronic term 'people with a mental health diagnosis'. The highly inexact term 'issue' reflects and compounds a lack of clarity about our focus of concern. Also, it sounds very odd to speak of 'people with a physical health diagnosis', so why is this verbal strategy used about our topic? These semantic somersaults and tentative euphemisms suggest a particular conceptual fuzziness about our topic; a dilemma created and compounded by its causes being highly contested and its consequences being typically negative.

Extending this point about ambiguity, we talk about 'mental health services' in a large and undifferentiated conceptual lump but we are much more specific about services for those with a diagnosis of diabetes or stroke, for example.

This suggests a particular uncertainty about what is being referred to and the range of people implicated. Is it only about risky people in touch, voluntarily or under duress, with statutory 'mental health services'; maybe what, with more justification (because of medical dominance), used to be called 'psychiatric services'? If not, then does it include the vast number of people seen only by their General Practitioner, but on repeat prescriptions of antidepressants for year after year? (Once benzodiazepines were discredited, these drugs became a blunderbuss medical response to any form of distress in community settings.)

Given that most of us at some time in our lives are distressed or dysfunctional and have incorrigible quirks that affect our relationships with others, then should we all be part of this undifferentiated conceptual lump? But if no distinctions can feasibly be made in reality, then why are we talking unendingly about our topic at all? Arguably, we could just give up on a hopeless or irresolvable area of inquiry. Moreover, if attributions about psychological differences in society include crime, sexuality and identity (to name three key controversies in recent times), should they be discussed in the same breath as 'mental health' or not?

We will all answer these questions in our own way but posing them highlights the ambiguity of the topics addressed in this book. This ensures an unending discourse about proper scientific definitions, which may or may not map readily and satisfactorily onto daily reality. Moreover, if we are honest, few simple policy or professional answers can be offered to humanity's social and existential complexity. Many of us are 'tired of living and scared of dying' and we are coping with that (or not) in our idiosyncratic ways. Indeed, I wonder whether the reason that 'mental health' is discussed so often by politicians and professionals, without resolution, is that in truth we are all confused about how to talk about the topic and what to do in practice, once the talking is over.

The certainties that are sometimes offered by government ministers, neuroscientists, biological psychiatrists or psychotherapeutic gurus might be a sort of whistling in the dark. The 'more resources' mantra from the first of these, and those lobbying them, would only be persuasive if we already had genuine proven answers about coherent policies and effective interventions. The implication of this logic is that 'more of the same' is a future solution when it is not, given that so much confusion, ignorance and practical failure have been evident to date.

What we do have are evidence-based clues about how wellbeing could be improved in the general population and how individuals who are distressed, unintelligible or dysfunctional might be helped in a compassionate way (although 'cure' tends to remain largely a pipedream). This more modest picture should come through in several of the entries in this book. I, like others, have no simple answers but I still make decisions in the midst of the confusion. Arguably, the part of the book headed 'Mental Abnormality' is an outmoded and offensive term. However, I have opted to retain it deliberately in order to highlight a social scientific point about norms.

Societies vary in the content of their norms. However, citizens who are sane by common consent always make some sort of distinction between those transgressing them and those who do not. An aspect of norms is that we largely tend to notice our everyday social world when 'things go wrong' (note my point above about the 'breakdown' of mental health being when it tends to come to our attention). This is one reason why the sociology of deviance has been recurrently interested in mental disorder, with the word 'disorder' really connoting not minds but conduct in its social context. To confirm this point, we do not habitually discuss 'mental order' because when rules are followed and role expectations fulfilled then life tends to go on unnoticed. As guardians of that implied 'mental order', professionals face a range of challenges, which can be *angst* ridden in their daily work. I have put a new entry at the end of Part 3: 'Challenges for Practitioners', to reflect this point.

Returning to the matter of language, I have altered some diagnostic terminology in the entry titles. For example, what was 'Personality Disorders' has been replaced by 'Challenging Conduct in Children and Adults'. This phrasing is not euphemistic but deliberately connotes again the normative character of psychiatric labelling. People can be and sometimes are both distressed and distressing to others (or if you prefer, 'troubled and troubling'). Alongside the new entry on 'Challenging Conduct in Adults and Children' in Part 2, I have also included: 'Temporo-Spatial Aspects of Mental Abnormality'. This subsumes the entry on 'Cross-Cultural Psychiatry', which was in the previous edition. Finally, in light of the recent policy discussion about the topic, I have included a new entry in Part 4: 'The Mental Health Impact of Social Media'.

To be clear, a recognition that our social context is a source of both causes and judgements about distress, dysfunction and incorrigibility does not imply for me a completely open-ended cultural relativism. Fear and sadness are part of the human condition in all times and places and non-conformity of some variety in any society *ipso facto* is ever present. Similarly, there have always been those acting in an unintelligible manner to their fellows. Responses of some sort 'from above and below' to deviations from expectations of psychological normality are evident in some way or other, on a continuum from sacralisation, admiration and tolerance to gentle paternalistic correction, strict authoritarian control and even murder. For example, we can contrast recent libertarian campaigns to remove legal controls over psychiatric patients (and opposing arguments from paternalists) to a period in Germany in the early 1940s, when they were systematically exterminated on the grounds that they were 'life devoid of meaning'. Thus, differences in norms about what is, or is not, mentally healthy, and what to do in response to transgressions, are certainly varied but they are by no means unlimited. Consequently, we can spot patterns of resemblance, not just unending difference, over time and place.

Some of the above points will be repeated and elaborated in several entries but they are offered by way of introduction to provide a context to the subject's complexity for any readers new to the topic of 'mental health'. I hope that all of these edits have improved the relevance of this book for a general readership.

Part I
Mental Health

Mental Health

DEFINITION

Mental health is used positively to indicate a state of psychological wellbeing, negatively to indicate its opposite (as in 'mental health problems') or euphemistically to indicate facilities used by, or imposed upon, people with mental health problems (as in 'mental health services').

KEY POINTS

- Three different uses of the phrase 'mental health' are examined.
- Reasons for the use of 'mental health' in preference to other terms, such as 'mental illness', are discussed.

Alternative connotations of the term 'mental health' indicated in the above opening definition will be discussed below, in relation to positive mental health, mental health services and mental health problems.

- *'Mental health' as a positive state of psychological wellbeing* A sense of wellbeing is considered to be part of health, according to the World Health Organization (WHO), which in 1951 described it as: 'the capacity of the individual to form harmonious relations with others and to participate in, or contribute constructively to, changes in his social or physical environment' (WHO, 1951: 4). This has been built on over time (see entry on Mental Health Promotion). Various attempts have been made to describe mental health positively by psychoanalysts (Kubie, 1954) and social psychologists (Jahoda, 1958). The latter reviewer described the term 'mental health' as being 'vague, elusive and ambiguous'. The range of definitions offered can be challenged on a number of grounds, related to their compatibility with one another and their internal consistency (Rogers and Pilgrim, 2014). Existential psychologists such as Maslow (1968) developed the idea of 'self-actualisation', which refers to each person fulfilling their human potential. But what if a person self-actualises at the expense of the wellbeing of others? Similarly, a statistical norm can be used to define mental health, but what of a society which contains unjust and destructive norms? One recurrent difficulty with defining positive mental health is the same one that dogs the definition of mental illness or mental disorder: it is not easy to draw a clear line between normal and abnormal mental states. Differences in norms over time and place are the main undermining factors in such attempts. What is normal in one society may not be so in another. Similarly, definitions of psychological normality and abnormality can vary over time in the same society. Is homosexuality a mental abnormality? Are hallucinations indicative of a spiritual gift or a mental illness? Posing these sorts of questions highlights the impermanent dividing line between mental health and mental abnormality.

- *'Mental health' as a prefix to describe one part of health services* Since the Second World War, the term 'mental health services' has now replaced that of 'psychiatric services' (although the latter is still sometimes used). Prior to the Second World War, there were hospitals, clinics and asylums. These were either under parochial control, with a 'voluntary' or charitable history, or they served a specialist regional or national function. At that time, though, they were not called 'services'. As Webster (1988) notes, prior to the NHS in Britain, there was an admixture of charitable hospitals and medical relief offered to those in the workhouse system. This is why many of the older general hospitals were adapted poorhouse buildings. However, a major exception to this mixed picture was the network of dedicated mental illness and mental handicap hospitals which, since the Victorian period, had been funded and run by the state (Scull, 1979). The notion of a 'health service', post-1948, when the NHS was founded, reflects a shift towards a coherent system of organisation and a notion of a publicly available resource (at the 'service' of the general population). Currently in Britain, most specialist mental health services are within the NHS. In addition, there are privately run mental health facilities. These vary from small nursing homes to large hospitals which receive NHS patients who cannot be accommodated by local NHS mental health services. With devolution in the UK, specific policies about mental health service organisation now vary from one country to another (Department of Health, 1998, 1999; Scottish Office, 1997; Welsh Assembly Government, 2002).

- *'Mental health' as a prefix to 'problems'* Just as the term 'mental health services' has probably carried a euphemistic value for those responsible for them (managers and politicians), the same is true of the term 'mental health problems'. By adding 'problems', to invert a notion of 'mental health', a less damning and stigmatising state can be connoted. The professional discourse of diagnosis ('schizophrenia', 'bipolar disorder', and so on) is stigmatising. Indeed, sometimes psychiatrists simply do not communicate diagnoses such as these to their patients because of their negative connotations. In this context, the term 'mental health problems' may be less offensive to many parties. However, this might simply be a diversionary euphemism and perhaps not persuasive as a tactic to avoid stigma for those with the label.

The terms 'mental health services' and 'mental health problems' may have been encouraged for additional reasons to those noted above. During the 19th century in Britain, all patients were certified under lunacy laws. That is, the state only made provisions for the control of madness. The fledgling profession of psychiatry (this term was first used in Britain in 1858) was singularly preoccupied with segregating and managing lunatics (Scull, 1979). With the onset of the First World War in 1914, soldiers began to break down with 'shell shock' (now called 'post-traumatic stress disorder') (Stone, 1985). From this point on, psychiatry extended its jurisdiction from madness to versions of nervousness provoked by stress or trauma.

Later, in the 20th century, more abnormal mental states came within its jurisdiction, such as those due to alcohol and drug abuse and personality problems.

Today, 'mental health services' may be offered to, or imposed upon, people with this wide range of problems, although madness or 'severe mental illness' still captures most of the attention of professionals. In this context, 'mental illness service' would be too narrow a description of the range of patients under psychiatric jurisdiction. The more accurate description, of 'mental disorder services', would be more inclusive. However, this term has not emerged in the English-speaking world. Also, the term 'psychiatric service' does not accurately reflect the multidisciplinary nature of contemporary mental health work. So, for now, the term 'mental health service' serves as a compromise description. It avoids some inaccuracies but, in some respects, it is also mystifying.

Another aspect of the term 'mental health problems' is that some people, critical of psychiatric terminology, would object on scientific or logical grounds to notions like 'mental illness' or 'mental disorder'. An acceptable alternative for these critics is 'mental health problems', although another, currently favoured alternative is 'mental distress'. Thus, use of the term 'mental health problems', and the even more vague 'mental health issues', sidesteps the potential offence created by psychiatric diagnoses, given that the latter do not have scientific or personal legitimacy for everyone.

See also: *mental health promotion; psychiatric classification; wellbeing*.

FURTHER READING

de Swaan, A. (1990) *The Management of Normality*. London: Routledge.
Rose, N. (1990) *Governing the Soul*. London: Routledge.
Shephard, B. (2002) *A War of Nerves: Soldiers and Psychiatrists, 1914–1994*. London: Pimlico.

REFERENCES

Department of Health (DH) (1998) *Modernising Mental Health Services*. London: DH.
Department of Health (DH) (1999) *A National Service Framework for Mental Health*. London: DH.
Jahoda, M. (1958) *Current Concepts of Positive Mental Health*. New York: Basic Books.
Kubie, S. (1954) 'The fundamental nature of the distinction between normality and neurosis', *Psychoanalytical Quarterly*, 23: 167–204.
Maslow, A.H. (1968) *Toward a Psychology of Being*. Princeton, NJ: Princeton University Press.
Rogers, A. and Pilgrim, D. (2014) *A Sociology of Mental Health and Illness* (5th edn). Maidenhead: Open University Press.
Scottish Office (1997) *A Framework for Mental Health Services in Scotland*. Appendix to NHS MEL (1997) SODD Circular 30/97. Edinburgh: Scottish Office.
Scull, A. (1979) *Museums of Madness: The Social Organization of Insanity in 19th Century England*. Harmondsworth: Penguin.
Stone, M. (1985) 'Shellshock and the psychologists', in W.E. Bynum, R. Porter and M. Shepherd (eds), *The Anatomy of Madness*, Vol. 2. London: Tavistock.
Webster, C. (1988) *The Health Services since the War*. London: HMSO Books.
Welsh Assembly Government (2002) *Adult Mental Health Services: A National Service Framework for Wales*. Cardiff: Welsh Assembly Government.
World Health Organization (WHO) (1951) *Technical Report Series No. 31*. Geneva: WHO.

mental health

Wellbeing

DEFINITION

*Wellbeing (or well-being) is now a common term and yet it defies a simple defini-
tion. It can be conflated with contentment, the common good, quality of life, mental
health or even health as a whole. Various permutations of cognitive elements (especially about meaning) and affective elements (especially about happiness) are connoted when the word is used.*

KEY POINTS

- Wellbeing can be defined in a range of ways.
- It has become an important priority for politicians in the developed world as
  an alternative or additional goal to economic prosperity.
- It is now an opportunity for the political advancement of the mental health
  professions.
- The derivation and nature of wellbeing are discussed in a variety of ways by
  religious and secular disciplines.

The ambiguities noted in the definition above are unpacked below in summary.
When we look at the psychological literature on wellbeing, we find a range of
authorities with overlapping concerns about how humans can live their lives to the
full (Ryff and Singer, 1998). For example, we find preferred terms such as 'self-
actualisation' (Maslow, 1968); 'individuation' (Jung, 1933); 'the will to meaning'
(Frankl, 1958); 'personal development' (Erikson, 1950); 'basic life tendencies'
(Buhler, 1972); 'the fully functioning person' (Rogers, 1962); and 'maturity'
(Allport, 1961).

HEDONIC AND EUDEMONIC ASPECTS OF WELLBEING

Since antiquity, the concerns of the above writers have broadly focused on positive
mood (being happy in a predominant or sustained way in life) or on positive meaning and fulfilment. The former are 'hedonic' and the latter 'eudemonic' aspects of
wellbeing. Hedonism was a philosophy that emphasised the pursuit of pleasure,
whereas eudemonia (or 'eudaimonia') from Aristotle emphasised the pursuit of a
meaningful life (Ackrill, 2006). The two can go together in our experience but not
always. For example, we might find meaning in suffering in various forms, such as
being depressed (Andrews and Thomson, 2009).

Our chances of subjective wellbeing are at their best if we live peaceably with
a network of good friends and have enough money to avoid poverty. People with
a faith also tend to fare better (Myers, 2000). Faith provides us with both social
capital and 'existential ordering' in our lives. Thus, for those without faith (for

example, atheists and humanists), these matters of social capital and existential ordering remain particularly important to reflect on as they have to be reinvented contingently in human life.

Some psychologists emphasise the objective aspects of the good life, for example Skinner's utopian vision of Walden Two in which our world contains predominantly positive reinforcement to ensure peaceful harmony in society (Skinner, 1948). Others (most of the authors noted above) tend to use more subjectivist or experiential criteria. Within American humanistic psychology, we find a convergence about the pursuit of positive wellbeing within the 'human growth movement'. In the American tradition of individualism, we find Carl Rogers echoing Aristotle's emphasis on eudemonia:

> for me, adjectives such as happy, contented, blissful, enjoyable, do not seem quite appropriate to any general description of this process I have called the good life, even though the person in this process would experience each one of these at the appropriate times. But adjectives which seem more generally fitting are adjectives such as enriching, exciting, rewarding, challenging, meaningful. ... It means launching oneself fully into the stream of life. (Rogers, 1962: 5)

Whereas Rogers focuses on the inner life of individuals and Skinner on the outer world of positive contingencies, both convey important aspects of our current public policy agenda about wellbeing.

POLITICAL INTEREST IN WELLBEING

The current interest of politicians in wellbeing suggests that the leaders of developed societies are exploring a measure of progress beyond the economic. There is little point in people being richer if they are no happier and even the latter term begs a question about its relationship with values and meanings (Layard, 2005). Happiness is an emotional state, which is transitory and can even be artificially induced (by drugs and other forms of consumption). It may or may not be linked in the lives of people with a long-term sense of fulfilment, inner peace and contentment or with giving and receiving support and affection.

But beyond this recent political interest in the topic, the disciplinary perspective of those studying it frames its nature. For example, through the lens of comparative religion, we can explore what the great faiths have said about wellbeing. This is relevant today because of the world distribution of faith groups that encourage particular ways of thinking about wellbeing. Deistic religions emphasise fulfilment in life though serving God and so eschew homocentric definitions of the good life. However, the latter is often defined by striving for peace, love and understanding in our dealings with others. Non-deistic traditions like Buddhism emphasise compassion, authenticity, the transitory nature of life, the acceptance of suffering and the futility of the individual ego grasping for either possessions or permanence.

More secular approaches to the topic in human science are divided between those that privilege social relationships and those that privilege the individual mind. For example, sociologists have mainly emphasised the link between well-being and social networks or social capital. By contrast, psychologists are more likely to emphasise 'mental capital', rather than social capital. The recent political emphasis has thus provided an opportunity for disciplinary advancement. For example, Cary Cooper, who led a team of psychologists and psychiatrists investigating wellbeing for the British government, made the point that:

> This is wonderful for psychology. It's showing the real importance of psychologists: I'm talking educational psychologists, clinical psychologists, occupational psychologists and health psychologists. There's recommendations for every single one of them in this report, about early detection, about treatment, it's all there. This is a blueprint for how psychology can improve the mental capital and well-being of our population. We've been given a real fillip in this work. (Cooper, 2008: 1010)

Note how wellbeing (an existential matter for us all) soon collapses into its opposite, which then becomes a site for professional expertise. Thus, the language of 'early detection' and 'treatment' immediately creeps in, when it is wellbeing (not pathology) that is supposed to be its focus.

Those involved in the Mental Capacity and Wellbeing Project publicised their findings in *Nature* (Beddington et al., 2008). The summary opening statement of the article emphasised that: 'Countries must learn how to capitalize on their citizens' cognitive resources if they are to prosper, both economically and socially. Early interventions will be key.' The main findings of the report were summarised as follows in the list, which gives a small nod to social context (the allusion to 'social risk factors such as debt'):

- *Boosting brain power in young and old* There is huge scope for improving mental capital through different types of intervention. The genetic contribution to mental capital is well below 50 per cent in childhood, rising to more than 60 per cent in adulthood and old age.
- *What science could do in the early years* Cognitive neuroscience is already uncovering neural markers, or biomarkers, that can reveal learning difficulties as early as in infancy.
- *Early detection of mental disorders* The challenge of tackling mental ill health is considerable. There is great potential in improving diagnosis and treatment, and in addressing social risk factors such as debt.
- *Learning must continue throughout life* This can have a direct effect on mental health and wellbeing across all age groups, and has particular promise in older people.
- *Changing needs for a changing workplace* The workforce is changing both in demographics and in the demands placed on it. Workers' mental wellbeing is an important factor when attempting to improve the mental capital of economies and societies (Beddington et al., 2008: 1058).

Alongside this psychological focus, a recurring aspect of wellbeing policy discussions is whether the concept should really be conflated in principle simply with positive health. The grounds for this are quite strong. Most of the social factors shaping mental health also shape physical health. For example, the very poor have both poor physical and mental health. Both of the latter (together and apart) affect reported subjective wellbeing. It is useful, then, when we are discussing wellbeing to consider general public health models, which are holistic in their conceptual ambition. An example is given diagrammatically in Figure 1.1 from Dahlgren and Whitehead (1993).

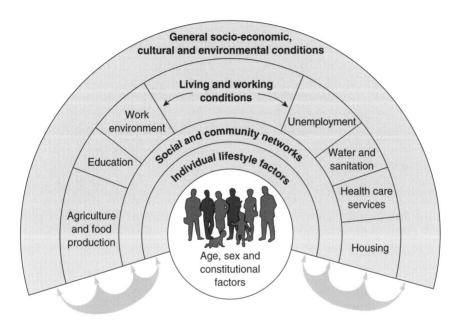

Figure 1.1 The main determinants of health (Dahlgren and Whitehead, 1993)

Note that an approach to wellbeing which is purely psychological only focuses on the inner tiers of this diagram. In developed countries, where material needs are largely met (with some more than others with adequate welfare safety nets), the outer circles are taken for granted – hence, the norms in these societies focus more on the psychological aspects of wellbeing.

WESTERN HUMANISTIC AND POSITIVE PSYCHOLOGY

A full-bodied psychological focus on wellbeing can be found in the growth of 'positive psychology' (Peterson and Seligman, 2004; Rogge, 2011). This explores psychological strengths and virtuous human action – the converse of the study of psychopathology. It has many resonances with both Buddhism and the existential approach to a meaningful existence offered by Maslow (1968), with his emphasis on self-actualisation, which is possible beyond the fulfilment of our basic needs

(Ryan and Deci, 2001). Also, Frankl (1958) emphasised that people are born seekers after meaning. This is expressed by us engaging actively in life, developing positive mutuality in our relations with others, and accepting that life brings with it disappointment and suffering. These cannot be avoided but they can be sources of new forms of activity and relationships.

Frankl argued that we become alienated and distressed when we do not orientate ourselves towards meaning in life. Meaning, not happiness, defined wellbeing for existential therapists and psychologists like Frankl and Maslow (although neither was opposed to happiness). This more philosophical approach to wellbeing is somewhat removed from the model described above about 'mental capital', which is more economistic in its logic.

In between these two positions about wellbeing (one about mental capital and the other about existential meaning) can be found the study of comparative health within populations. Here we find a strong interdisciplinary consensus on the importance of relationships (Pilgrim et al., 2009), as well as on the injuries of class placing limits on our capacity for wellbeing. The latter come not just from the direct impact of poverty but also from the relative deprivation of being excluded from status and meaningful engagement as citizens (Sennett and Cobb, 1972; Wilkinson, 2005).

This middle position about wellbeing suggests that it is best understood as a psychosocial phenomenon, which certainly implicates objective conditions; it is easy to rejoice in the tent of plenty and understandable if we feel miserable when having little in life. But it also implicates subjective meanings, which are internal states (attitudes, values, beliefs) derived from relationships, so they are negotiated intersubjectively.

THE GLOBAL CONTEXT OF WELLBEING

One common aspiration of public policy within developed societies has been to promote wellbeing. The very prospect of such an aspiration immediately throws into relief Skinner's environmental emphasis. For example, absolute poverty and war conditions affecting the general population pre-empt such an aspiration. In the past few decades, ongoing wars in Africa and the Middle East have simply negated wellbeing for the majority. The policy aspiration is meaningful in North America, Australasia or Western Europe because: (a) they have developed economies; and (b) they have been free of warfare on their own soil, although, with sporadic terrorist attacks, this picture is now changing to some extent.

However, we cannot assume that measures of wellbeing applied cross-nationally form a neat linear pattern in which peace and increased wealth lead to improvements in reported wellbeing. For example, in repeated studies conducted globally, Inglehart and his colleagues have found a curvilinear relationship between wealth and subjective wellbeing, as shown in Figure 1.2 (Inglehart et al., 2008).

One of the richest countries in the world, the USA, is not the happiest, being well outperformed by much poorer Latin American countries and those in Scandinavia with a social democratic tradition in which boasting about one's wealth is culturally eschewed. This trend is mainly because of differences in status inequalities and poor welfare provision in the USA, which generates envy (in the first case) and insecurity (in the second case). Basically, peaceful and more equal societies are happier societies (Wilkinson and Pickett, 2009).

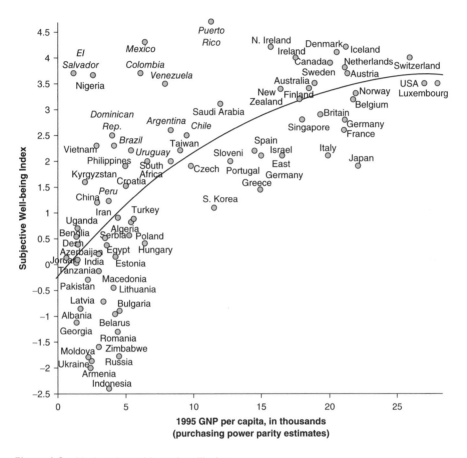

Figure 1.2 National wealth and wellbeing

CRITICS OF THE PURSUIT OF HAPPINESS

Some writers have offered us sustained critiques of wellbeing defined by the pursuit of happiness; note that it is a fundamental component of the American constitution. One criticism from non-theistic philosophies such as Buddhism is that grasping for goals is counterproductive. This is summarised from empirical psychology by Martin (2013: 31) thus: 'to get happiness forget about it: then with any luck, happiness will come as a by-product in pursuing meaningful activities and relationships'.

Critics of consumer capitalism, such as Barber (2007), have pointed out that constant consumption does not make us happier but it does render us more immature in our expectations about life and constantly envious of those who have more than us. This creates a 'hedonic treadmill', in which we consume more and more because something better is always promised by the next purchase or the new model of what we have already. Studies of GNP (gross national product) have shown that as it increases, it is not then necessarily reflected in raised levels of subjective wellbeing (Layard, 2005).

Some feminist critics, such as Ahmed (2010), have argued that our current developed world preoccupation with happiness is not freeing but oppressive. She utilises case studies of 'feminist killjoys', 'unhappy queers' and 'melancholic migrants' to demonstrate her argument. Echoing the Buddhist point (and from Rogers and Martin above), she notes that we should focus on 'happenstance' not happiness.

See also: *mental health; pleasure; spirituality.*

FURTHER READING

Delle Fave, A. (ed.) *The Exploration of Happiness*. London: Springer.

Pilgrim, D. (2015) *Understanding Mental Health: A Critical Realist Exploration*. London: Routledge.

REFERENCES

Ackrill, J.L. (2006) 'Aristotle on eudaimonia', in O. Höffe (ed.), *Aristoteles: Nikomachische Ethik*. Berlin: Akademie Verlag.

Ahmed, S. (2010) *The Promise of Happiness*. Durham, NC, and London: Duke University Press.

Allport, G. (1961) *Pattern and Growth in Personality*. New York: Holt, Rinehart & Winston.

Andrews, P.W. and Thomson, J.A. (2009) 'The bright side of being blue: depression as an adaptation for analyzing complex problems', *Psychological Review, 116* (3): 620–54.

Barber, B.R. (2007) *Consumed: How Markets Corrupt Children, Infantilise Adults and Swallow Citizens Whole*. New York: W.W. Norton.

Beddington, J., Cooper, C.L., Field, J., Goswami, U., Huppert, F.A., Jenkins, R., Jones, H.S., Kirkwood, T.B.L., Sahakian, B.J. and Thomas, S.M. (2008) 'The mental wealth of nations', *Nature, 455*: 1057–1060.

Buhler, C. (1972) *Introduction to Humanistic Psychology*. Belmont, CA: Wadsworth.

Cooper, C.L. (2008) 'Interview: a blueprint for mental capital and well-being', *The Psychologist, 21* (12): 1010–11.

Dahlgren, G. and Whitehead, M. (1993) Tackling inequalities in health: what can we learn from what has been tried? Working paper prepared for the King's Fund International Seminar on Tackling Inequalities in Health, September 1993, Ditchley Park, Oxfordshire. London, King's Fund. Accessible in: Dahlgren, G. and Whitehead, M. (2007) *European Strategies for Tackling Social Inequities in Health: Levelling up Part 2*. Copenhagen: WHO Regional Office for Europe. Available at: www.euro.who.int/__data/assets/pdf_file/0018/103824/E89384.pdf (accessed 15 November 2016).

Erikson, E. (1950) *Childhood and Society*. New York: W.W. Norton.

Frankl, V. (1958) *Man's Search for Meaning*. New York: Pocket Books.

Inglehart, R.F., Foa, R., Peterson, C. and Welzel, C. (2008) 'Development, freedom, and rising happiness: a global perspective (1981–2007)', *Perspectives on Psychological Science, 3* (4): 264–85.

Jung, C.G. (1933) *Modern Man in Search of a Soul*. San Diego, CA: Harcourt Brace Jovanich.

Layard, R. (2005) *Happiness*. London: Penguin.

Martin, M.M. (2013) 'Paradoxes of happiness', in A. Delle Fave (ed.), *The Exploration of Happiness*. London: Springer.

Maslow, A. (1968) *Toward a Psychology of Being*. New York: Van Nostrand.

Myers, D.G. (2000) 'The faith, friends and funds of happy people', *American Psychologist*, 55: 56–67.

Peterson, C. and Seligman, M. (eds) (2004) *Character Strengths and Virtues: A Handbook and Classification*. Oxford: Oxford University Press.

Pilgrim, D., Rogers, A. and Bentall, R. (2009) 'The centrality of personal relationships in the creation and amelioration of mental health problems: the current interdisciplinary case', *Health*, 13 (2): 237–56.

Rogers, C. (1962) *Toward Becoming a Fully Functioning Person*. Washington, DC: A.W. Combs.

Rogge, B. (2011) 'Mental health, positive psychology and the sociology of the self', in D. Pilgrim, A. Rogers and B. Pescosolido (eds), *The SAGE Handbook of Mental Health and Illness*. London: Sage.

Ryan, R.M. and Deci, E.L. (2001) 'On happiness and human potentials: a review on hedonic and eudaimonic wellbeing', *Applied Review of Psychology*, *52*: 141–66.

Ryff, C.D. and Singer, B. (1998) 'The contours of positive human health', *Psychological Inquiry*, 9: 1–28.

Sennett, R. and Cobb, J. (1972) *The Hidden Injuries of Class*. New York: Vintage Books.

Skinner, B.F. (1948) *Walden Two*. New York: Hackett.

Wilkinson, R.G. (2005) *The Impact of Inequality: How to Make Sick Societies*. London: Routledge.

Wilkinson, R.G. and Pickett, J. (2009) *The Spirit Level: Why More Equal Societies Almost Always Do Better*. London: Allen Lane.

Philosophical Aspects of Mental Health

DEFINITION

All of the entries in this book contain implicit or explicit philosophical assumptions or aspects. Three concerns of philosophy are especially important: the study of being (ontology); the study of knowledge (epistemology); and the study of values in human affairs (ethics).

KEY POINTS

- All academic topics, including that of mental health, rest on philosophical assumptions.

- That includes those relating to what is assumed to exist, what is assumed to be a persuasive form of knowledge and those that arise from values.
- These three sets of assumptions are described in relation to three branches of philosophy: ontology, epistemology and ethics.

In light of the above definition, we can think of any topic in human science in terms of the relationship between what exists (ontological matters), how we understand ourselves and the world (epistemological matters) and values (ethical matters). This relationship is provided in the triangle diagram in Figure 1.3.

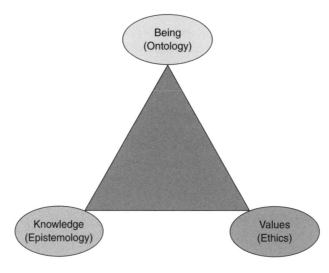

Figure 1.3 Ontology, epistemology and ethics

ONTOLOGY, EPISTEMOLOGY AND ETHICS

The previous entries on mental health and wellbeing indicate that it might be possible to study their relatively stable aspects across time and place (an ontological matter). For example, if a person reports that their life is fulfilling and they relate well to others and have daily activities that are meaningful, then they *are* mentally healthy. The counter-example would be that if a person is dissatisfied with life, they have no trusting relationships with others and their daily life lacks meaning, then they *are not* mentally healthy.

In both cases, we could develop different ways of *understanding* these people and their existence. For example, we could discuss the first case in terms of eudemonia (from Aristotle), or of having strong and healthy ego functions (from Freud), or because of their faith in God (from the Abrahamic traditions). In the second case, we could discuss the person in terms of alienation (from Marx), or mental illness (from Kraepelin). These are epistemological aspects of wellbeing, theorised or understood in different ways.

Other ontological matters relate to reason and emotion. Mentally healthy people could be described *as being* reasonable in their dealings with others and the world and not being overly governed by their emotions. Indeed, *being unreasonable* is the overarching hallmark of what we, for now, tend to describe as 'mental disorder' (Pilgrim and Tomasini, 2012). This ontological matter at that point becomes an ethical one. How should we respond to people in our midst who are miserable, unintelligible or incorrigible? (Broadly, these forms of conduct describe those suffering from what modern psychiatry tends to call 'neurosis', 'psychosis' and 'personality disorder'.) The way in which we answer the question of responding to the lack of reason in our midst reveals both our own moral expectations and our taken-for-granted assumptions about what it is to be mentally healthy. We see here how epistemology and value judgements interweave in practice for us.

Aristotle called our acculturated assumptions about life and how to live it 'doxa' – hence, the words 'orthodoxy', 'heterodoxy' and 'unorthodox': those deemed to be mentally abnormal in a particular time and place or thus unorthodox in their conduct. That conduct might be accounted for by sin or mental illness. These different accounts reflect both epistemological matters (the way in which unorthodox conduct is interpreted) and ontological matters (the way in which that conduct is described consensually and then explained causally). The constant role of norms and values becomes evident when we consider what tends to get labelled as mentally abnormal.

We only tend to notice conduct when it goes wrong – when it goes right (according to current shared norms and mores), our acts and those of others are unremarkable. Those judgements are ones made in the context of the culture we come to know well in a time and place. For example, a hundred years ago, talking to oneself in a church was deemed to be normal (praying) but speaking to oneself in the street was not (a sign of insanity). Today, though, with hands-free mobile phones, the latter judgement is made less often. We can see, then, that just one form of conduct will vary in its normality or abnormality over time and place. In this case, once praying and phone explanations are excluded, an attribution of 'hearing voices' might be made.

Another ethical aspect of mental health relates to paternalism and coercion. If people are deemed to be reasonable, then an ethical assumption we operate is that the autonomous citizen should be respected and left to do as they please (provided that it is not a crime). On the other hand, once we encounter people behaving unreasonably, that assumption can break down. The abnormal action might seem to warrant both the need to care for and control the rule-breaking person. If their conduct is deemed a particular threat to a moral order, this might even warrant coercive control. The philosopher John Stuart Mill, who himself suffered from mental health problems, considered that adult citizens should be free to speak and act without constraint unless they were either 'lunatics' or 'idiots'.

This question about whether the state *should* intervene in the lives of 'lunatics' or 'idiots' remains with us today and remains an ethical question. The ethical response of 'parens patriae' (agents of the state acting paternalistically towards some citizens but not others) then elevates ethical considerations into legal codes in two senses. First, the transgressive conduct of the identified patient is operationalised in some way to be discerned and assessed by psychiatric experts. In this sense, the latter are rule assessors and (if they act coercively) they are rule enforcers. Second, the use of force by agents of the state to control mental abnormality has ethical consequences. In other circumstances, such action would be deemed to be false imprisonment and assault. Mental health legislation protects agents of the state (mental health professionals) from these charges.

These difficult ethical considerations have both ontological and epistemological aspects. The risky behaviour under consideration is real enough: the notion of risk to self or others is at the centre of legal decisions about the detention and treatment of people diagnosed with a mental disorder. If we deem those who are assessed as risky to be out of control because they are mentally ill (an epistemological assumption), then their moral autonomy is deemed to be impaired and the paternalism of others ethically warranted. On the other hand, if we do not consider them to be ill, their moral autonomy should be respected and they should be held morally responsible for their actions. The latter position was argued by the controversial psychiatrist Thomas Szasz. Various positions on autonomy and responsibility can be rehearsed between these poles.

See also: *psychiatric classification.*

FURTHER READING

Barker, P. (ed.) (2011) *Mental Health Ethics: The Human Context.* London: Routledge.
Pilgrim, D. (2015) *Understanding Mental Health: A Critical Realist Exploration.* London: Routledge.

REFERENCE

Pilgrim, D. and Tomasini, F. (2012) 'On being unreasonable in modern society: are mental health problems special?', *Disability and Society,* 27 (5): 631–46.

Work

DEFINITION

In English, 'work' is used as a noun (to describe a role with a specific range of actions and skills) or a verb (to describe how effort is exerted or productivity achieved).

KEY POINTS

- Work is required in all societies to ensure basic need satisfaction for human beings.
- Both unemployment and poor employment are threats to mental health.
- The shift from an emphasis on production to consumption has also had major implications for mental health.

The above definition offered of work signals our expectations about roles, effortful activity and the rewards the latter may bring. It might also imply a division of labour (between mental and physical labour) and a relationship of employment (working for others or working for oneself). All societies require some or most in their midst to work some or most of the time for the basic necessities of food, water, shelter and warmth. Societies vary, however, in who is expected to work in this regard and variable patterns of work are linked to age, gender and disability. In some cases, particular races or classes are more likely to be literally owned by others for the purpose of work (slavery).

After basic necessities are supplied by productivity, other needs, actual or imagined, are then the concern of complex societies. These 'service industries' function to support the efficiency of basic need satisfaction (for example, food production and supply, water supply, building and repairs, heating, responses to illness, crisis or disaster).

Over and above this, functions not required for human survival but important for social order, such as wealth, efficiency, repair and citizens' quality of life, are also arenas for work and employment (such as cleaning, lighting, leisure, transport systems and infrastructure, financial systems, sport and entertainment). In complex societies with central state powers, these two functions and arenas of work are regularly underpinned by work directed at social order, wealth expansion and societal survival. Mental labour is important here as education is the focus of social reproduction (the young learning to adopt their society's norms, mores and values), skills training for differentiated forms of physical labour, and research and development to improve efficiency and status for states and nations. In relation to social control, policing and other emergency services, health services (including mental health services) and the armed services all play a role. All of these then become large arenas of employment.

Finally, we have the production and retailing of goods that are not required for either of the other two functions but whose consumers believe they require for need satisfaction. This third arena of work activity affects the style and content of the other two and is an activity in its own right. More will be said on consumption below.

The link between work and mental health was made explicit by Freud, who defined it for adults by two activities in their life (work and love). If work is one pathway to mental health, this also implies that if that route is unrewarding or too difficult, then it may harm wellbeing. This Freudian assumption also implies that the absence of access to work will be detrimental to mental health. Those following

Freud, even those dismissive of his theories more generally, have confirmed his assumptions about the importance of work.

Thus, work is a potential source of both personal satisfaction and needed income and of personal stress. The ratio, of the former to the latter, tends to increase with the amount of financial reward (objective income) and the subjective sense of reward and control enjoyed by workers (job satisfaction and task control). When the balance is tilted towards low wages and poor task control, then mental health is affected negatively. Job satisfaction is also a function of the quality of working relationships (this is why human resources departments in public and private employing organisations are concerned about matters such as team work, morale and bullying).

Therefore, while the absence of work can be a source of poor mental health, this is also the case, but more so, with insecure employment. Indeed, studies looking at the correlation between work and mental health suggest that the worst mental health scores are not found in the unemployed but in those in insecure employment (low wages, poor task control, poor job security). This may well reflect the predictable pattern of life out of work being a source of ontological security. By contrast, the poorly employed suffer ontological insecurity (Rogers and Pilgrim, 2003).

Consumption is a source of employment for retail and other support staff but it has been the focus for criticism from many commentators on late capitalism. These observations made before the recent world recession, which was triggered by unsustainable debt encouraged by financial organisations and created by persuaded consumers, make two important points about work consumption and mental health. The first, from Layard (2005), notes that the richer we get and the more we consume, the less happy we become. He calls this the 'hedonic treadmill'. The second point, from Barber (2007), is that the obsession with consumption infantilises citizens and corrupts and displaces the process of fulfilling democratic affiliation with our fellows. This process of individualised consumerism undermines social capital. Barber is clear, then, that the assumed ideological conflation of capitalism with democracy (with its openness to and encouragement of social capital) applied in its phase of production. However, in its later and more recent development of consumption, democracy is now grossly flawed.

Thus, modern-day capitalist societies, which have shifted from production to consumption in their emphasis, are a threat to mental health. They offer false dawns of happiness for consumers, cutting them off from the reward of relating to others and substituting this with their relationship with things. People develop what Marx called 'imagined needs', which are manipulated by those producing goods and services that people do not really need but believe they do.

As the recent world recession also indicates, consumer capitalism poses a second and critical threat to add to the ongoing one just noted. Once the socio-economic arrangements put consumption and not production for basic need satisfaction at the centre, then rising debt levels and diminishing trust within the financial service sector affect workers and consumers alike (and, of course, many are both). Once the system rapidly contracts or collapses, all of the roles involved are then jeopardised – jobs in service industries are lost and wages depressed. Consumers are left less able or unable to consume. In relation to mental health, this might imply the need for things to get worse before they get better.

See also: *economic aspects of mental health; social class; wellbeing.*

FURTHER READING

De Witte, H. (1999) 'Job insecurity and psychological well-being: review of the literature and exploration of some unresolved issues', *European Journal of Work and Organizational Psychology*, 8 (2): 155–77.

Stansfeld, S. and Candy, B. (2006) 'Psychosocial work environment and mental health: a meta-analytic review', *Scandinavian Journal of Work, Environment & Health*, 32 (6): 443–62.

REFERENCES

Barber, B.R. (2007) *Consumed: How Markets Corrupt Children, Infantilize Adults and Swallow Citizens Whole*. New York: W.W. Norton.

Layard, R. (2005) *Happiness*. London: Penguin.

Rogers, A. and Pilgrim, D. (2003) *Mental Health and Inequality*. Basingstoke: Palgrave Macmillan.

Neuroscience

DEFINITION

Neuroscience is an interdisciplinary field of inquiry that investigates the nervous system and its role in human life.

KEY POINTS

- The interdisciplinary rationale of neuroscience is explained and cautions about its reductionist excesses noted.
- Attention is drawn to the commercial and ideological interests at play that encourage a naive commitment to biological reductionism. The latter reflects an over-enthusiasm from some interest groups, for using neuroscience to explain the origins of mental health problems.

As the above definition indicates, the nervous system attracts the interest of a variety of academic disciplines. These have included neurology, biochemistry, psychology, physiology, philosophy and psychiatry. The clinical professions have been particularly interested in learning from and contributing to its topics of investigation. The interdisciplinary range of interest emerged, and was subsequently consolidated during, the 1960s with the arrival of a variety of august bodies: the International Brain Research Organisation (1960); the International Society for Neurochemistry (1963); the European Brain and Behaviour Society (1968); and the Society for Neuroscience (1969).

The role of neuroscience in the field of mental health has been widespread since then and the focus for both evangelical hopes and profound scepticism. Some psychiatrists and psychologists have adopted the epistemological starting point that all behaviour and experience are *reducible* to brain functioning. A less reductionist view (and probably one strongly endorsed by most psychologists and psychiatrists) is that brain functioning is *implicated* in all experience and behaviour, whether the latter is deemed to be normal or abnormal.

By and large, the disputes about neuroscience in the field of mental health have been in relation to this problematic question of what the philosopher of psychology Wolman (1981) has called 'hoped-for-reductionism'. This axiomatic, rather than empirical, position has been adopted in the past 150 years by a range of experts, including Freud and Kraepelin. Both of these 'founding fathers' of modern psychiatry assumed that eventually the source of all mental illness would be identifiable in the neural substrate of the patient. For Kraepelin, it was already self-evidently the case in the late 19th century. By contrast, Freud thought that such discoveries resided in a distant future time, and offered psychology as a preferred interim explanatory and clinical framework.

The recent consensus noted now about brain functioning being *implicated* in psychological functioning has emphasised the interaction of the nervous system with all aspects of the human context, especially in the developmental environment of the child. This consensus has been a way of avoiding the reduction of our biology to our genetics, leading to the interest in 'epigenetics': the ways in which our inherited genetic tendencies are modified for good or bad by our early experience. Some psychologists also point out that our experience is itself then important. Our memories of our past and the meanings we attach to them become determinants of our thoughts, feelings and actions in the present. Those particular events, and the meanings we give them, contribute to our particular and current sense of human agency (Archer, 2000). With the reality of human agency in mind, it is fair to say that the brain affords our capacity to experience life and to conduct ourselves but it does not explain our inner life or our actions (Tortorello, 2017).

Accordingly, our actions and interests alter our brain functioning. For example, when we smile or stroke a beloved pet, our brain chemistry changes. These everyday examples show that interactive models are required if we are to avoid biological reductionism while not excluding the important role of our nervous system. This point has become evident when we look at the evidence on the impact of childhood adversity on neurobiological development (Anda et al., 2006; Read et al., 2014). Another obvious and common demonstration of this point is the consumption of alcohol and other substances. These are taken in (our planned action) knowing (our cognition) that they will make us feel good (our emotions). The simple and common folly of inebriation is thus an interesting neuroscientific topic and it implicates wider contextual factors, from alcohol pricing policies to the particular biographical circumstances of the person seeking comfort in forms of self-medication. This interactive view about emotions and brain functioning is explored by Fox (2008).

Critiques of neuro-reductionism have come from neuroscientists themselves. For example, the physician and poet Raymond Tallis (2011) has attacked the arrogance and naivety of his colleagues, who explain away culture and human conduct by referring to neural functioning alone. Tallis calls this academic tendency 'neuromania'. Other scientists are more concerned to expose the ideological and commercial motives within this tendency. An example of this is the work of Steven Rose, a neurobiologist who is sceptical of the descent of neuroscience into simplistic expectations of the triumph of bio-reductionism (Rose and Rose, 2012). The psychiatrist and psychopharmacologist David Healy (2002) has also noted that neuroscience has increased in popularity, alongside the pharmaceutical companies' interest in defining mental health problems in categorical somatic terms. This process permits new 'magic bullets' to be sold profitably, which attack putative disorders in the brain (see the entries on Psychiatric Classification and The Pharmaceutical Industry). Thus, commercial interests promote the reductionist wing of neuroscience.

This promotion of neuro-reductionism is also evident from politicians, who might prefer to deal with assumed or putative biological problems inside individuals, rather than concede their cultural, social and fiscal origins, which would render governments politically culpable. Recent governmental confidence in neuroscience has been reflected in large-scale funded initiatives. These have included US presidents George Bush (Senior's) 'Decade of the Brain' in the 1990s (Jones and Mendell, 1999) and Barak Obama's more recent (2013) Brain Research through Advancing Innovative Neurotechnologies (BRAIN) initiative.

This political tendency to rely on neuroscience as a source of solutions to complex psychosocial problems has also been evident this side of the Atlantic, with the European Union's Human Brain Project (HBP) (HBP-PS Consortium, 2012). The reductionist risks of these projects are evident in the latter, with its explicit methodological boast about de-coupling the brain from its social context:

> The evolutionary function of a brain is to control the organisms' behaviour in their environment. In principle, therefore, the only way to test or characterise the high-level behavioural or cognitive capabilities of a brain model is to create a closed loop between the model and a body acting in an environment and to interrogate the model through well-designed experiments … Once a set-up has successfully replicated, we can then identify causal mechanisms by lesioning or manipulating specific brain regions, transmitter systems, types of neuron, etc. (HBP-PS Consortium, 2012: 49)

This is an articulation of the scientific justification for closed system reasoning. By contrast, the critics of neuro-reductionism, noted above, have been keen to highlight its dangers and the competing need to address the role that both human agency and supra-personal factors play dynamically in open systems. Moreover, not only is neuroscience biased heavily towards closed, not open, systems investigations, for reasons of its own methodological convenience noted in the cited passage above, it also assumes that functional psychiatric disorders are self-evidently brain disorders. For example, the HBP report designates mood disorders, psychotic disorders, anxiety disorders and addiction as being brain diseases (alongside the traditional designations of dementia and 'other neurological disorders') (HBP-PS Consortium, 2012: 98). Such a highly contestable assumption indicates why neuroscience is likely to be the focus of substantial contention for the foreseeable future.

See also: *causes and consequences of mental health problems; creativity; psychiatric classification; spirituality; the myth of mental illness.*

FURTHER READING

HBP-PS Consortium (2012) *The Human Brain Project: A Report to the European Commission.* Lausanne: HBP-PS Consortium.
Healy, D. (2002) *From Psychopharmacology to Neuropsychopharmacology.* Budapest: Animula.
Pilgrim, D. (2019) *Critical Realism for Psychologists.* London: Routledge.
Rose, N. (2019) *Our Psychiatric Future.* Bristol: Polity Press.

REFERENCES

Anda, R., Felliti, B., Bremner, J.D., Walker, J., Whitfield, C. and Perry, B. (2006) 'The enduring effects of abuse and related adverse experiences in childhood: a convergence of evidence from neurobiology and epidemiology', *European Archives of Psychiatry and Clinical Neuroscience,* 265 (3): 174–86.
Archer, M. (2000) *Being Human: The Problem of Agency.* Cambridge: Cambridge University Press.
Fox, E. (2008) *Emotion Science.* Basingstoke: Palgrave Macmillan.
HBP-PS Consortium (2012) *The Human Brain Project: A Report to the European Commission.* Lausanne: HBP-PS Consortium.
Healy, D. (2002) *From Psychopharmacology to Neuropsychopharmacology.* Budapest: Animula.
Jones, E.G. and Mendell, L.M. (1999) 'Assessing the "decade of the brain"', *Science, 284* (5415): 739.
Read, J., Fosse, R., Moskowitz, A. and Perry, B. (2014) 'The traumagenic neurodevelopmental model of psychosis revisited', *Neuropsychiatry,* 4 (1): 64–79.
Rose, S. and Rose, H. (2012) *Genes, Cells and Brains: Bioscience's Promethean Promises.* London: Verso.
Tallis, R. (2011) *Aping Mankind: Neuromania, Darwinitis and the Misrepresentation of Humanity.* London: Acumen.
Tortorello, F. (2017) 'What is real about reductive neuroscience?', *Journal of Critical Realism 16* (3): 235–54.
Wolman, B.B. (1981) *Contemporary Theories and Systems in Psychology.* Amsterdam: Plenum.

Subjective and Objective Aspects of Mental Health

DEFINITION

The subjective aspects of mental health refer to inner experiences and personal communications about them. The objective aspects of mental health refer to descriptions of it from the outside by lay people or experts, but especially the latter. The subjective methodological tendency in human science is personal and intensive (traditionally called an 'idiographic' form of inquiry) and the objective tendency is impersonal and extensive, though individual subjective data can be aggregated to inform these objective ('nomothetic') psychological descriptions.

KEY POINTS

- The case for forms of subjectivism and objectivism is rehearsed.
- The limitations of an imbalanced emphasis in either direction in mental work are explored.

Human science has been highly contested. On the one hand, it has had to deal with the challenge of us being language users with idiosyncratic inner lives and particular biographical contexts, making us unique givers of, or searchers for, meaning in our lives. How can we truly respect these unique inner lives: the challenge of subjectivity? On the other hand, with the risk that the answer to the latter might end in nihilism and solipsism, how can we communicate, and generalise, about aspects of human existence in a valid and agreeable way from the outside: the challenge of objectivity? The tension in psychology between idiographic and nomothetic forms of inquiry was noted above.

Answers to these questions have been diverse and for our subject we find a range of extremes (Wann, 1964). For example, in psychology, radical behaviourism favoured limiting scientific data to objective descriptions of the contingent relationships between an organism's environment and its responses to it, so-called 'stimulus-response psychology' (Skinner, 1972). In the other direction, there have been those who have favoured forms of deep subjectivity. These include 'depth psychology', which is a broad term to describe all of the variants emerging in the wake of Freudian theory, as well as phenomenology and existentialism. The Freudian tradition emphasises the ubiquity of interpretative procedures in human life and then utilises these for therapeutic ends. (The science of interpretations is called 'hermeneutics' and so psychoanalysis is a hermeneutic method to understand the human mind, as well as a treatment method for mental health problems.)

Phenomenology is a method for studying consciousness developed by Husserl (1913/1982). It has been highly influential in mental health, particularly in purer forms such as the person-centred work of Rogers (1961) but also in personal construct theory (Kelly, 1955) and Maslow's notion of 'self-actualisation' (Maslow, 1968). Husserl's work also influenced existential philosophers like Sartre (1957) and the clinical application of existential psychotherapy (Frankl, 1946; May, 1969). The blurring of influences within this subjectivist trend is exemplified by the work of Laing, a psychoanalyst influenced heavily by Sartrean existentialism, whose warning here about the risks of an unbalanced interest in objectivity and an evasion of subjectivity in mental health work clarifies the contention we are dealing with in this entry:

> The relation between experience and behaviour is the stone that the builders will reject at their peril. Without it the whole structure of our theory and practice must collapse. (Laing, 1967: 17)

This crisp description of our dilemma from Laing has been clouded by different nuances of the notion of phenomenology. For subjectivists, the latter is very clearly about giving personal authority to ordinary people (or, in the case of psychotherapy, to patients). However, a seminal work in psychiatry from Jaspers (1912/1968) on phenomenology has provided a claimed authority for the latter at times, but sometimes it is also used to emphasise *the diagnostician's authority* in taking the detail of symptom presentation seriously. This has meant, for example, that Jasper's 'descriptive psychopathology' can be used to defend the symptom-based emphasis of *DSM* (Mullen, 2007). This ambiguity highlights the choice that exists for us between privileging the experience of the patient non-judgementally and privileging instead the subjective authority of the *diagnostician* in pronouncing upon the patient's symptoms (Laing, 1967; Berrios, 1989; Broome, 2002).

From a philosophical perspective, when we turn to the offer and risks of objectivism about our topic, we find examples of *positivism*: theory building in science from the systematic observation of reality (empiricism), aimed at discerning lawful relationships, which are assumed to really exist (they have an ontological certainty) in nature and society (they are mind-independent). The notion of 'mind-independence' distinguishes realist from anti-realist positions in human science (for example, found in some forms of social constructivism or constructionism). Does the world exist independently of the way we see it and can it be validly described and explained? And, alternatively, is the world only *ever* knowable via the way we apprehend and represent it? These questions highlight the competing position of realists and anti-realists.

The strength of a realist position is that it can offer us the caution of fallibility: we can agree in consensus, and incrementally, whether a knowledge claim is repeatedly and demonstrably true or not as a statement about the world we share. In other words, it is about ontology (what exists) and not just epistemology (our knowledge). A criticism of subjectivism is that it cannot be subjected to proper falsification, when and if everyone's perspective is deemed to be sovereign and beyond question or judgement. This is the contentious matter of 'epistemological privileging': who has a right to claim a perspective that is superior to another, and how do we draw that conclusion? Subjectivism is highly respectful of individuality but it runs the risk of solipsism. Objectivism is respectful of democratic transparency, agreed interpersonally, but it runs the risk of being insensitive to personal experiential nuances.

A problem for positivism, as a form of realism, is that it always incorporates assumptions and these assumptions will vary from one scientist to another. As a consequence, the subjectivity of the scientist cannot really be bracketed or ignored: the futile ideological aspiration of being 'disinterested', when objectivity is being pursued. For example, Skinner's viewpoint of pure objectivism is based largely on logical positivism, which focused on pure empirical descriptions and operationalised definitions about a topic of interest. But, for example, for our purposes, operationalised definitions of mental health problems are based tautologically on social norms, which reflect shared values from the psychologist's immediate host society, about what is worthy and acceptable conduct and what is not. Values cannot be extracted from human science; they are embedded and inevitable.

In contrast to Skinner's behaviourism, psychiatric positivism is largely based on medical naturalism: the assumption that mental disorders exist, 'ready-made' and 'out there' in nature, awaiting discovery in patients by clinicians or epidemiologists. Psychiatric positivism assumes that the patients they encounter are embodied examples, or carriers, of objective disease structures and their underlying pathological processes. This is why systems like *DSM* and *ICD* are about the privileging of *a priori* agreed categories, which individual patients are then fitted into, thereby acquiring the label for that category. It is easy to see, then, why this process is offensive to subjectivists. Moreover, psychiatric positivism confuses its preferred descriptions of reality (for example, in *ICD* and *DSM*) with reality itself. But the map is not the territory. This error of reasoning is called the 'epistemic fallacy' by critical realists: a cue for the final point in this entry.

One compromise between strong subjectivism and these forms of flawed positivism has been offered by critical realism (Bhaskar, 1989) and applied to mental health work (Pilgrim and Bentall, 1999; Pilgrim, 2015). This approach accepts that *both* subjective and objective factors are relevant to consider together for our topic. This respects the aspirations of phenomenology and hermeneutics but also draws attention to their ultimate limits. For example, a focus on meanings alone, when privileging the experiential perspective of the patient, will limit our assumptions about causation to personal (psychological) factors. In fact, it is more than possible that both biological (sub-individual) and social (supra-individual) features can in part and variably determine our mental health. At the same time, the meanings we attach to our experiences are very important and so positivism, whether medical or behaviourist, has the limitation of not accepting or working respectfully and modestly with that importance. It is also self-deceiving when claiming that values can be bracketed in human science, when this is an impossible aspiration.

For critical realism, positivism, whether it is psychological or psychiatric, is a form of 'naive realism', because it cannot accommodate the due importance of subjectivity in human science, except when turning it into aggregate data or comparisons within it, for example in psychometric testing. Positivism also wrongly tries to exclude values from consideration in scientific research. This is futile for all science but is particularly problematic in human science. 'Disinterested and objective' knowledge claims are completely impossible in human science because experts are *part of the cultural* context in which mental health problems are embedded. They share the assumptions of all others in that context about what is, and is not, a problem and what aspects of reality should be researched and which should be ignored; the matter of a shared normativity in society by all citizens including scientists and clinicians. We can do our best to be methodologically consistent and honest about what we find, but values will always guide which research questions are asked and which are not. Values will always inflect our interpretative judgements and the conclusions we draw from those findings.

See also: *anti-psychiatry; causes and consequences of mental health problems; psychiatric classification; psychological formulations; the myth of mental illness*.

FURTHER READING

Meichenbaum, D. (1977) *Cognitive-Behaviour Modification*. New York: Plenum.
Wann, T.W. (ed.) (1964) *Behaviorism and Phenomenology: Contrasting Bases for Modern Psychology*. Chicago, IL: University of Chicago Press.

REFERENCES

Berrios, G.E. (1989) 'What is phenomenology?', *Journal of the Royal Society of Medicine, 82*: 425–8.
Bhaskar, R. (1989) *Reclaiming Reality: A Critical Introduction to Contemporary Philosophy*. London: Verso.
Broome, M. (2002) 'Explanatory models in psychiatry', Correspondence, *British Journal of Psychiatry, 181*: 351–2.
Frankl, V. (1946) *Man's Search for Meaning*. New York: Beacon Press.
Husserl, E. (1913) *Ideas Pertaining to a Pure Phenomenology and to a Phenomenological Philosophy – First Book: General Introduction to a Pure Phenomenology*, trans. F. Kersten (1982). The Hague: Nijhoff.
Jaspers, K. (1912) 'Zeitschrift für die gesamte Neurologie und Psychiatrie', English translation (1968) 'The phenomenological approach in psychopathology', *British Journal of Psychiatry, 114*: 1313–23.
Kelly, G. (1955) *The Psychology of Human Constructs*. New York: W.W. Norton.
Laing, R.D. (1967) *The Politics of Experience and the Bird of Paradise*. Harmondsworth: Penguin.
Maslow, A.H. (1968) *Towards a Psychology of Being*. New York: Wiley.
May, R. (1969) *Love and Will*. New York: W.W. Norton.
Mullen, P. (2007) 'A modest proposal for another phenomenological approach to psychopathology', *Schizophrenia Bulletin, 33* (1): 113–21.
Pilgrim, D. (2015) *Understanding Mental Health: A Critical Realist Exploration*. London: Routledge.
Pilgrim, D. and Bentall, R.P. (1999) 'The medicalisation of misery: a critical realist analysis of the concept of depression', *Journal of Mental Health, 8* (3): 261–74.
Rogers, C. (1961) *On Becoming a Person: A Therapist's View of Psychotherapy*. London: Constable.
Sartre, J.-P. (1957) *The Transcendence of the Ego: An Existentialist Theory of Consciousness*, trans. and ed. F. Williams and R. Kirkpatrick. New York: Noonday.

Skinner, B.F. (1972) *Beyond Freedom and Dignity*. New York: Vintage Books.

Wann, T.W. (ed.) (1964) *Behaviorism and Phenomenology: Contrasting Bases for Modern Psychology*. Chicago, IL: University of Chicago Press.

Sadness

DEFINITION

Sadness is a state of mournful sorrow.

KEY POINTS

- Sadness and depression are discussed.
- The problem of cultural relativism in describing emotional states is outlined.
- Criticisms of the psychiatric diagnosis of depression are summarised.

In the *Oxford English Dictionary*, one of the meanings of 'depression' is described as: '(Psych.) state of morbidly excessive melancholy, mood of hopelessness and feelings of inadequacy often with physical symptoms.' Here, deliberately, we start not with depression but with sadness. Because the word 'depression' has now entered the vernacular, even though the dictionary indicates it to be a technical term from psychiatry, sadness will be explored first. A discussion of the meaning of depression will then follow.

Feelings of any sort are experienced and then possibly expressed with words. Words themselves shape what it is legitimate to feel and not feel. As words reflect thoughts, once they are learned after infancy, they typically merge with feelings in a person's experience. The words available to describe feelings vary from culture to culture. In English, there are about 2,000 words to describe feelings, although only about 200 are in common use (Wallace and Carson, 1973). By contrast, the Ifalukians of Micronesia have only 58 words to describe transient internal states (Lutz, 1980) and the Chewong of Malaysia have only seven words which translate into English words about emotions (Howell, 1981). Russell (1991) found that in some African languages, a single word is used to mean both 'anger' and 'sadness' in an English translation.

When asked to look at emotional expressions in human faces, North American and Japanese subjects agree on 'sadness' and 'surprise' but not on 'anger' or 'fear'. These differences should lead us to be cautious about assuming that technical terms in Anglo-American psychiatry, related to mood states, have universal applicability.

Because of the richness of the English language, we may also assume that other languages are more restricted in their emotional descriptions, but this is not always the case. For example, we do not have good words in English to capture the German notions of *angst* or *Schadenfreude*, hence our tendency to leave them untranslated while having a general sense of their meaning.

With this caution about cultural differences in mind, Russell (1991), in his cross-cultural comparisons, concluded that there were, indeed, some universal emotional states. These can be roughly translated into this emotional circumflex based on two dimensions using ordinary words of the English language, with equivalents in the majority of others (see Figure 1.4).

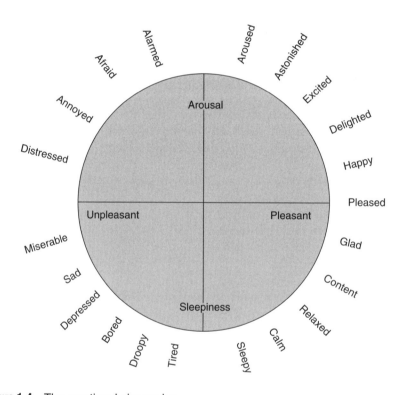

Figure 1.4   The emotional circumplex

For our purposes here, it should be noted that being sad seems to be a universal state. It is probably also fair to assume that the state is not peculiarly human. All higher mammals seem to show signs of sadness under conditions of loss or learned helplessness (Seligman, 1975).

Because it is an unpleasant state, a related matter is whether distressing sadness should be suppressed or simply left to persist or disappear without intervention. Here again, cultural differences come into play. Cultures vary in their expectations of how long and how profoundly we should mourn the loss of others. Buddhists argue that suffering (with sadness being one of its manifestations) is inherent to the human condition. Likewise, existentialists argue that we should stay with discomforting feelings (like sadness and anxiety) in order to confront their source and meaning in our lives. By technicalising this form of suffering as an illness and invoking medical paternalism to remove it (for example, by using 'antidepressant' drugs), arguably we are party to a form of rationalistic arrogance and cultural imperialism (Horwitz and Wakefield, 2007; Summerfield, 2008; Watters, 2010). Also, even when sadness is accepted as a form of mental illness, it is often coterminous with a field of experience that determines levels of loneliness and support, and so the context and emotional state of the person may be inextricably entwined (Kawachi and Berkman, 2001; Fujiwara and Kawachi, 2008).

Turning then to the term 'depression', its meaning is not consistent in Western psychiatry, nor is it preferred by psychiatrists universally. For example, in China, both psychiatrists and lay people use the notion of 'neurasthenia' in preference to 'depression'. The term 'neurasthenia' was used in English psychiatry in the 19th century to describe nervous fatigue but is now obsolete in the West (Kleinman, 1988). Anglo-American psychiatry currently agrees that depression is its 'common cold' – the diagnosis of greatest prevalence – but it still does not consistently agree on its meaning. Pilgrim and Bentall (1999) reviewed a variety of authoritative psychiatric texts and found the following:

- Some major texts do not even define depression (e.g. Beck et al., 1979; Golden and Janowsky, 1990). This may imply that the concept has self-evident validity for the authors and requires no formal description.
- Some texts argue that depression is primarily a disturbance of *mood* with all other features (cognitive symptoms like negativism and somatic ones like poor appetite) being secondary to this (e.g. Becker, 1977).
- Other texts argue that it is primarily defined by *cognitive* features – a negative view of self, the world and the future (e.g. Beck et al., 1979).
- There is no agreement on whether depression is an illness, a syndrome, a mood or a symptom (cf. Montgomery, 1990).
- While *DSM-IV* (American Psychiatric Association, 1994) demands the presence of depressed mood plus four other symptoms for a diagnosis of major depression, some other North American authorities offer a wider range of symptoms but argue that none, *not even depressed mood*, is essential for the diagnosis (e.g. Willner, 1985).
- A final complication is that mild to moderate ('neurotic') depression is often co-present with anxiety, with some texts consequently arguing that a unified diagnosis of a 'general neurotic syndrome' should replace both (e.g. Tyrer, 1990).

Thus, what starts as an apparently obvious consensus, that depression is the commonest of all mental disorders and that it is now understood well by lay people as well as mental health professionals, turns out to be problematic. We cannot assume that our Western view of depressive illness has universal applicability. Nor can we assume that psychiatrists have a strong agreement about what they mean by 'depression'. Claims that 'clinical depression' is categorically different from 'dysphoria', or 'everyday unhappiness', cannot be demonstrated readily. Despite the difficulties surrounding the conceptual validity of 'depression' (or maybe in part because of its woolly inclusiveness), epidemiologists now record it as being the fourth largest contributor to the global burden of disease – a role that is considered to be rising (Murray and Lopez, 1995).

None of the above critical discussion is to argue that people cannot be profoundly sad and that this experience is not life-diminishing or even at times life-threatening. However, it does query whether the use of the word 'depression', as a medical codification of 'sadness' or 'misery', offers us clarity or improves our understanding of a universally experienced and extremely common aspect of human suffering.

See also: *causes and consequences of mental health problems; fear; madness; neuroscience.*

FURTHER READING

Horwitz, A.V. and Wakefield, J.C. (2007) *The Loss of Sadness: How Psychiatry Transformed Normal Sorrow into Depressive Disorder.* Oxford: Oxford University Press.
Seligman, M.E.P. (1975) *Helplessness: On Depression, Development and Death.* San Francisco, CA: Freeman.

REFERENCES

American Psychiatric Association (APA) (1994) *Diagnostic and Statistical Manual of Mental Disorders* (4th edn) (*DSM-IV*). Washington, DC: APA.
Beck, A.T., Rush, A.J., Shaw, B.F. and Emery, G. (1979) *Cognitive Therapy of Depression.* New York: Guilford Press.
Becker, J. (1977) *Affective Disorders.* Morristown, NJ: General Learning Press.
Fujiwara, T. and Kawachi, I. (2008) 'A prospective study of individual-level social capital and major depression in the United States', *Journal of Epidemiology and Community Health,* 62: 627–33.
Golden, R.N. and Janowsky, D.S. (1990) 'Biological theories of depression', in B.B. Wolman and G. Stricker (eds), *Depressive Disorders.* New York: Wiley.
Horwitz, A.V. and Wakefield, J.C. (2007) *The Loss of Sadness: How Psychiatry Transformed Normal Sorrow into Depressive Disorder.* Oxford: Oxford University Press.
Howell, S. (1981) 'Rules not words', in P. Heelas and A. Lock (eds), *Indigenous Psychologies: The Anthropology of the Self.* San Diego, CA: Academic Press.
Kawachi, I. and Berkman, L.F. (2001) 'Social ties and mental health', *Journal of Urban Health,* 78: 458–67.
Kleinman, A. (1988) *Rethinking Psychiatry.* New York: Free Press.
Lutz, C. (1980) 'Emotion words and emotional development', PhD dissertation, University of Harvard, Cambridge, MA.
Montgomery, S. (1990) *Anxiety and Depression.* London: Livingstone.
Murray, C.J.L. and Lopez, A.D. (eds) (1995) *The Global Burden of Disease.* Cambridge, MA: Harvard University Press.

Pilgrim, D. and Bentall, R.P. (1999) 'The medicalisation of misery: a critical realist analysis of the concept of depression', *Journal of Mental Health*, 8 (3): 261–74.

Russell, J.A. (1991) 'A circumflex model of affect', *Journal of Personality and Social Psychology*, 45: 848–56.

Seligman, M.E.P. (1975) *Helplessness: On Depression, Development and Death*. San Francisco, CA: Freeman.

Summerfield, D. (2008) 'How scientifically valid is the knowledge base of global mental health?', *British Medical Journal*, 336: 992–4.

Tyrer, P. (1990) 'The division of neurosis: a failed classification', *Journal of the Royal Society of Medicine*, 83: 614–16.

Wallace, A.F.C. and Carson, M.T. (1973) 'Sharing and diversity in emotional terminology', *Ethos*, 1: 1–29.

Watters, E. (2010) *Crazy Like Us: The Globalization of the American Psyche*. New York: Free Press.

Willner, P. (1985) *Depression: A Psychobiological Synthesis*. New York: Wiley.

Fear

DEFINITION

Fear is the behaviour and experience provoked in humans and other animals by real or perceived threats.

KEY POINTS

- Fear and anxiety are described.
- The psychiatric codification of anxiety-based problems is discussed.

Fear is a normal physiological and behavioural response to threat, evident in most animals. The term 'anxiety' is usually described as 'irrational fear', but the experience is still one of fear. Anxiety is manifested directly in humans in a range of symptoms. These include cognitive disturbances (such as poor concentration, irritability, a sense of impending doom or 'free floating anxiety'), autonomic arousal (such as sweating, dry mouth and palpitations), muscle tension, hyperventilation and sleep disturbances. The permutation of these various symptoms varies from one anxious person to another.

Traditionally, anxious and depressed patients are described as 'neurotic' personalities if their symptoms are chronic, or as having 'neurotic reactions' if not. In the vernacular, neurotic reactions are often called 'nervous breakdowns'. Neurotic patients are distressed and conscious of, or even preoccupied with, their symptoms. In all other respects, they are deemed to be rational and coherent and they are able to relate successfully to others. This traditionally differentiates the neuroses from the psychoses.

However, the boundary between neurosis and other states is not fixed. At times, neurotic patients may be deemed to lack insight and they may become asocial in their behaviour. Also, when neurotic symptoms become chronic and resistant to treatment, the patient may be reclassified as being 'personality disordered'. For example, those with chronic obsessive-compulsive symptoms who fail to respond to treatment may be reclassified as suffering from 'obsessive-compulsive personality disorder'. Similarly, the chronic social phobic might be thought of as suffering from an 'anxious avoidant personality disorder'.

Current psychiatric classification systems like *DSM* and *ICD* divide the broad field of anxiety neurosis into three groups, which subsume types:

- Phobic anxiety disorders (agoraphobia, with or without panic disorder, social phobia and specific phobias).
- Panic disorder (without agoraphobia).
- Anxiety disorder (generalised; obsessive-compulsive – under *DSM* but *ICD* places it as a separate disorder – mixed with depression (*ICD* only)).

Sigmund Freud distinguished between objective anxiety (a function of external threat) and subjective anxiety, which was derived from internal conflicts. In the latter case, he pointed in a general sense to the conflict between the instincts (sexual energy or libido, to which he later added the death instinct) and the socially required rationality and morality demanded of civilised adults.

The term 'anxiety' tends to be limited to humans but can be created experimentally in other mammals. The earliest demonstration of this was by Ivan Pavlov, who gave shocks to dogs unpredictably under conditions in which they could not escape. This began a behaviourist tradition of viewing anxiety as a conditioned fear response.

However anxiety is explained, in the field of mental health it is seen as the core common characteristic of neurotic presentations, if depression is excluded. Moreover, both the psychoanalytical and behaviourist traditions view anxiety as developmentally derived and pervasive. Freud considered that we are all, to some degree, neurotic. Psychoanalysis views us all as ill, with anxiety neurosis being the price we pay for living in a rule-bound, civilised world. Similarly, behaviourists would argue that we are all frightened of something to some degree.

Eventually, behaviourists conceded that anxiety and other emotions implicated thoughts, not just behaviour (reducing the gap between the objective emphasis in behaviourism and the subjective emphasis in psychoanalysis). This has led to a modification of the treatment of neurosis, within the behaviourist tradition. Previously, the emphasis was narrowly on the modification of fearful behaviour – an example of this was the gradual exposure of the person to the object evoking their fear ('systematic desensitisation'). Now, behavioural methods have been overtaken by cognitive-behavioural therapy, which works with the inner life as well as external responses.

Existential therapists take a different view of anxiety. Rather than seeking to remove it as a form of distress (the behavioural view) or establish a common understanding with the patient about its historical source (the psychoanalytical view), the existentialist would ask the patient to tolerate it, rather than remove or explain it. From this process, the patient is offered an opportunity to discover meaning in the ambiguity of the anxious experience. Existentialists view anxiety, like Buddhists view suffering, as integral to the human condition rather than as an exceptional state (what Søren Kierkegaard called 'sickness unto death').

The sociological questions that arise from these general psychological statements relate to why some people experience this or that form of anxiety in a particular context. Take the example of agoraphobia – panic or strong insecurity when away from a patient's home base. In the wake of industrialisation, this emerged in crowded urban areas with the new threats this brought, especially to women. The diagnosis is still given to twice as many women as men. Public spaces are more risky in complex urban areas than in quiet rural villages. All forms of anxiety symptoms increase in probability in the wake of social stress or specific trauma. As a consequence, the social antecedents of an anxious presentation are important to understand. For example, domestic violence and other violent crimes predict the development of panic disorder in victims.

The preference of the medical profession for drug treatments and the high prevalence of anxiety symptoms in the general population gave rise to problems about their use. Drugs targeting anxiety are called anxiolytics and the largest group of these, the benzodiazepines, dominated the market between the 1960s and the 1980s. These were very addictive and ineffective at symptom reduction after a few weeks. This created an iatrogenic epidemic of addiction with no long-term mental health gain for the patients receiving the drugs. Professionally led and self-help groups then had to be set up to help people come off these drugs. Since then, low-dose antidepressants have been used as an alternative, as well as drugs altering autonomic nervous system activity such as beta-blockers.

The descriptions given under *DSM* and *ICD* above focus only on those diagnoses in which anxiety is directly experienced and overtly expressed by the patient. Apart from *ICD* separating obsessive-compulsive disorder (OCD), both systems deal with other indications of the role of anxiety, even if they are formally described outside the domain of the anxiety disorders. Freud's original interest in hysteria (now described as 'histrionic' reaction or personality and 'somatisation' and 'hypochondriasis'), as a pure form of neurosis, raises an important question: is anxiety at the heart of *all* forms of mental abnormality?

Certainly, psychological theories of psychosis are now emphasising the role of underlying trauma and anxiety (for example, see Richard Bentall's (2003) *Madness Explained*). Some psychoanalysts, like Ronald Fairbairn and Harry Guntrip, have suggested that all psychopathology is about the anxious struggle to preserve the ego. Others, like John Bowlby, have also focused on the role of actual or anticipated loss or separation being a recurrent source of anxiety as well as depression in human beings. While these views about the role of anxiety in depressive, psychotic and schizoid phenomena remain contentious, in the cases of OCD, histrionic behaviour and hypochondriasis, the patient is involved in barely veiled attempts to deal with the pain of anxiety.

The professional jurisdiction over anxiety disorders has shifted over the years. During the late 19th century, as the psychiatric profession established itself, it took very little interest in neurosis and was preoccupied with lunacy. The problem of shell shock from the First World War altered this focus. However, the treatment of neurosis remained split off in the private consulting world of the psychotherapist, military treatment centres or metropolitan specialist facilities like the Tavistock Clinic.

After the Second World War, mental health professionals in the NHS began to take more and more interest in anxiety problems, with clinical psychologists, nurse therapists and some psychiatrists championing their treatment using psychological therapies. The treatment of anxiety problems is now common in mental health services but most patients presenting with these difficulties are not referred to specialist services, with the demand for the latter well outstripping supply. As a result, experiments with community-based, self-help and computerised systems of treatment are becoming more common, particularly as confidence in drug treatments has been undermined by the benzodiazepine-dependence problem noted earlier.

See also: *causes and consequences of mental health problems; challenging conduct in adults and children; psychiatric classification; sadness.*

FURTHER READING

Bentall, R.P. (2003) *Madness Explained: Psychosis and Human Nature*. London: Allen Lane.
Bowlby, J. (1988) *A Secure Base*. London: Routledge.
de Swaan, A. (1990) *The Management of Normality*. London: Routledge.
Feltham, C. (ed.) (1997) *Which Psychotherapy? Leading Exponents Explain Their Differences*. London: Sage.
Goldberg, D. and Huxley, P. (1992) *Common Mental Disorders: A Bio-social Model*. London: Routledge.
Guntrip, H. (1961) *Personality Structure and Human Interaction*. London: Hogarth Press.
Noyes, R. and Hoehn-Saric, R. (1998) *The Anxiety Disorders*. Cambridge: Cambridge University Press.

REFERENCE

Bentall, R.P. (2003) *Madness Explained: Psychosis and Human Nature*. London: Allen Lane.

Physical Health

DEFINITION

In its simplest terms, physical health refers to soundness of the body. It is often defined negatively, though, by the absence of disease. A person may be healthy but

KEY POINTS

- The interplay between physical and mental health is discussed and examples given.
- Cautions about the notion of 'somatisation' are rehearsed.

This entry appears in a book on mental health for two reasons. First, a person's physical health status predicts their mental health status and vice versa. For example, psychiatric patients have high rates of physical morbidity. They are four times more likely to die of cardiovascular and respiratory disease, and five times more at risk of becoming diabetic. Second, some abnormalities of the body (particularly of the nervous system) lead to psychological, as well as physical, symptoms. The separation of mind and body is called 'Cartesian dualism' by philosophers, following the trend begun by Descartes of discussing these separately. In some cultures, this dualism does not exist, which is reflected in the way in which words are used to describe health and illness.

The interplay of physical and mental health has led to a group of mental health professionals ('liaison psychiatrists' and 'clinical health psychologists') working in areas of physical medicine and surgery. A number of points can be summarised about the enmeshment of physical and mental health:

- *The treatment of mental disorders using psychotropic drugs has physical consequences for patients* Psychiatric drugs have a blunderbuss impact on the central nervous system and have a range of adverse bodily consequences. These include dry mouth, acute dysphoria, movement disorders, constipation, sleep disturbaces, weight gain, sedation and blood disorders. These risks increase with higher doses ('megadosing') and with the prescription of several drugs at the same time ('polypharmacy'). These iatrogenic impacts of treatment have been a longstanding basis for critiques of psychiatry.
- *Physical disease can have direct psychological consequences* An example here is diabetes, where the physiological fluctuations can affect the degree of experienced distress (anxiety and low mood). In addition, diabetics have the concept of control (balancing carbohydrate intake, insulin use and exertion) imposed on their lives after the diagnosis. This ongoing process is stressful for patients.
- *Psychosomatic illnesses* These are physical illnesses to which psychological functioning makes a causal contribution. For example, gastrointestinal disturbances in an anxious person may lead to chronic dyspepsia or ulceration of the stomach or gut. At one time, ulcers of this sort were thought of, overwhelmingly, as being of psychological origin but, more recently, bacterial causes have also been identified. A more common and clear-cut example is the link between anxiety and hypertension. The latter is an immediate risk factor for

cardiovascular disease and a long-term risk factor for vascular dementia (see below). Psychosomatic illnesses are sometimes called 'psychogenic' but, as the next point indicates, the latter term is wider and so is not a synonym.

- *Psychogenic disorders* These include psychosomatic illnesses and other conditions in which minor symptoms of illness are exaggerated in a distressed fashion by the patient ('hypochondriasis' or 'hypochondriacal overlay') or the person has dramatic symptoms with no apparent physical evidence of cause ('hysterical conversion disorders'). Even more dramatically, some people inflict harm on themselves to receive emergency medical treatment ('Munchausen's Syndrome'). In very rare cases, an extension of this are parents or care staff who harm children to seek medical attention ('Munchausen's Syndrome-by-Proxy'). Psychiatrists use the term 'somatisation' to describe the expression of psychological distress in bodily terms.

- *Somato-psychological reactions* This is when a physical disease or acquired disability leads to psychological distress. An example of this is the way in which people differ in their psychological adaptation to losing, or losing the use of, limbs. Some people develop a prolonged grief reaction to the loss or their personality becomes irritable, whereas others do not react in these ways.

- *Neurological diseases* These invariably have psychological consequences. In dementia, the person becomes disorientated in time and space and short-term memory problems are evident. Amnesia predominates in those who chronically abuse alcohol and these patients may also experience visual hallucinations ('Korsakoff's psychosis'). As another example of the mutual influence of mind and body, cardiovascular functioning can be affected negatively by chronic stress and behavioural factors, such as poor diet and a low-exercise lifestyle. In turn, these effects can create chronic hypertension, which increases the risk of one form of dementia. In the case of those diagnosed with parkinsonism and multiple sclerosis, there are high rates of associated depression and lethargy.

- *Drug reactions and withdrawal* Some drugs create temporary psychological effects. This largely describes the effects of psychoactive drugs like caffeine, heroin, benzodiazepines and hallucinogens. Occasionally, psychotic reactions occur in the wake of amphetamine and cannabis use. Some prescribed medications for physical illness have behavioural effects (for example, some oral antihistamines can cause sedation and an increased risk of accidents, and psychotic reactions have been recorded in the use of some anti-malarial agents). Drug withdrawal also has psychological consequences. For example, nicotine withdrawal produces agitation in the smoker.

- *The psychological benefits of physical exercise* Physical exercise creates mental health gain for two reasons. First, it alters the biochemical functioning of the brain to raise mood. Second, the sense of control, which exercise bestows, raises self-esteem. For these reasons, physical exercise can be used successfully in the treatment of 'mild to moderate' presentations of generalised anxiety and depression.

- *The psychological impact of multiple illnesses* This is particularly relevant in older people because the probability of multiple illness increases with age, but it can apply at any age in an individual case. Multiple illnesses create pain and pain is demoralising. It also creates functional deficits (around movement and access to routine daily activities). The latter create a sense of loss and loss of control in the patient, which is saddening for them.
- *The ambiguity of pain* Neuroscientists studying pain note that it has sensory, cognitive and emotional aspects (experienced concurrently by the patient in a 'pain matrix'). The traditional distinction between physical and psychological pain is that the latter has no obvious sensory source (such as a tumour, scald or wound). However, experientially, some very depressed patients describe a form of physical pain and they may have very strong beliefs about their body being diseased. Also, some forms of illness, such as fibromyalgia and irritable bowel syndrome, which include a dominant symptom of acute pain, are correlated with distressing psychological histories (of trauma or abuse). Again, this highlights the ambiguities surrounding the experience of distress in a social context, which maintains the Cartesian split between mind and body.
- *The physical correction of healthy bodies for intended mental health gain* This is contentious in relation to both the behaviour of professionals and their patients. On the one hand, under *DSM-IV* (American Psychiatric Association, 1994), patients who complain unreasonably that some part of their anatomy requires correction are diagnosed as suffering from 'body dysmorphic disorder'. On the other hand, cosmetic surgeons are kept in business by the needs of patients, with no obvious disease, demanding and acquiring corrective intervention, such as facelifts and breast enlargement. Another example in this controversial area is the intervention of surgeons, physicians and psychiatrists in the treatment of transgenderism. Outside the domain of sex-change negotiations between lay people and professionals, body modification is also common now in a range of unilateral decisions made by adult citizens – body piercing, tattooing and scarification. All of these activities are aimed, among other things, at some form of mental health gain via individual expression, group identity and resistance to conformity. In the case of transgenderism, recent policy options about self-identification have brought key questions to the fore. Is it right or wrong for adults to block puberty in gender-variant children? Should transmen have resources allocated to their maternity services? Is transgenderism a mental disorder or a self-identified existential state and how should healthcare professionals respond to this ambiguity? These debates continue at the time of writing.

Psychogenic illnesses have also been surrounded by disputes. By definition, hypochondriacal patients are chronically disaffected with the medical profession. Under *DSM*, hypochondriasis is a 'somatoform disorder'. To the embarrassment of their treating psychiatrist, some patients with this label may transpire to have an unrecognised physical pathology. For this reason, the medical profession is increasingly using the more cautious description of 'medically unexplained symptoms'. Some other patients, described as 'somatisers', have been involved in a collective opposition movement. An example is those with 'chronic fatigue syndrome', who sometimes resent their problems being ascribed to underlying psychological causes.

A final example of a controversy about the 'somatisation' thesis is that in some cultures, the presentation of physical illness has a different significance from that applying in the norms of Western medicine. For example, a common medical assumption is that South Asian patients, who are 'really' depressed, present with bodily complaints. This diagnostic tendency has not escaped without criticism.

See also: *causes and consequences of mental health problems; substance misuse.*

FURTHER READING

Banks, J. and Prior, L. (2001) 'Doing things with illness: the micro-politics of the CFS clinic', *British Journal of Sociology*, 52 (2): 11–23.

Breggin, P. (2008) *Brain-Disabling Treatments in Psychiatry*. New York: Springer.

Feinstein, A., Magalhaes, S., Richard, J.-F., Audet, B. and Moore, C. (2014) 'The link between multiple sclerosis and depression', *Nature Reviews Neurology*, 10: 507–17.

Fenton, S. and Sadiq-Sangster, A. (1996) 'Culture, relativism and mental distress', *Sociology of Health and Illness*, 18 (1): 66–85.

Kirmayer, L.J. and Young, A. (1998) 'Culture and somatization: clinical, epidemiological, and ethnographic perspectives', *Psychosomatic Medicine*, 60 (4): 420–30.

Krause, I.B. (1989) 'Sinking heart: a Punjabi communication of distress', *Social Science & Medicine*, 29 (4): 563–7.

MacLachlan, M. (1997) *Culture and Health*. London: Wiley.

Manu, P. (1998) *Functional Somatic Syndromes*. Cambridge: Cambridge University Press.

Moncrieff, J. (2008) *The Myth of the Chemical Cure: A Critique of Psychiatric Drug Treatment*. Basingstoke: Palgrave

Moncrieff, J. (2013) *The Bitterest Pills: The Troubling Story of Antipsychotic Drugs*. Basingstoke: Palgrave.

Pearce, R. (2018) *Understanding Trans Health: Discourse, Power and Possibility*. Bristol: Policy Press.

Pilgrim, D. (2018) 'Reclaiming reality and redefining realism: the challenging case of transgenderism', *Journal of Critical Realism*, 17 (3): 308–24.

Riva, de la P., Smith, K., Xie, X.S. and Weintraub, D. (2014) 'Course of psychiatric symptoms and global cognition in early Parkinson disease', *Neurology*, 83 (12): 1096–103.

Rogers, A.E. and Allison, T. (2004) '"What if my back breaks?" Making sense of musculoskeletal pain among South Asian and African-Caribbean people in the North West of England', *Journal of Psychosomatic Research*, 57 (1): 79–87.

Shreffler, K.M., Johnson, D.R. and Scheuble, L.K. (2014) 'Ethical problems with infertility treatments: attitudes and explanations', *Social Science Journal*, 47 (4): 731–46.

Sorkin, D.H., Ngo-Metzger, Q., Kaplan, S.H., Reikes, R. and Greenfield, S. (2015) 'Mental health symptoms and patient-reported diabetes symptom burden: implications for medication regimen changes', *Family Practice*, 32 (3): 317–22.

REFERENCE

American Psychiatric Association (APA) (1994) *Diagnostic and Statistical Manual of Mental Disorders* (4th edn) (*DSM-IV*). Washington, DC: APA.

Pleasure

DEFINITION

'A feeling of satisfaction or joy; sensuous enjoyment as an object of life.' (The Concise Oxford Dictionary)

KEY POINTS

- The relevance of pleasure to the topic of mental health is examined and examples given.
- The importance of the denial of pleasure in religious and psychological systems of thought is discussed.

Pleasure is not discussed at length in most of the literature of mental health professionals. The experience contains the fluid interplay of closely related emotions on the emotional circumplex (see the entry on Sadness and Figure 1.4). These are at one end of the pleasant–unpleasant dimension and are experienced subjectively as being: 'content', 'glad', 'pleased', 'happy', 'delighted' and 'excited'. In everyday language, pleasure implies a state of being: it is constituted by thought and action, not just a feeling state. The two aspects of the dictionary definition point to pleasure as being both an emotion and a motivation or an intention.

Despite the relative lack of discussion about it in the literature, pleasure-seeking does have implications for mental health in a number of ways:

- *The pursuit of pleasure is a civil right in modern democracies* In this sense, the achievement of pleasure can be seen as being close to the World Health Organization's definition of psychological wellbeing. Human behaviour includes a number of pleasure-seeking activities. If pursued with due caution, they can increase wellbeing, buffer the person against mental health problems and create no long-term risk to the individual or others. Examples here would include satisfying work and sexual activity, moderate intoxication, telling jokes or listening to comedy, listening to or playing music, watching or playing sport, preparing or eating food, reading or writing, watching television, going to the theatre, walking and doing other exercise, and so on. Freud defined work and love as the two touchstones of positive mental health. He emphasised the tension between the pleasure principle, our natural tendency to avoid pain, and its modification by the demands of civilisation (the reality principle). The first was about infantile wish fulfilment, whereas the second was about adult adaptation. Other analysts, such as Wilhelm Reich, were more emphatic that free and pleasurable sexual expression was a prerequisite of avoiding both mental and physical health problems. His view was that pleasure was positive and healthy and Reich elevated erotic love to a special health-giving position. He not only argued that mandatory monogamy was an impediment to mental health, but also held that pornography and prostitution were oppressive and unhealthy expressions of sexual need.

- *Short-term access to a state of pleasure can lead to long-term mental health problems* The most obvious example of this is in relation to intoxication. As drunks with hangovers know, intoxication is a fleeting form of pleasure but also one that seductively re-engages the victim. Heroin addicts describe hours of intense warm pleasure after the initial 'rush' of an intravenous injection. These transient experiences in those who misuse substances are so overwhelmingly addictive that they are sought repeatedly, often at the expense of all other social obligations or personal needs. Other examples of pleasure-as-danger include the risk of HIV infection in unguarded sexual activity and the risk of death or injury from fast driving.

- *Pleasure can be a precarious or absent state in some mental health problems* The clearest example of this is in relation to bipolar disorder. However, the periods of exuberance, grandiosity and industry in 'high' phases are not inevitably experienced as pleasurable; sometimes patients express distress when they are manic. Also, unrestrained mania can lead to exhaustion and even death. The depressive collapse that ensues after a manic episode is certainly not a pleasurable state. The inability to experience pleasure may also be indicative of other problems, such as those with diagnoses of schizoid personality disorder and schizophrenia (where it is a 'negative symptom'). A lack of pleasure appears in psychiatric texts as 'loss of libido' or 'anhedonia'.

- *Humanistic psychology takes a permissive view of pleasure* Examples of this can be found in the humanistic psychology literature of the 1960s (sometimes called the 'human potential' or 'growth' movement) and the more recent study of positive psychology. In the first case, in reaction to the negative emphasis of psychoanalysis, with its focus on the abandonment of wish fulfilment and the need for the growing child to rescind its wishes, the 'growth movement' was permissive and positive. People were encouraged to elaborate and pursue their fantasies. However, the human potential movement was not merely hedonistic, as it also encouraged people to find meaning in all forms of experience, not just pleasure. In the case of positive psychology, there is an emphasis on the study of how people achieve and succeed, rather than on studying their defects. It studies the promotion of positive personal traits, such as interpersonal effectiveness and self-determination. This is a recent elaboration of the work of American humanistic psychologists, such as Carl Rogers and Abraham Maslow. Positive psychology puts personal wellbeing at the centre of the benign interpersonal processes of support and tolerance. The experience of pleasure in this view of mental health is not an end in itself but a permitted outcome or experience.

The notion that people should be able to achieve and sustain pleasure is at odds with some philosophical and scientific positions about the human condition (although hedonism has always had its philosophical advocates). For example, Buddhism and existentialism tend to emphasise suffering and angst as being integral to the human condition, and that striving against this truth is futile. Paradoxically, they also argue that pleasure may be achieved for periods of time by not striving for it.

The major deistic faiths tend to emphasise the denial of pleasure as a prerequisite of salvation or spiritual experience. For example, celibacy and frugality are emphasised in the Catholic Church, in its clergy and other religious members (nuns and monks). All Christian and Jewish groups demand that sexual pleasure is limited to monogamous relationships. Islam is less clear about the latter demand, as it sometimes tolerates polygamy, but it concurs with the other two faiths about the taboo on premarital and extramarital sexual activity.

Most faiths restrict access to types of food and encourage periods of restraint and abstinence. Muslims and Mormons are not permitted alcohol and the latter are denied caffeine. Sexual abstinence and fasting are also associated with deeper spiritual understanding in Hinduism. Some young male Hindus even seek castration as a path to religious fulfilment.

Evolutionary psychology suggests that humans and other animals are not driven by pleasure but by the need to survive and to pass on their genes. This would suggest that aggression and sexual promiscuity (in heterosexual males) are the real drivers of human action, not pleasure-seeking. If pleasure occurs, it is a by-product, not a primary goal. Taken to its logical conclusion, the aggressive psychopath represents an evolutionary success.

As an indication of Freud's ambivalence about the role of pleasure, not only did he emphasise the reality principle, but he also introduced the competing death instinct 'Thanatos' into his theory about the human condition. In doing this, he emphasised the role of aggression rather than pleasure in normal psychology and so came near to the evolutionist position.

See also: *challenging conduct in adults and children; creativity; fear; sadness; substance misuse; wellbeing.*

FURTHER READING

Freud, S. (1920/1955) 'Beyond the pleasure principle', in the *Collected Works of Sigmund Freud*, Vol. 18. London: Hogarth Press.

Kopp, S. (1973) *If You Meet the Buddha on the Road, Kill Him*. New York: Sheldon Press.

Maslow, A.H. (1968) *Toward a Psychology of Being*. Princeton, NJ: Princeton University Press.

Reich, W. (1961) *The Function of the Orgasm*. New York: Farrar, Straus and Giroux.

Rogge, B. (2011) 'Mental health, positive psychology and the sociology of the self', in D. Pilgrim, A. Rogers and B. Pescosolido (eds), *The SAGE Handbook of Mental Health and Illness*. London: Sage.

Ryan, R.M. and Deci, E.L. (2001) 'On happiness and human potentials: a review on hedonic and eudaimonic wellbeing', *Applied Review of Psychology*, 52: 141–66.

Seligman, M. and Csikszentmihalyi, M. (2000) 'Positive psychology', *American Psychologist*, 55 (1): 5–14.

pleasure

Creativity

DEFINITION

An act of imagination that leads to a solution to a problem or a novel form of artistic expression.

KEY POINTS

- The link between mental abnormality and creativity is explored.
- Psychological and sociological accounts for this link are examined.

Retrospective analyses of successful historical figures, from different fields, highlight the creative potential that has come to be associated with their distress or madness. This is particularly true of painters, composers and writers but scientists also have high rates of reported psychopathology. Of the many poets and writers cited are Ezra Pound and William Styron, as well as Sylvia Plath and Anne Sexton (both of whom committed suicide). Vincent van Gogh also committed suicide and would probably now be seen as suffering from bipolar disorder, although he appears in older psychiatric texts as a 'creative psychopath'. This defunct diagnosis (also given to Joan of Arc and T.E. Lawrence) was used in relation to personality disorder.

Many classical composers were noted for their social conformity and for being emotionally unremarkable (for example, Bach, Mendelssohn, Haydn and Schubert). However, collectively, composers have had high rates of mental health problems compared to those for the general population. Mozart is now thought to have suffered from Gilles de la Tourette's Syndrome (a mixture of nervous tics and obsessive-compulsive symptoms). Handel and Schumann were noted for their dramatic mood swings, with Schumann's work only appearing when he was manic. Schumann was diagnosed retrospectively as suffering from schizophrenia by Eugen Bleuler, the psychiatrist who invented that diagnosis. Some of the best work of Beethoven, including his Ninth and arguably finest symphony, appeared after he became depressed because of his hearing difficulties. Debussy transformed a period of ill health and depression into bursts of creativity. Of the Russian Romantics, Tchaikovsky and Scriabin were noted for their tortured mental states.

In common parlance today, the term 'artistic temperament' is sometimes a code for 'mentally unstable' and the examples given above suggest that depression can be either an impediment to creativity or its source. A whole musical genre emerged from the depressive state – 'the blues'. The term may be traceable to the skin hue of cold and dejected slaves but it now connotes depression. During the

20th century, many popular creative artists were described as having a range of psychological problems, including substance misuse, psychosis and suicidal depression, for example, Ernest Hemingway, Brendan Behan, Dylan Thomas, Brian Wilson and Nick Drake. The list of famous *performing* artists who have lived recklessly (often abusing substances) and died young is long and includes Judy Garland, Elvis Presley, Janis Joplin, Jimi Hendrix, Brian Jones, Keith Moon, Gram Parsons, Jim Morrison, Amy Winehouse and Kurt Cobain.

It is a moot point whether performers are artists or technicians. However, they are obliged to bring to life an artistic event each time they perform and so, in that basic sense, they are creative. Famous performing artists often have the pressures and pleasures of an erratic lifestyle on the road ('sex and drugs and rock and roll') and the omnipotence and self-indulgence triggered by fame and fortune. Also, the *desire* in performers to be famous might reflect a form of pathological narcissism. Frustration, unhappiness and self-indulgence may accrue, whether or not fame is actually achieved. Descriptions of people with narcissistic and histrionic personality disorder emphasise their unending need for dramatic performance and admiration.

Another field in which the confluence of psychopathology and creativity has been evident is in comedy. Examples here in living memory are Spike Milligan, Tony Hancock and Peter Cook. Humour and wit are good examples of creative reasoning and were the basis of a whole piece of work for Sigmund Freud (*Jokes and Their Relation to the Unconscious* (1905)). Similarly, depth psychologists such as Jung and Winnicott have seen play and playfulness as being healing expressions of unconscious life.

Psychological accounts of the coexistence of mental health problems and creativity suggest several factors to consider. Some mental health problems affect the motivational level and focus of the individual involved. People who are manic have unusually high levels of energy, which can be converted into industry. Similarly, conditions in which asocial features predominate allow a person's attention to be sustained in a project. Creative people tend to work very hard at their art or science and can be obsessive, often to the exclusion or detriment of their personal relationships.

Depth psychology would suggest that the unconscious is the source of *both* creativity *and* mental abnormality. Freudians view unconscious impulses as being 'sublimated' into socially acceptable products and that 'regression at the service of the ego' can be observed in some patients. Freud considered the imagination to be neurotic daydreaming. Later psychoanalysts, like Melanie Klein, suggested that creativity represents fixation at infantile stages of development. Fixation at the depressive stage involves a person creatively using their destructive fantasies in a reparative or guilt-ridden way. Fixation at the schizoid phase suggests that the person operates just this side of madness and uses their fantasies to avoid people. This frees or compels them to explore their inner world, intensively and extensively. Klein's emphasis on the role of destructive forces operating in both the imagination and the creative act points up a paradox noted by many.

Thus, ambivalence exists in depth psychology about whether creative people have ever properly grown up (fixation) or whether they are simply prone to regression. An example of the latter is the Freudian view that painting is a regressed sublimation of the smearing of faeces. The notion that creativity is linked to psychological immaturity is indicated by the study of poets and popular song-writers, who tend to be at their best in adolescence and young adulthood. However, this trend is not evident in other fields.

Some existential therapists, like Rollo May, argue that neurosis is blocked crea-tivity and that to provide therapy to imaginative people might rob them of their achievements. May (1972) cites Rilke, who left psychotherapy after discovering its goals: 'If my devils are to leave me, I am afraid my angels will take flight as well.' The emphasis in existentialism is on a state of being, which resists narrow rationality and remains open to all experience. For existential therapists (and some psychoanalysts), the poet John Keats is often quoted favourably by this insight: 'negative capability is when a man is capable of being in uncertainties, mysteries, doubts, without any irritable reaching after fact and reason'. This mod-ern existential view of creativity can be found in the older religious traditions of Christian mysticism and Buddhism. For example, St John of the Cross was of the view that: 'to come to the knowledge you have not, you must go by a way which you know not'.

A more recent psychological approach to creativity can be found (seemingly oddly) in the study of computers, their use of rules and their ability to be pro-grammed to generate new forms of jazz, symphonic music and drawings. This has been championed by Margaret Boden and is more appealing to those studying cognitive science who eschew the older depth psychology and existentialism.

A social, rather than psychological, framing of creativity suggests other possible accounts. The first, already noted about slavery and 'the blues', is that creativity may be stimulated by collective adversity. Desperate circumstances can ensure that 'necessity is the mother of invention'. The second is to do with consequences rather than causes. Creativity involves transgression – a break with convention. People with mental health problems transgress rules with or without reflection and insight. Creativity can thus be framed as one version of transgression, which happens to find social approval. By contrast, madness is a form of transgression that invites perplexity, pity, fear or ridicule.

The social framing of creativity suggests that it is context dependent and so cannot be described abstractly, as the essential characteristics of individuals (their particular skills of invention and ingenuity in all contexts). The sources of the acts of transgression might be psychological (as discussed earlier), biological (inherited aptitude) or social (we may learn to be imaginative in the family or at school), or some combination of these. However, whatever the source, judgements about the *outcome* are always social, as they require others to place a positive or negative value on the creative act.

A good example of the contingent nature of creativity is the reaction to the destruction by fire, in London in May 2004, of many expensive warehoused works of modern art. Some mourned their loss, whereas others thought it comical because they thought the works were trivial and without particular merit. To take a different example, a scientific inventor might produce many prototypes, which are cast aside until one is found which has some practical application. The same industry and imagination went into all versions but only one found approval, because of its use-value. The willingness to experiment with the absurd (avoiding the trap of Keats's 'fact and reason') means that creative people, like mad people, risk ridicule and social marginalisation.

If a fine line might exist between the obsessive crank and the creative genius, depending on whether or not others approve of the acts or products, this is also true of religious innovations. Christ wandered in the desert and claimed that he was the son of God. He went berserk in the temple and ranted and raved. The Buddha abandoned his regal existence and wandered aimlessly in the forest. On observing a sick man, an old man and a corpse, he became certain of the possibility of enlightenment about human existence. The prophet Mohammed felt compelled to retreat into a cave near Mecca, where a command hallucination kept telling him to cry. These religious leaders are now venerated by the majority of the world's population. All of them behaved in a way that would invite a retrospective diagnosis of schizophrenia. They now have excessive credibility, whereas the vast majority of those with a current diagnosis of schizophrenia have little or none.

See also: *madness; spirituality; wellbeing*.

FURTHER READING

Andreasen, N. (1980) 'Mania and creativity', in R.H. Belmaker and H.M. van Praag (eds), *Mania: An Evolving Concept*. New York: Spectrum.

Boden, M. (2004) *The Creative Mind: Myths and Mechanisms*. London: Routledge.

Freud, S. (1905) *Jokes and Their Relation to the Unconscious*, Vol. 8 of *The Standard Edition of the Complete Psychological Works of Sigmund Freud, 1953–1974*. London: Hogarth Press.

Jamison, K.R. (1993) *Touched with Fire: Manic Depressive Illness and the Artistic Temperament*. New York: Free Press.

May, R. (1972) *Love and Will*. London: Fontana.

Nettle, D. (2001) *Strong Imagination: Madness, Creativity and Human Nature*. Oxford: Oxford University Press.

Post, F. (1994) 'Creativity and psychopathology: a study of 291 world famous men', *British Journal of Psychiatry*, 165: 22–34.

REFERENCES

Freud, S. (1905) *Jokes and Their Relation to the Unconscious*, Vol. 8 of *The Standard Edition of the Complete Psychological Works of Sigmund Freud, 1953–1974*. London: Hogarth Press.

May, R. (1972) *Love and Will*. London: Fontana.

Spirituality

KEY POINTS

- The relationship between spirituality and mental health is ambiguous in a number of ways.
- Spirituality, like madness and creativity, is one aspect of the non-rational dimension to human existence.
- Religious faith predicts wellbeing.

Not too long ago, 'religiosity' was typically viewed as symptomatic of mental disorder but recent debates in the field of mental health have altered this bias. It is certainly the case that mad people are sometimes preoccupied with religion and understand their idiosyncratic experiences in spiritual terms and sometimes their recovery. However, madness might be experienced as an existential turning point, not just as a period of personal catastrophe or alienation. Spirituality, like creativity, invites us to consider positive aspects of non-rationality in our lives, instead of it being framed singularly as psychopathology ('irrationality').

While all religions are rooted in and celebrate spirituality, many people report a spiritual dimension to their lives without any declared allegiance to a faith group. Thus, a distinction can be made between spiritual *experience* and religious *belief*, even if, for many people, these may remain subjectively intertwined. Spiritual experience is subjectively focused and typically has few or no behavioural implications, beyond the subtle and idiosyncratic. In contrast, religious beliefs manifest themselves objectively in a range of ways: sacred buildings; codified knowledge (scriptures); moral strictures; dietary habits; small and grand devotional rituals and obligations; and prayer, contemplation or meditation. Warfare and other forms of violence might also be justified on religious grounds, as might self-harm and sacrifice.

It may be worth noting that of the faith systems, Buddhism, a non-theistic approach to existence and its problems, is the one which has been most strongly associated with the *experiential* rather than the faith emphasis of spirituality. However, other religions also have sub-traditions with this emphasis, such as the Sufi version of Islam as well as the Jewish and Christian versions of mysticism.

A third ambiguity is that religious affiliation can have mental health consequences, which may say more about group membership than spirituality *per se*.

Take the example of radicalised Muslims who become suicide bombers. It is clear that their political disaffection with Western materialism and their strong small group affiliation reinforce a coherent and meaningful sense of identity. Religion is a common system of meaning for this process of identity formation and existential commitment to self-sacrifice. In other words, in this case, religion, not spirituality, seems to have a positive psychological function for the individuals, about a proud identity, even if the consequence for others is lethal. And, although major faiths do not argue that mass murder is a noble expression of spiritual life, historically violence has been justified recurrently by religious grievance or crusading evangelism.

A more benign example of this point about religion and personal identity and self-respect comes from evidence about the link between faith and wellbeing. Faith groups provide a double advantage to people: they offer a framework of meaning and that framework occurs in an interpersonal field of comforting rituals and supportive social contact. Studies of psychological distress suggest that the better ratings of religious people cannot be accounted for by social capital alone (the common framework of meaning is also important). Health benefits flow from this – religious affiliation is linked to measurable reductions in both morbidity and mortality.

Thus, religion provides purpose and comfort, about the vagaries of life and death, and offers one source of social capital. It is not very surprising, then, that religious faith brings with it a buffer against distress and increases the probability of conformity to norms (both indicators of the absence of mental disorder). By contrast, spirituality does not necessarily implicate social capital – indeed, it may be associated with social isolation. For example, some of the most dramatic accounts of spiritual experience are about people in their own idiosyncratic existential space. Their relationship is not with others but with a great Being or whole ('the Oneness'), which transcends time and space.

This transcendental or mystical realm is what Freud, a materialist and atheist, called the 'Oceanic Experience', when the boundaries of the ego dissolve in dreams and madness or in spiritual experiences. It is in this realm of idiosyncratic mystical experience that the blurred boundary between madness (an interpersonal attribution) and spiritual experience (a personal attribution) becomes apparent. Was the Buddha enlightened or mad? When the prophet Mohammed heard a voice that made him cry, was this a symptom of schizophrenia or a command from God? Was Jesus God-made-flesh or was he suffering from a delusion of grandeur? As far as hallucinatory experiences are concerned, we can add Paul on the road to Damascus and Moses seeing the burning bush. Collective hallucinations are also present in religious traditions (those witnessing the resurrection of Christ and the group sightings since then of the Virgin Mary). A number of Christian sects (the Quakers, Shakers, Mormons and Seventh Day Adventists) have been led by people who had such experiences.

Since the time of 'anti-psychiatry', and in particular with the writings of Laing and Grof, the ambiguous relationship between psychosis and spirituality has been a matter of much debate. Both involve an alternative consciousness, though in the first case this can go on for months or years, whereas spiritual experiences tend to be fleeting. Also, psychosis emerges often without apparent warning, whereas the conditions of possibility for spiritual experience involve deliberate elicitation rituals of emotional arousal, extraordinary social isolation or drug use. These create conditions of 'liminality', which is the threshold between everyday thoughts and feelings and a full-blown 'Oceanic Experience' or state of transcendence. These out-of-the-ordinary experiences may lead to altered views of the world, which are then incorporated back into routine daily life. By contrast, the psychotic patient may or may not come back from this journey of crossing liminality.

Social isolation, deliberate or imposed, connects the conditions associated with both psychosis and transcendental experience. In the first case, psychotic patients often eschew others and others may shun them in turn, creating a vicious circle of personal alienation. In the case of the mystical aspects of religion, social isolation is created more deliberately and is even ritualised. The disciplinary regimes of nuns and monks demand degrees of physical isolation from open society and its norms. This isolation creates a disconnection from regular expectations about sexual intimacy and attachments to egocentric material goals, which typically link work and consumption – hence the recurring focus in religious life on chastity and poverty. Itinerant Hindu holy men put themselves outside routine family attachments and Buddhist monks go with their begging bowl to their local communities.

These routines create social constriction. Within that constriction, depending on the extent of the rituals required, the individual becomes further isolated during periods of silent contemplation, prayer or meditation. These create the personal context for extraordinary experiences, as social isolation increases the probability of hallucinations and strengthens the commitment to a belief system, unchallenged by contrary viewpoints in open society.

A final point to note about spirituality is that it offers a fourth dimension to mental health. The first three (the biological, psychological and social dimensions of mental health) are sufficient for materialists and atheists. For others, a consideration of spirituality is also required. Spirituality and religious affiliation offer a potential source of hope for those with mental health problems and protect many people from these problems or reduce their experienced impact.

See also: *creativity; madness; social and cultural capital; wellbeing.*

FURTHER READING

Awara, M. and Fasey, C. (2008) 'Is spirituality worth exploring in psychiatric out-patient clinics?', *Journal of Mental Health*, 17 (2): 183–91.

Barker, P. and Buchanan-Barker, P. (eds) (2004) *Spirituality and Mental Health: Breakthrough.* London: Whurr.

Clarke, I. (2001) *Psychosis and Spirituality: Exploring the New Frontier.* London: Whurr.

Donat, J.G. (1988) 'Medicine and religion: on the physical and mental disorders that accompanied the Ulster Revival of 1859', in W.F. Bynum, R. Porter and M. Shepherd (eds), *The Anatomy of Madness*, Vol. 3. London: Tavistock.

Grof, S. (1998) *The Cosmic Game.* Dublin: Newleaf.

Koenig, H.G. (2008) 'Religion and health: what should psychiatrists do?', *Psychiatric Bulletin*, 32: 201–3.

Laing, R.D. (1968) *The Politics of Experience and the Bird of Paradise*. Harmondsworth: Penguin.

Myers, D.G. (2000) 'The faith, friends and funds of happy people', *American Psychologist*, 55: 56–67.

Saxena, S. (2006) 'A cross-cultural study of spirituality, religion, and personal beliefs as components of quality of life', *Social Science & Medicine*, 62 (6): 1486–97.

Schieman, S. (2011) 'Religious beliefs and mental health: application and extension of the stress process model', in D. Pilgrim, A. Rogers and B. Pescosolido (eds), *The SAGE Handbook of Mental Health and Illness*. London: Sage.

Public Mental Health

DEFINITION

The combination of values and evidence to generate measures that could create a mentally healthy society.

KEY POINTS

- The rationale of public mental health is outlined.
- Improvements in wellbeing and the prevention of mental health problems are discussed.

A public mental health agenda is concerned with how individuals, families, organisations and communities think and feel, individually and collectively, and the attendant impact that this may have on overall mental health and wellbeing in society. In the past, public health has been dominated by epidemiology and disease control, in line with an early interest in mortality and physical morbidity (see the entry on Psychiatric Classification in Part II). Concerns about public mental health have arrived relatively late on the policy scene, but in the past decade wellbeing and the prevention of mental disorders have acquired more political interest. With this has come an interest in gauging the cost-effectiveness of political interventions to alter measured population-level mental health.

During, and contributing to, this recent interest, economists, psychiatrists and psychologists have introduced the notion that happiness should be a central political concern. The notion that happiness is a form of positive mental health is arguably a paradox given that some have argued it is a form of mental abnormality: 'it is statistically abnormal, consists of a discrete cluster of symptoms, is associated with a range of cognitive abnormalities, and probably reflects the abnormal functioning of the central nervous system' (Bentall, 1992: 94). Bentall's (1992) article notes that realistic predictions about life arise from a slightly depressive rather than happy personal outlook.

Notwithstanding this paradox, we can consider the following policy aspects of our new public mental health agenda, which are dealt with in the entries in the 'See also' section noted at the end of this entry:

- The prevention of mental disorder and promotion of positive mental health.
- The promotion of full citizenship for those who have experienced mental health problems.
- The promotion of wellbeing and the reduction in inequalities about it.
- The interaction of physical and mental health.

Economic appraisals of policy-driven interventions across the above list show mixed results. These are summarised in Table 1.1.

Table 1.1 Economic estimates of mental health promotion interventions

Context	Intervention	Cost impact
Health-visiting to reduce post-natal depression	Post-natal screening and psychologically informed sessions	No cost savings: benefits outweighed by training and higher staff costs
Parenting to prevent persistent conduct disorders	Parenting-style programmes targeting parents of children at risk of conduct disorders	Cost savings of 8:1 over 25 years mainly to the criminal justice system and the NHS
School-based social and emotional learning programmes	Programmes to help children recognise and manage emotions and relationships, set goals, aid decision-making	Lower conduct problems drive net savings from crime and NHS-related impact and wider benefits
Reducing bullying	Anti-bullying programmes in schools	Good value for money based on improved future earnings
Early detection and intervention for psychosis	Early detection and treatment service (CBT, medication)	NHS cost savings initially from avoidance of suicide psychotic episodes but reduced savings over time
Primary Care Screening, prevention for alcohol misuse	Screening by GPs and five-minute advice session	Robust economic case for intervention increased savings by use of practice nurses, rather than GP and targeting
Workplace screening for anxiety and depression	Screening and six sessions of CBT for those at risk	Cost saving for business relates to reduction in absenteeism
Promoting wellbeing in the workplace	Wellbeing programmes including risk appraisal, personalised information advice, online and workshop resources	Costs reduced for business and public sector employers and NHS
Debt and mental health	Mixture of debt-reduction advice models, telephone, internet and face-to-face advice	Better outcomes compared to no action

Context	Intervention	Cost impact
Population-level suicide awareness	GP suicide-prevention education	Highly cost-effective for healthcare system
Bridge safety measures for suicide prevention	Construction of bridge safety barriers	Substantial cost savings but risk of diversion to other lethal means
Primary Care Collaborative care for depression in type II diabetes	Case management by nurse and liaison with GP over and above routine care	Cost-effective after two years but high net additional costs due to implementation
Tackling medically unexplained symptoms	CBT for somatoform conditions	Cost saving estimated for the long term from reduced utilisation
Befriending of older adults	Weekly befriending contact for an hour for isolated and lonely people	Unlikely to be cost-effective to public purse but improved quality of life at low cost

Source: Rogers and Pilgrim (2014)

The summary in Table 1.1 was of interventions collated by Knapp et al. (2011). They examined the returns on investment in interventions which focused on economic pay-offs (for every pound spent). They concluded that not all interventions were cost-effective but three 'big hits' were identifiable: the prevention of dysfunctional conduct through social and emotional learning programmes; suicide prevention through bridge safety barriers; and suicide training in primary care. The three least cost-effective interventions were: early intervention for depression in diabetes; befriending of older adults; and health visitor interventions to reduce post-natal depression.

The other consideration to these micro techno-centric interventions is at the macro level: what cultural and economic factors affect population-level mental health? The answer to this broadly is that public mental health increases with stable periods of security (i.e. freedom from want and violence) and that the more equal a society is the greater is its level of wellbeing. Put differently, war-torn countries and those subject to either absolute or relative poverty tend to be mentally unhealthy. Also, recovery rates from mental health problems are affected by economic cycles (Warner, 1985). Thus, the particular social conditions of a particular country or region at a particular point in time determine prospects for improving mental health at the population rather than individual level (Herrman, 2011).

The logic of public mental health has little to do with mental health services. The latter are about containment and treatment (or at best tertiary prevention, which is the attempt to prevent relapse in identified patients). Primary prevention (reducing the stressors in society that prompt symptom formation) and secondary prevention (providing early interventions to reduce the prospects of mental health problems becoming chronic) arise from the resources available in wider society rather than funded mental health services. All public policies affecting peace, stability, social cohesion, child rearing, relative inequality and personal security can affect the success of public mental health as a political aspiration.

See also: *mental health promotion; mental health policy; physical health; social models; warfare; wellbeing.*

FURTHER READING

Goldie, I. (2010) *Public Mental Health Today: A Handbook.* London: Pavilion/Mental Health Foundation.

Lenzer, J. (2004) 'Bush plans to screen whole US population for mental illness', *British Medical Journal*, 328 (7454): 1458.

Rogers, A. and Pilgrim, D. (2014) *A Sociology of Mental Health and Illness* (5th edn). Maidenhead: Open University Press.

Walker, P. and John, M. (eds) (2012) *From Public Health to Wellbeing.* Basingstoke: Palgrave Macmillan.

REFERENCES

Bentall, R.P. (1992) 'A proposal to classify happiness as a psychiatric disorder', *Journal of Medical Ethics*, 18: 94–8.

Herrman, H. (2011) 'Promoting mental health', in D. Pilgrim, A. Rogers and B. Pescosolido (eds), *SAGE Handbook of Mental Health and Illness*. London: Sage.

Knapp, M., McDaid, D. and Parsonage, M. (eds) (2011) *Mental Health Promotion and Mental Illness Prevention: The Economic Case.* London: Department of Health.

Rogers, A. and Pilgrim, D. (2014) *A Sociology of Mental Health and Illness* (5th edn). Maidenhead: Open University Press.

Warner, R. (1985) *Recovery from Schizophrenia: Psychiatry and Political Economy.* London: Routledge.

Childhood Adversity

DEFINITION

Childhood adversity refers to challenges to development created by stressors outside the family (such as poverty, warfare and stranger assaults) and within it (such as neglect and sexual, physical and emotional abuse).

KEY POINTS

- There is a strong consensus that childhood adversity has an adverse impact on mental health in both the short and long term.
- Survivors of childhood maltreatment are over-represented in prison and psychiatric populations.

The relationship between childhood adversity and mental health is now well demonstrated and appears in lay accounts as well as in the professional literature (Rogers and Pilgrim, 1997). Developmental theories about mental health have been drawn from both behaviourism (Watson and Rayner, 1920) and psychoanalysis (Winnicott, 1965). One psychoanalyst, John Bowlby, formed a bridge between these two forms of psychology when developing his 'attachment theory'. Disruptions in attachments during childhood were shown by him to be linked to a wide range of short-term and long-term problems of anxiety, depression and delinquency (Bowlby, 1969).

Childhood adversity includes extra-familial stressors (such as warfare, poverty and stranger assaults) and abuse and neglect within families, which entail dysfunctional parent–child–environment relationships (Cichetti, 1987; Wurtele, 1998). Children who are physically abused or neglected suffer poor stimulation, poor diet and sometimes direct neurological damage from trauma to the head. These can lead to emotional withdrawal and intellectual developmental delays, expressed through poor comprehension and expressed language for age. Victims may go on to manifest impulsivity, aggression, oppositional challenges to authority and later criminality, as well as a range of symptoms of distress, including depression, anxiety, nightmares and flashbacks.

Sexual victimisation in childhood raises the risk of sexual precocity ('traumatic sexualisation'), teenage pregnancy and later sexual dysfunction and confusion about victims' sexuality (Kendall-Tackett et al., 1993). Intra-familial abuse increases the risk of chaotic adult behaviour involving suicidal action, self-harm, substance misuse, mood swings, dissociation (hysterical fugue states) and dramatic panic about abandonment in intimate relationships (Browne and Finkelhor, 1986). This pattern might be labelled by professionals as 'borderline personality disorder' in adulthood. In high-income countries, up to 5 per cent of boys and 10 per cent of girls are subjected to penetrative sex, 10 per cent of children suffer emotional abuse (being repeatedly humiliated and derided) and up to 16 per cent suffer physical attacks (Gilbert et al., 2008). Survivors of maltreatment in childhood are over-represented in both psychiatric and prison populations. Sexual abuse alone increases the risk in survivors of diagnoses of eating disorders, depression, anxiety, substance misuse, somatisation and personality disorders (Polusny and Follette, 1995). It also shapes the capacity of survivors to adapt to the stresses of later intimate relationships (Roberts et al., 2004).

Although there is a dominant discourse about stranger assaults from paedophiles, most abuse takes place inside families. Thus, intra-familial abuse is different from impersonal trauma and so it is a moot point whether its consequences are adequately described by the notion of 'post-traumatic stress disorder' alone. Ussher and Dewberry (1995), in their large survey of female survivors, found that: 'a range of long-term psychological effects was significantly related to … abuse perpetrated by father or step-father, abuse which was repeated or prolonged, presence or threats of violence, blaming the child, saying that disclosure would split the family and a younger age of onset'.

Psychotic and not just neurotic symptoms are traceable to childhood adversity. Apart from trauma, 'communication deviance' in families raises the risk of psychotic experiences (Neria et al., 2002; Read et al., 2003; Janssen et al., 2004; Anda et al., 2006; Read and Bentall, 2012; Varese et al., 2012). Children deemed to be at genetic risk of psychosis raised by adoptive parents are more likely to become psychotic only if the adoptive parents showed communication deviance (Wahlberg et al., 1997). This suggests the importance of a benign early environment in the primary prevention of mental health problems, including 'severe mental illness'.

See also: *age; attachment theory; causes and consequences of mental health problems; mental health promotion; warfare.*

FURTHER READING

Read, J. and Bentall, R.P. (2012) 'Negative childhood experiences and mental health: theoretical clinical and primary prevention implications', *British Journal of Psychiatry*, 200: 89–91.

Varese, F., Smeets, F., Drukker, M., Lieverse, R., Lataster, L.,Viechtbauer, W., Read, J., van Os, J. and Bentall, R.P. (2012) 'Childhood adversities increase the risk of psychosis: a meta-analysis of patient-control, prospective- and cross-sectional cohort studies', *Schizophrenia Bulletin*, 38: 661–71.

REFERENCES

Anda, R., Felliti, B., Bremner, J.D., Walker, J., Whitfield, C. and Perry, B. (2006) 'The enduring effects of abuse and related adverse experiences in childhood: a convergence of evidence from neurobiology and epidemiology', *European Archives of Psychiatry and Clinical Neuroscience*, 265 (3): 174–86.

Bowlby, J. (1969) *Attachment*. London: Hogarth Press.

Browne, A. and Finkelhor, D. (1986) 'The impact of child sexual abuse: a review of the research', *Psychological Bulletin*, 99: 66–77.

Cichetti, D. (1987) 'Developmental psychopathology in infancy: illustration from the study of maltreated youngsters', *Journal of Consulting and Clinical Psychology*, 55: 837–45.

Gilbert, R., Widom, C.S., Browne, K., Fergusson, D., Webb, E. and Janson, S. (2008) 'Burden and consequences of child maltreatment in high-income countries', *The Lancet*, 3 December: 61706–7.

Janssen, I., Krabbendam, L., Bak, M., Hanssen, M., Vollebergh, W., De Graaf, R. and van Os, J. (2004) 'Childhood abuse as a risk factor for psychotic experiences', *Acta Psychiatrica Scandinavica*, 109: 38–45.

Kendall-Tackett, K.A., Williams, L.M. and Finkelhor, D. (1993) 'Impact of sexual abuse on children: a review and synthesis of recent empirical studies', *Psychological Bulletin*, 113: 164–80.

Neria, Y., Bromet, E.J., Silevers, S., Lavelle, J. and Fochtmann, L.J. (2002) 'Trauma exposure and posttraumatic stress disorder in psychosis: findings from a first-admission cohort', *Journal of Consulting and Clinical Psychology*, 70: 246–51.

Polusny, M. and Follette, V. (1995) 'Long-term correlates of child sexual abuse: theory and review of the empirical literature', *Applied and Preventive Psychology*, 4: 143–66.

Read, J., Agar, K., Argyle, N. and Aderhold, V. (2003) 'Sexual and physical abuse during childhood and adulthood as predictors of hallucinations, delusions and thought disorder', *Psychology and Psychotherapy: Theory, Research and Practice*, 76: 1–22.

Read, J. and Bentall, R.P. (2012) 'Negative childhood experiences and mental health: theoretical clinical and primary prevention implications', *British Journal of Psychiatry*, 200: 89–91.

Roberts, R., O'Connor, T., Dunn, J. and Golding, J. (2004) 'The effects of child sexual abuse in later family life: mental health, parenting and adjustment of offspring', *Child Abuse and Neglect*, 28 (5): 535–45.

Rogers, A. and Pilgrim, D. (1997) 'The contribution of lay knowledge to the understanding and promotion of mental health', *Journal of Mental Health*, 6 (1): 23–36.

Ussher, J. and Dewberry, C. (1995) 'The nature and long-term effects of childhood sexual abuse: a survey of adult women survivors in Britain', *British Journal of Clinical Psychology*, 34: 177–92.

Varese, F., Smeets, F., Drukker, M., Lieverse, R., Lataster, L., Viechtbauer, W., Read, J., van Os, J. and Bentall, R.P. (2012) 'Childhood adversities increase the risk of psychosis: a meta-analysis of patient-control, prospective- and cross-sectional cohort studies', *Schizophrenia Bulletin*, 38: 661–71.

Wahlberg, K.-E., Wynne, L.C., Oja, H., Keskitalo, P., Pykalainen, L., Lahti, I., Moring, J., Naarala, N., Sorri, A., Seitamaa, M., Laksy, K., Kolassa, J. and Tienari, P. (1997) 'Gene–environment interaction in vulnerability to schizophrenia: findings from the Finnish Adoptive Family Study of Schizophrenia', *American Journal of Psychiatry*, 154: 355–62.

Watson, J.B. and Rayner, R. (1920) 'Conditioned emotional reactions', *Journal of Experimental Psychology*, 10: 421–8.

Winnicott, D.W. (1965) *The Maturational Process and the Facilitating Environment: Studies in Theories of Emotional Development*. London: Hogarth.

Wurtele, S.K. (1998) 'Victims of child maltreatment', in A.S. Bellack and M. Hersen (eds), *Comprehensive Clinical Psychology*, Vol. 9. New York: Pergamon.

Attachment Theory

DEFINITION

Attachment theory emphasises that consistent benign care in infancy predicts good mental health. The corollary to this assumption is that disruptions to optimal care will lead to immediate and long-term distress and dysfunction.

KEY POINTS

- The features of attachment theory are outlined and its origins traced.
- The relevance of the theory for public policy and mental health practice is explored.

Attachment theory has had an important role in health and social policy and especially in family casework and childcare policies (Rutter and O'Connor, 1999). Moreover, it forms a good case study of a wider phenomenon: the impact of warfare on policy.

At first, the theory was developed predominantly by John Bowlby, in parallel with some of his British psychoanalytical colleagues sharing an environmentalist perspective. Freud's early circle contained those, such as Otto Rank and Sandor Ferenczi, who had already emphasised the importance of trauma in infancy and its adult legacy. In the 1950s, Bowlby came to similar conclusions to Donald Winnicott and Ronald Fairbairn, with their emphasis on the infant's early internalisation of relationships with significant others, particularly the mother (Fairbairn, 1950; Winnicott, 1958). However, Bowlby also incorporated more behavioural theorisations from animal studies (Bretherton, 1992).

Bowlby was trained as a psychoanalyst just before the Second World War and practised as an army psychiatrist. After the war, he became Deputy Director of the Tavistock Clinic in London and was asked by the World Health Organization to provide advice on displaced children (see below). His work prior to, during and shortly after the war together provided a particular insight into child development, especially in relation to symptoms of distress and their link to separation from parents, or their link to dysfunctional forms of parenting (Bowlby, 1940). Prior to the war, he had worked in a child guidance clinic observing many cases and he was also witness to the psychological impact of the Kindertransport of Jewish children coming to Britain from Nazi Germany. In 1949, Bowlby's known earlier work on delinquent and affectionless children and the effects of hospitalised and institutionalised care led to the WHO commission. This work, *Maternal Care and Mental Health*, was the most important early mark of his global policy impact (Bowlby, 1951).

In that report, the seeds of attachment theory were growing. Bowlby emphasised that the infant needed a secure base of consistent warm benign care. This conclusion was built not only on his clinical observations, but also on other key sources. The latter included the work of Anna Freud on child analysis and studies of institutional care, such as those of Spitz (1946) and Goldfarb (1945). It also resonated with another psychoanalyst, Erik Erikson, who was developing the view that critical periods of development in childhood shaped later mental health (Erikson, 1950).

At odds with the purely human focus of psychoanalysis, Bowlby incorporated findings from a growing sub-discipline of zoology: ethology. The latter is the study of animal behaviour in its natural environment. Ethology suggests that certain aspects of behaviour, particularly those related to mating and parenting, are biologically inherited, creating instinctive bonds and fixed patterns of action in *all* animals, although their diversity and flexible expression increase with evolution (Lorenz, 1935; Tinbergen, 1951). These patterns are not just about the acts of individual organisms, but are also pointedly about *relations between* individuals in the species. For example, the newborn lamb must nuzzle for the teat, just as much as the ewe, having just given birth, must stand patiently and receptively. Mutuality and interdependence are adaptive for the survival of the species.

Empirically, attachment theory was built up after the war, with findings from the naturalistic filmmaker James Robertson, under Bowlby's supervision (Robertson, 1953). The film *A Two-Year-Old Goes to Hospital* graphically showed the distress experienced and expressed by young children in conditions of separation, which added to the evidence also on film from Spitz in 1947 (*Grief: A Peril in Infancy*). Here, the methodological link to note with ethology was naturalistic observation: conduct as it was witnessed in actual lived settings, which was neither genetic presumption nor psychotherapeutic speculation. Both of the latter were *post hoc* forms of theorising. By contrast, anyone watching the films could see distress live and *in situ*. When Bowlby reported to the World Health Organization, two points were clear for him: first, that mothers were central to our mental health for life, and, second, that social progress will come from a political commitment to support the role of positive parenting:

> Just as children are absolutely dependent on their parents for sustenance, so in all but the most primitive communities, are parents, especially their mothers, dependent on a greater society for economic provision. If a community values its children it must cherish their parents. (Bowlby, 1951: 84)

The report in 1951 led to actual changes of policy in practice to minimise the distress of children when entering hospital, for example in the shift to encourage a parental presence whenever possible. Nevertheless, it did not bring an end to lengthy periods of institutional separation in children's homes and forms of schooling.

By the end of the 1950s, attachment theory was fleshed out, with the invaluable assistance of Mary Ainsworth, whom Bowlby supervised (Bowlby et al., 1956). A number of elements were emphasised that were at odds with classical psychoanalysis, for example in arguing that the infant tendency to cling was more important psychologically than sucking, implying that the direct individual relationship was even more fundamental than food. That view was confirmed experimentally about primates by Harlow (1961). And, rather than dwelling on Freud's oral, anal and phallic phases of development, Bowlby was interested in the dynamics of attachment, separation and loss (Bowlby, 1969, 1973, 1980). He proposed three phases of separation response. First, the child protests: this arises from separation anxiety. Second, when the lost parent does not return, the child experiences despair: namely, a form of grief or mourning. Third, after a period the child becomes detached and goes into denial about the loss: this Bowlby aligned to Freud's ideas about repression and other defence mechanisms.

Not only did attachment theory go on to shape the theory and practice of family casework, but it also influenced social policy at the other end of the life span. Those studying bereavement and compassionate dying in the hospice movement were influenced directly by attachment theory (Parkes, 1972). It has also been evident in family and marital therapy and rehabilitation work with perpetrators of domestic violence (Weiss, 1977; Byng-Hall, 1985; Doumass et al., 2008). Subsequent psychosocial theories of both depression and psychosis have relied heavily upon arguments about the quality of early parenting in predicting adult mental health problems (for example, Brown and Harris, 1978; Schore, 2001; Ross, 2004).

Attachment theory has, however, had its detractors (see, for example, Contratto, 2002). Feminists have been concerned that being overly focused on the mother can lead to her being glibly blamed for mental disorder. It was a normative assumption on the part of Bowlby in the mid-20th century that optimal parental care was maternal, rather than being gender neutral. It is easy to see how the maternal focus could be used to rationalise conservative policy demands to keep women at home and out of the labour force. Notwithstanding this form of legitimate criticism, attachment theory has retained a strong presence in advocates across a range of health and social policies.

See also: *causes and consequences of mental health problems; mental health policy; mental health promotion; public mental health; warfare.*

FURTHER READING

Bretherton, I. (1992) 'The origins of attachment theory: John Bowlby and Mary Ainsworth', *Developmental Psychology*, 28: 759–75.
Contratto, S. (2002) 'A feminist critique of attachment theory and evolutionary psychology', in M. Ballou and L.S. Brown (eds), *Rethinking Mental Health and Disorder: Feminist Perspectives.* New York: Guilford Press.

REFERENCES

Bowlby, J. (1940) 'The influence of early environment in the development of neurosis and neurotic character', *International Journal of Psycho-Analysis*, 21: 1–25.
Bowlby, J. (1951) *Maternal Care and Mental Health*. Geneva: World Health Organization.
Bowlby, J. (1969) *Attachment and Loss*, Vol. 1: *Attachment*. New York: Basic Books.
Bowlby, J. (1973) *Attachment and Loss*, Vol. 2: *Separation*. New York: Basic Books.
Bowlby, J. (1980) *Attachment and Loss*, Vol. 3: *Loss, Sadness and Depression*. New York: Basic Books.
Bowlby, J., Ainsworth, M., Boston, M. and Rosenbluth, D. (1956) 'The effects of mother–child separation: a follow-up study', *British Journal of Medical Psychology*, 29 (2): 211–47.
Bretherton, I. (1992) 'The origins of attachment theory: John Bowlby and Mary Ainsworth', *Developmental Psychology*, 28: 759–75.
Brown, G. and Harris, T. (1978) *Social Origins of Depression*. London: Tavistock.
Byng-Hall, J. (1985) 'The family script: a useful bridge between theory and practice', *Journal of Family Therapy*, 7: 301–5.
Contratto, S. (2002) 'A feminist critique of attachment theory and evolutionary psychology', in M. Ballou and L.S. Brown (eds), *Rethinking Mental Health and Disorder: Feminist Perspectives.* New York: Guilford Press.
Doumass, D., Pearson, C. and Elgin, J.M. (2008) 'Adult attachment as a risk factor for intimate partner violence: the "mispairing" of partners' attachment styles', *Journal of Interpersonal Violence, 23* (5): 616–34.
Erikson, E. (1950) *Childhood and Society*. New York: W.W. Norton.
Fairbairn, W.R.D. (1950) *Psychoanalytic Studies of the Personality*. London: Hogarth.
Goldfarb, W. (1945) 'Psychological privation in infancy and subsequent adjustment', *American Journal of Orthopsychiatry*, 15: 247–55.
Harlow, H.F. (1961) 'The development of affectional patterns in infant monkeys', in B.M. Foss (ed.), *Determinants of Infant Behaviour*. London: Methuen.
Lorenz, K.Z. (1935) 'Der Kumpan in der Umwelt des Vogels', *Journal für Ornithologie, 83:* 137–213.
Parkes, C.M. (1972) *Bereavement: Studies of Grief in Adult Life*. New York: International Universities Press.

Robertson, J. (1953) 'Some responses of young children to loss of maternal care', *Nursing Care*, 49: 382–6.

Ross, C. (2004) *Schizophrenia: An Innovative Approach to Diagnosis and Treatment*. London: Haworth Press.

Rutter, M. and O'Connor, T.G. (1999) 'Implications of attachment theory for child care policies', in J. Cassidy and P.R. Shaver (eds), *Handbook of Attachment: Theory, Research, and Clinical Applications*. New York: Guilford Press.

Schore, A. (2001) 'The effects of early relational trauma on right brain development, affect regulation and infant mental health', *Infant Mental Health Journal*, 22 (1): 201–79.

Spitz, R.A. (1946) 'Anaclitic depression', *Psychoanalytic Study of the Child*, 2: 313–42.

Tinbergen, N. (1951) *The Study of Instinct*. Oxford: Clarendon Press.

Weiss, R.S. (1977) *Marital Separation*. New York: Basic Books.

Winnicott, D.W. (1958) *The Child and the Family*. London: Tavistock.

Mental Health Promotion

DEFINITION

Like mental health, mental health promotion has been defined in a variety of ways. Common or recurring strands include the promotion of happiness, the right to freedom and productivity, the absence of mental illness, and the fulfilment of an individual's emotional, intellectual and spiritual potential.

KEY POINTS

- The relationship between mental health promotion and the primary prevention of mental illness is considered.
- The range of factors which are implicated in both of these closely related concepts is outlined.

The promotion of mental health is closely linked to the primary prevention of mental health problems. The subtle distinction is that in the former case, positive mental health has to be defined as one or more desired outcomes. In the latter case, there needs to be a demonstration that the probability of diagnosed mental illness is reduced. A danger of conflating mental health promotion with the primary prevention of mental illness is that it may maintain a restricted focus on a limited clinical population and not address the population's needs as a whole (Tudor, 1996).

The World Health Organization (1986) has offered a view of mental health promotion – the ability of individuals to 'have the basic opportunity to develop and use their health potential to live socially and economically productive lives'. In 1986, WHO launched a campaign to implement a charter for action to achieve health for all by 2000 and beyond. Later, it emphasised that: 'the concept of health potential encompasses both physical and mental health and must be viewed in the context of personal development throughout the life span' (World Health Organization, 1991: 3).

The primary prevention of mental illness can be distinguished from secondary and tertiary prevention. Secondary prevention refers to nipping mental health problems 'in the bud' following early detection. Tertiary prevention refers to lowering the probability of relapse in those with chronic mental health problems.

The distinction, but also the relationship between promotion and primary prevention, was also made clear by Albee (1993), who used two versions of an equation using similar factors (see Figure 1.5).

$$1\ \text{Incidence of mental illness} = \frac{\text{stress} + \text{exploitation} + \text{organic factors}}{\text{support} + \text{self-esteem building} + \text{coping skills}}$$

$$2\ \text{Promotion of mental health} = \frac{\text{coping skills} + \text{environment} + \text{self-esteem}}{\text{stress} + \text{exploitation} + \text{organic factors}}$$

Figure 1.5 Preventing mental illness and promoting mental health

The factors in the two equations can be addressed one by one:

- *Stress* In the entry on Social Class, it is noted that stress accounts for some of the differences in diagnosis between poorer and richer people. While both groups have adverse and positive experiences, the ratio between the two is different, with the richer group having more buffering positive experiences. Those exposed to lower levels of personal and environmental stress are more likely to be mentally healthy. Conversely, the higher the level of stress, be it acute and severe (trauma) or chronic and low level, the higher the probability of a person developing a mental health problem.
- *Exploitation* The exploitation of individuals, whether it is financial or related to physical, sexual or emotional abuse, increases the risk of mental health problems. Conversely, a person not exposed to these versions of exploitation is more likely to maintain their mental health. The discourse of exploitation is not common in the psychiatric and psychological literature (Sartorius and Henderson, 1992). This may reflect the tendency of the two disciplines to avoid the language of politics, which might bring accusations of unscientific bias and risk undermining professional credibility. However, a problem for the human sciences is that they are intrinsically about human relationships. Exploitation and other expressions of power differentials are part of the landscape, in some form or other, at all levels of all human societies.

Another reason that professionals do not typically address the question of exploitation is that it is beyond their immediate control. The scope of their interventions is limited to the micro level. This refers to the coping strategies of individuals (as in the use of social skills training or cognitive-behavioural therapy), family interventions (Dwivedi, 1997) and, at its most extensive, local community psychology initiatives (Rappaport et al., 1984). By contrast, political factors, which manifestly affect the possibility of developing mental health for all, in line with the World Health Organization's expectation noted earlier, are outwith the direct and privileged control of professionals. These include measures to prevent starvation and warfare and to ensure that all citizens are well housed and educated and protected from the prejudicial actions of others (Sartorius, 2001).

- *Organic factors* These refer to environmental toxins and stressors and to biological susceptibility. (The entry on Causes and Consequences of Mental Health Problems discusses the latter.) The former refers to poisons (such as lead and petrochemicals) that damage the nervous system. They also refer to behavioural stressors, which are then mediated by physiological mechanisms to produce brain damage. The most common example of this is in relation to raised blood pressure increasing the risk of stroke and dementia. The stressors here include insecure work conditions, noisy and dangerous living environments, and lifestyle habits such as quality of diet and exercise levels.
- *Social support* This is a crucial buffer against mental health problems. Chronic personal isolation increases the risk of both depression and psychosis. Both are reduced in probability in those people who are part of a supportive social network or primary group (be it close friends or family).
- *Self-esteem building* This refers to early family life and its capacity for developing confidence in the growing child. It also refers to the presence of benign and affirming current relationships – linking back to the above points about exploitation and social support.
- *Coping skills* The ingenuity in coping with adversity varies from person to person and probably links back to personal styles learned in the family and at school. Much of the work of cognitive therapists is devoted to enabling patients lacking these coping skills normally to learn new ones. Conversely, those studying positive psychology have identified those of us who excel at being positive across a range of social contexts.

These factors demonstrate that positive mental health and the primary prevention of mental illness implicate a wide range of factors – political, social, psychological and biological (Herrman, 2011). Strategically, mental health promotion requires changes in both public policies (NB plural) and public education (Tones and Tilford, 1994). For example, a number of apparently separate policies can affect mental health related to, among others: environmental pollution, child protection, employment, leisure, street cleaning, traffic levels, parenting, schooling, diet and exercise.

The approach taken to mental health promotion and primary prevention reflects the constructs used by those intervening (be they politicians or health and welfare professionals). The public policy implications for mental health, noted in the list above, reflect a social model of mental health. Those who emphasise psychological determinism would limit their interest to individual and family life. Those who emphasise biodeterminism would highlight biological interventions (such as genetic counselling and early intervention for psychosis). At its most extreme, this might culminate in a eugenic policy to prevent mental illness.

See also: *causes and consequences of mental health problems; eugenics; mental health; physical health; warfare; wellbeing.*

FURTHER READING

Goldie, I. (2010) *Public Mental Health Today: A Handbook.* London: Pavilion/Mental Health Foundation.
Walker, P. and John, M. (eds) (2012) *From Public Health to Wellbeing.* Basingstoke: Palgrave Macmillan.
Young, L.E. and Hayes, V. (eds) (2002) *Transforming Health Promotion Practice.* Philadelphia, PA: F.A. Davis.

REFERENCES

Albee, G. (1993) 'The fourth revolution', in D. Trent and C. Reed (eds), *Promotion of Mental Health*, Vol. 3. London: Avebury.
Dwivedi, K.N. (ed.) (1997) *Enhancing Parenting Skills.* Chichester: John Wiley.
Herrman, H. (2011) 'Promoting mental health', in D. Pilgrim, A. Rogers and B. Pescosolido (eds), *The SAGE Handbook of Mental Health and Illness.* London: Sage.
Rappaport, C., Swift, C. and Hess, R. (eds) (1984) *Studies in Empowerment: Steps towards Understanding and Action.* New York: Haworth Press.
Sartorius, N. (2001) 'Primary prevention of mental disorders', in G. Thornicroft and G. Szmukler (eds), *Textbook of Community Psychiatry.* Oxford: Oxford University Press.
Sartorius, N. and Henderson, A.S. (1992) 'The neglect of prevention in psychiatry', *Australian and New Zealand Journal of Psychiatry*, 26: 550–3.
Tones, K. and Tilford, S. (1994) *Health Education: Effectiveness, Efficiency and Equity.* London: Chapman Hall.
Tudor, K. (1996) *Mental Health Promotion: Paradigms and Practice.* London: Routledge.
World Health Organization (WHO) (1986) *Health Promotion: Concepts and Principles in Action.* Copenhagen: WHO European Regional Office.
World Health Organization (WHO) (1991) *Implications for the Field of Mental Health of the European Targets for Attaining Health for All.* Copenhagen: WHO European Regional Office.

Part II
Mental Abnormality

Psychiatric
Classification

DEFINITION

Psychiatric classification today is offered in two overlapping systems. One is from the American Psychiatric Association, specifying its descriptions of mental disorders: the Diagnostic and Statistical Manual of Mental Disorders *(DSM). The other is part of a wider classification of health and illness offered by the World Health Organization called the* International Classification of Diseases *(ICD). These vary slightly but they have developed over time in tandem and so their content converges strongly.*

KEY POINTS

- A brief history of the modern classification of mortality and morbidity is outlined.
- Problems of introducing mental disorders into this global tradition are introduced.

In the 18th century, the Scottish physician Cullen suggested a classificatory system of what he called the 'neuroses'. This very wide notion, which today would subsume most mental disorders, contained the aetiological premise that madness and misery reflect damage to the nervous system and the alteration of nervous energy (hence the remaining notion of 'nervousness'). This assumption persevered in dominant ideas from German psychopathology noted below. In late 18th-century France, de Sauvages offered a general classification of diseases of ten broad categories, the eighth of which was 'insanity' (Pilgrim, 2007). However, in the early days of modern medical epidemiology, only physical diseases were emphasised: the first extensive medical deliberations about diagnosis were mainly from statisticians about causes of death.

Conferences of the International Statistical Institute (ISI) met regularly at the turn of the 20th century, with a narrow focus on producing an 'International Classification of Causes of Death'. This mortality focus began to alter, boosted by concerns from the Health Organisation of the League of Nations (LoN). The latter was formed after the First World War to encourage international cooperation and as such was the precursor of the United Nations (UN, established in 1945), with its Health Organisation wing similarly the precursor of the World Health Organization (WHO). The WHO was endorsed in 1946 by 61 UN members and launched in 1948.

A so-called 'mixed commission' of representatives from the ISI and LoN was created in the 1920s and its findings about medical classification were published in 1928 (Knibbs, 1929). This mixed commission put forward proposals for revisions of the *International List of Causes of Death* both then and in 1938. At this stage, the shift towards morbidity, as well as a retained interest in mortality, was emphatically *physical*, with such 'Lists of Diseases'. Forms of the latter had existed from country to country, reflecting cultural emphases on, and variations in the presence of, types of disease. The intention now was to agree on an international consensus about standardised diagnostic criteria. It should be noted, however, that this international consensus-building was dominated by Western European and North American representatives. This is particularly relevant in the case of psychiatric morbidity because of marked cultural variations in the norms that define psychological normality.

This work in progress was then incorporated by the WHO when it issued its first classification document, called *ICD-6*, with the number used being in compliance with the revisions since the 19th century of the older ISI system of classification. The full title adopted then was *Manual of the International Statistical Classification of Diseases, Injuries, and Causes of Death* (WHO, 1949). *ICD-6* introduced psychiatric diseases for the first time.

Such a late inclusion is itself noteworthy because it represented a softening of the epidemiology over time. Starting with a preference for hard data on mortality (death is certain for us all), a shift was evident towards physical morbidity and then only eventually was mental pathology considered. This ambivalence about psychiatric disease was understandable from 'hard-headed' statisticians. Cause of death and physical morbidity based upon measurable signs (visible changes to the body or laboratory tests) relied on objective confidence. That confidence could not be offered by psychiatry because its focus, overwhelmingly, was on symptoms (what patients said and did) and not hard signs. This is one reason why, in the case of so-called 'organic mental illnesses', critics of psychiatric diagnosis, such as the psychiatrist and psychoanalyst Thomas Szasz (see the entry on The Myth of Mental Illness), argue that they are not mental illnesses at all but physical (i.e. neurological) ones.

Functional psychiatric diagnoses therefore pose a logical and empirical problem for statisticians because medical epidemiology, which is the study of the distribution of diseases, is essentially useful because it tries to map *causal* pathways. For example, cancer maps linked to radiation sources or outbreaks of infectious disease linked to the presence of food or animal sources ('vectors') are offered to connect a disease to its aetiological source. Simply counting cases for its own sake, as is the case in 'psychiatric epidemiology', has a much more limited social administrative purpose and advances medical science very little, if at all. Put differently, it is difficult to credibly and precisely measure mental disorder beyond creating broad aggregate data sets (Wakefield, 1999). Moreover, functional diagnoses are only arrived at tautologically, which severely weakens their scientific credibility. For example:

Q: How do you know that this patient has schizophrenia?

A: Because she lacks insight into her strange beliefs and she experiences auditory hallucinations.

Q: Why does she have strange beliefs and experience hallucinations?

A: Because she suffers from schizophrenia.

Thus, the presence of functional mental disorders within *ICD* is contentious because their associated diagnoses *ipso facto* are based on symptoms and not biological signs, thereby undermining their scientific legitimacy. Given this, all that psychiatric epidemiology can do is provide putative maps of disease presence, with causes being bracketed or unknown. Some social scientists have tried, in the Meyerian tradition, to investigate the social patterning of psychiatric morbidity. This tradition of 'social psychiatry' has been an interdisciplinary and not narrowly a medical project, more interested in understanding the workings of a 'biopsychosocial model' of causation than exploring fine diagnostic considerations.

DEVELOPMENTS AFTER THE SECOND WORLD WAR

The first edition of *DSM* appeared in 1952 (Grob, 1991), but its origins can be traced to the First World War. In 1918, in response to the challenge of dealing with the acute symptoms of 'shell shock' (now 'post-traumatic stress disorder' or PTSD), the American Medico-Psychological Association, which was to become the American Psychiatric Association (APA) in 1921, produced the *Statistical Manual for the Use of Institutions of the Insane* (Salmon, 1929).

The first edition of the *DSM* reflected the dominance at the time of Freudian and Meyerian psychiatry in both the academy and clinic in the USA. Psychoanalytical ideas had gained a new legitimacy after 1918, and social psychiatric ideas also grew in popularity. Meyer's multi-factorial approach to explaining the emergence of mental health problems was popular among academic psychiatrists during the inter-war period (1918–39). The Meyerians were not opposed to diagnosis but assumed that it was a rough starting point from which to ask the question: 'Why is this particular person presenting with these particular problems at this particular time in their life?' Meyer was interested in the various forces, biological, psychological and social, that might impinge on particular patients to explain their presenting complaint (Meyer, 1952). Thus, three main factions within the APA were emerging after the Second World War, associated with biological psychiatry, psychoanalysis and social psychiatry. The first group upheld the tradition of Kraepelinian psychopathology, the second the work of Freud, and the last was an interdisciplinary group that adopted a flexible biopsychosocial approach to clinical work and academic research, encouraged by Meyer's intellectual leadership.

These German-speaking origins for *DSM* were integrated into an unstable mix by lobby groups in the APA, but during the 1950s and 1960s the first two traditions predominated (Wilson, 1993). This mixture was reflected in the *DSM* revision of 1968. However, that dominance of a biographical or psychosocial view of mental health problems was displaced during the 1970s by the older eugenic tradition that was traceable to Kraepelin and Griesinger. This tradition upheld the view that mental illnesses were essentially genetically caused or shaped diseases of the 'nerves and brains' (Shorter, 1997: 76). Scull (2011: 46) noted that, according to this 19th-century biomedical consensus, 'the mentally infirm were a biologically defective lot, their madness the product of deformed brains and inferior heredity'.

The positions adopted by the three groups about classification were different, though roughly aligned. For example, they all broadly distinguished between psychosis and neurosis and conceded that they all encountered patients with problems of chronic interpersonal dysfunction (now dubbed 'personality disorders'). But at the heart of the tension between the groups, which was substantial, was the question of aetiology or assumed causation. Also, the Freudian tradition accepted end-point descriptions about symptoms (such as anxiety, depression, obsessionality, and so on) but held that these were not discrete and fixed. Not only might they be co-present in different combinations from one patient to another, with different overall diagnoses, but they might also change over time ('symptom substitution').

Moreover, for psychoanalysis, we are all ill: it is only a matter of degree. This is an analogue approach to diagnosis (a 'more or less' approach), which implies that mental disorders are about continua, not categories. By contrast, the Kraepelinian tradition viewed mental illness, like physical illness, to be present or absent in patients and assumed that it was the result of an underlying neurological or neurochemical dysfunction. Diagnosis, then, was a digital matter (a 'present or absent' approach) about a putative underlying pathology of the brain. This tension between a categorical and a continuum approach to psychopathology still divides psychiatrists and psychologists to this day.

With these differing assumptions and approaches to diagnosis within US psychiatry, only two outcomes were possible for *DSM*. The first was the negotiation of compromises (reflected to some extent in the dropping of aetiological assumptions and the introduction of dimensions as well as categories), and the second was the political victory of one lobby over the others. During the 1970s, the latter outcome became more evident, when biological psychiatrists consolidated their relationship with the pharmaceutical industry in the wake of the putative 'pharmacological revolution' of the 1950s (Healy, 1997). This group of neo-Kraepelinians formed an 'invisible college' of like-minded researchers at Washington University, St. Louis and in New York. They captured the *DSM* apparatus within the APA (Blashfield, 1982; Bayer and Spitzer, 1985; Wilson, 1993). That biological lobby within the APA has since controlled the development of *DSM*, although this has also provoked political resistance from both inside and outside medicine.

In 2013, when the fifth edition of *DSM* was published, an extension of the logic of biomedical psychiatry caused problems for the APA from a range of critics (see below). Of particular concern to many was that the numbers of diagnoses had expanded unreasonably and the thresholds for pathology had been lowered. For example, bereavement, previously excluded from *DSM*, was now to be included as a disorder, and angry, grumpy people were to be considered as suffering from a 'temper dysregulation disorder'. In the UK, an editorial in the *Journal of Mental Health* warned of a post-2013, when 'the pool of "normality" would shrink to a mere puddle' (Wykes and Callard, 2010: 301). In the USA, Marcia Angell (former editor of the *New England Journal of Medicine*) likewise mused that: 'it looks as though it will be harder and harder to be normal' (Angell, 2011: 3). This sort of concern about *DSM-5* being too expansive was even expressed disparagingly by the Chair of the *DSM-IV* committee (Frances, 2013), as well as by other researchers of psychiatric diagnosis. They feared that ordinary emotional reactions such as sadness, and character features like shyness, would now be turned unfairly into forms of pathology (e.g. Horwitz and Wakefield, 2007; Lane, 2008).

DSM (like *ICD*) has included both organic and functional diagnoses as forms of mental disorder. With the dominance of biological psychiatry growing in the 1970s within the APA affecting its revisions since then, a form of unified biological aetiology was increasingly assumed. Formally, in a compromise with the older Freudian and Meyerian influence on *DSM-I* and *DSM-III*, aetiology had been dropped from the system. A reflection of this confidence was articulated by Guze:

> what is called psychopathology is the manifestation of disordered processes in various brain systems that mediate psychological functioning … By taking into consideration genetic codes and epigenetic development, guided and shaped by broad ranging environmental influences, only some of which are now recognized and understood, biology clearly offers the only comprehensive basis for psychiatry, just as it does for the rest of medicine. (Guze, 1989: 317–18)

Given this increasing confident presumptuousness from biological psychiatry since the 1970s, the controversy about *DSM-5* involved it being attacked from at least three distinct directions, with the first two of these being evident in an international campaign of opposition to *DSM-5* (see the online petition, 'Is the *DSM-5* safe?', at http://dsm5response.com). In the run up to, and on publication of, *DSM-5* in May 2013, three main reactive lobbies were discernible (Pilgrim, 2013).

First, there were the *medical revisionists*. Those like Frances, as noted above, were concerned about the diagnostic expansionism in *DSM-5* but they were not against diagnosis in principle, indeed they actively supported it. Whether or not this expansionism was seen as good or bad, it was empirically not in doubt. In 1917, the American Medico-Psychological Association recognised 59 psychiatric disorders but after that, the numbers have just kept rising through the years: 1952 (128), 1968 (159), 1980 (227) and 1987 (253). By the time that *DSM-IV* had emerged, it encompassed 347 categories.

Second, there were the *psychological antagonists*. For example, British psychologists reviewing the logic and trajectory of *DSM-5* were against diagnosis in principle and instead favoured context-specific formulations (British Psychological Society, 2011). This summarises the type of object:

> The putative diagnoses presented in *DSM-5* are clearly based largely on social norms, with 'symptoms' that all rely on subjective judgments, with little confirmatory physical 'signs' or evidence of biological causation. The criteria are not value-free, but rather reflect current normative social expectations … [taxonomic] systems such as this are based on identifying problems as located within individuals. This misses the relational context of problems and the undeniable social causation of many such problems. (British Psychological Society, 2011: 1)

These psychologists attacked psychiatric positivism for being both unscientific and unhelpful to patients, whereas the psychiatric revisionists were pro-diagnosis.

Third, there were the *biological reductionists*, who argued that *DSM-5* was not biological enough in its descriptions. This was the most embarrassing objection for the American Psychiatric Association, because it came from the National Institute of Mental Health (NIMH) in the USA. In earlier years, NIMH had co-sponsored the launch of the revision of *DSM*. Two weeks before the publication of *DSM-5*, Tom Insell, the Medical Director of NIMH, issued a sharp attack on it, arguing that *DSM* at best increased reliability (by encouraging clinicians to regularly agree on symptom checklists) (Insell, 2013). He held that *DSM* had no validity because its 'hotchpotch' (*sic*) criteria are not rooted demonstrably in biological research, a point that critics in the second group above would agree with but from which would also draw out some quite different epistemological and political conclusions. Insell proposed a laboratory-based approach to diagnosis: the NIMH's 'Research Domain Criteria'. These are predicated on the assumption that all mental disorders are self-evidently brain diseases.

DIFFERENCES BETWEEN *ICD* AND *DSM*

There is a very large overlap in content, with only a few gaps and nuances of naming between the two systems. For example, 'narcissistic personality disorder' has not appeared in *ICD* but it has in *DSM*. The former uses the term 'multiple personality disorder', not 'dissociative identity disorder', and 'anankastic personality disorder', not 'obsessive-compulsive personality disorder'. However, the symptom checklists that are offered as criteria to constitute these different names are more or less the same in both systems. Moreover, commonly used categories, such as 'schizophrenia', are utilised by both systems, despite their scientific validity now being fundamentally in question (see the entry on Madness).

The revisions of both systems were fairly separate for a while, although US psychiatrists played a role after the Second World War in informing *ICD-6* and subsequent revisions. By the 1980s, a strong convergence was evident as a symptom checklist approach was emphasised in both and assumptions about aetiology were dropped (Kendell, 1991). *ICD-10* (still in use at the time of writing) was published in 1990 (WHO, 1990).

In 2015 the WHO issued a new edition (*ICD-11*). The part referring to mental disorders was aligned closely with *DSM-5*. Two new features in common were that there was an expansion of the number of diagnoses, and aetiological assumptions were revisited in both *DSM* and *ICD*. Now there is an explicit assumption that diagnoses can be traced validly to either environmental stressors or to underlying neurobiological malfunctions. For example, *ICD-11* assumes that obsessive-compulsive problems arise from neurobiological factors. That question of aetiology (not just the traditional query about weak conceptual validity) will ensure that classification systems will remain controversial for the foreseeable future, as debates revolve around tracing the impact of external stressors and demonstrating the actual, rather than assumed, primary causal role of biological factors.

See also: *causes and consequences of mental health problems; neuroscience; psychological formulations; the myth of mental illness.*

FURTHER READING

Blashfield, R.K. and Burgess, D.R. (2007) 'Classification provides an essential basis for organizing mental disorders', in S.O. Lilienfield and W.T. O'Donohue (eds), *The Great Ideas of Clinical Science: 17 Principles that Every Mental Health Professional Should Understand.* New York: Routledge.

Division of Clinical Psychology (2011) *Good Practice Guidelines on the Use of Psychological Formulation.* Leicester: British Psychological Society.

Frances, A. (2013) *Saving Normal.* London: HarperCollins.

Johnstone, L. and Boyle, M., with Cromby, J., Dillon, J., Harper, D., Kinderman, P., Longden, E., Pilgrim, D. and Read, J. (2018) *The Power Threat Meaning Framework: Towards the Identification of Patterns in Emotional Distress, Unusual Experiences and Troubled or Troubling Behaviour.* Leicester: British Psychological Society.

Le Francois, B., Menzies, R. and Reaume, G. (eds) (2013) *Mad Matters: A Critical Reader in Canadian Mad Studies.* Toronto: Canadian Scholars Press.

Pilgrim, D. (2015) 'Influencing mental health policy: DSM-5 as a disciplinary challenge for psychology', *Review of General Psychology*, 18 (4): 293–301.

REFERENCES

American Psychiatric Association (APA) (1994) *Diagnostic and Statistical Manual of Mental Disorders* (4th edn) (*DSM-IV*). Washington, DC: APA.

American Psychiatric Association (APA) (2013) *Diagnostic and Statistical Manual of Mental Disorders* (5th edn) (*DSM-5*). Washington, DC: APA.

Angell, M. (2011) 'The illusions of psychiatry', *The New York Times Review of Books*, 14 July.

Bayer, R. and Spitzer, R.L. (1985) 'Neurosis, psychodynamics and *DSM-III*: a history of the controversy', *Archives of General Psychiatry*, 42: 187–96.

Blashfield, R. (1982) 'Feighner et al.: invisible colleges and the Mathew Effect', *Schizophrenia Bulletin*, 8: 1–12.

British Psychological Society (2011) 'Response to the American Psychiatric Association: *DSM-5* development'. Available at http://apps.bps.org.uk/_publicationfiles/consultationresponses/DSM-5%202011%20-%20BP

Frances, A. (2013) *Saving Normal.* London: HarperCollins.

Grob, G. (1991) 'Origins of *DSM-I*: a study in appearance and reality', *American Journal of Psychiatry*, 148: 421–31.

Guze, S. (1989) 'Biological psychiatry: is there any other kind?', *Psychological Medicine*, 19: 315–23.

Healy, D. (1997) *The Anti-Depressant Era.* London and Cambridge, MA: Harvard University Press.

Horwitz, A.V. and Wakefield, J.C. (2007) *The Loss of Sadness: How Psychiatry Transformed Normal Sorrow into Depressive Disorder.* Oxford: Oxford University Press.

Insell, T. (2013) 'Directors blog: transforming diagnosis'. Available at www.nimh.nih.gov/about/director/2013/transforming-diagnosis.shtmlS%20response.pdf

Kendell, R.E. (1991) 'Relationship between *DSM-IV* and *ICD-10*', *Journal of Abnormal Psychology*, 100 (3): 297–301.

Knibbs, G.H. (1929) 'The *International Classification of Disease* and causes of death and its revision', *Medical Journal of Australia*, 1: 2–12.

Lane, C. (2008) *Shyness: How Normal Behavior Became a Sickness.* New Haven, CT: Yale University Press.

psychiatric classification

Meyer, A. (1952) *The Collected Works of Adolf Meyer*. New York: Basic Books.

Pilgrim, D. (2007) 'The survival of psychiatric diagnosis', *Social Science and Medicine*, 65 (3): 536–47.

Pilgrim, D. (2013) 'The failure of diagnostic psychiatry and the prospects of scientific progress informed by critical realism', *Journal of Critical Realism*, 12 (3): 336–57.

Salmon, T.W. (1929) 'Care and treatment of mental diseases and war neurosis ("shell shock") in the British army', in T.W. Salmon and N. Fenton (eds), *The Medical Department of the United States Army in the World War*, Vol. *10: Neuropsychiatry*. Washington, DC: US Government Printing Office.

Scull, A.T. (2011) *Madness: A Very Short Introduction*. New York: Oxford University Press.

Shorter, E. (1997) *A Short History of Psychiatry: From the Age of the Asylum to the Age of Prozac*. New York: Wiley.

Wakefield, J.C. (1999) 'The measurement of mental disorder', in A.V. Horwitz and T.L. Scheid (eds), *A Handbook for the Study of Mental Health*. Cambridge: Cambridge University Press.

Wilson, M. (1993) '*DSM-III* and the transformation of American psychiatry: a history', *American Journal of Psychiatry*, 150 (3): 399–410.

World Health Organization (WHO) (1949) *Manual of the International Statistical Classification of Diseases, Injuries, and Causes of Death* (6th revision). Geneva: WHO.

World Health Organization (WHO) (1990) *International Statistical Classification of Diseases, Injuries, and Causes of Death* (10th edn) (*ICD-10*). Geneva: WHO.

Wykes, T. and Callard, F. (2010) 'Diagnosis, diagnosis, diagnosis: towards *DSM-5*', *Journal of Mental Health*, 19 (4): 301–4.

Lay Views of Mental Disorders

DEFINITION

Lay views of mental disorder refer to two sets of descriptions. The first are the accounts of people with mental health problems who speak from their experience. The second are the views of non-patients about the nature of mental disorder.

KEY POINTS

- The emergence of a lay perspective on mental health and illness is discussed.
- Themes from patients' accounts are summarised.
- Public views of mental health and illness are described.

The notion of a 'lay' view is traceable to the historical division in Western societies of expert and non-expert knowledge. A binary divide is implied with expertise on one side (seen as superior) and inexpert views on the other (deemed to be inferior). The notions of 'lay preacher' and 'the laity' in Christian churches distinguish clerical authority from its followers or flock. It was extended into secular medical scientific language. For example, when psychoanalysis took hold as a profession, from an early stage, a dispute broke out about whether those not qualified in medicine could practise. A liberal view prevailed, supported by Freud, but to this day these practitioners are still called 'lay analysts'.

A full research interest in what non-experts think about mental health and illness is fairly new, probably for two reasons. First, the study of health, whether it is physical or mental, is less easy and appealing to researchers than the study of illness (the patient's experience of disease). Second, without sociopolitical changes in the role of users of health services, mental health professionals showed very little spontaneous interest in the accounts of 'their' patients. (The term 'patient', like that of 'follower' or 'flock', implies passivity, with one party forever playing catch-up.)

However, these changes did take place. Managers of health and welfare bureaucracies, with political approval and encouragement, increasingly sought the views of service users in order to improve service quality. Moreover, new social health movements critical of professionally dominated models of care began to assert, in very clear terms, their 'lay view'. Below, two versions of the latter are summarised, one from patients and the other from non-patients:

The patient perspective Sources of knowledge about the patient perspective come from: user-led surveys (e.g. Read and Baker, 1996; Kokanovic et al., 2008); case studies using qualitative methods (e.g. Barham and Hayward, 1991); studies of users' views of mental health services (e.g. Rogers et al., 1993) or specific forms of treatment (e.g. Rose et al., 2004); and demands emerging from the mental health service users' movement (e.g. Chamberlin, 1993). This wide-ranging literature points to a number of themes. Patients view their experiences in a variety of ways, with only a minority embracing a model which mirrors a psychiatric diagnosis. Other accounts, based upon social explanations, biographical accounts or spiritual knowledge, are often preferred. These alternative accounts also emphasise the baggage created by a psychiatric diagnosis and patients are often fearful of the negative views this invokes in others. This is well justified as social exclusion is, indeed, encountered in practice. Complaints from patients are largely about the narrow biomedical service responses and the personal insensitivity that these create.

Lay views of mental health and illness There are a number of pathways into researching lay views of mental health and illness. The first is to look at legal decision-making under the control of juries. Jury verdicts reflect ambivalence about expert knowledge. For example, psychiatric expert witnesses may be believed sometimes but not others. Two famous cases here were of the British mass murderers Peter Sutcliffe and Dennis Nilsen. In these cases, psychiatrists argued that they suffered from mental disorder (paranoid schizophrenia and psychopathic disorder, respectively) but the juries held them to be personally responsible for their actions. These verdicts seem to reject medical paternalism and may reflect the lack of credibility of psychiatric expertise. In one of the cases (Sutcliffe), interventions from psychiatrists after the trial ensured that he was transferred from prison to a secure hospital, indicating that the lay view did not prevail in the legal process.

A second pathway of understanding is in the study of 'nimby' ('not in my back yard') campaigns (Sayce, 2000). Lay views about people with mental health problems are predictably hostile and distrustful. Stereotypes of mental health problems in antiquity focused on aimless wandering and violence (Rosen, 1968). Studies of stereotypes in modernity show that non-patients still mainly focus on deranged psychotic behaviour and do not mention the commonest of all psychiatric diagnoses: depression (Cochrane, 1983). Moreover, public hostility to psychiatric patients is not merely one of attitude. Read and Baker (1996) asked patients about their encounters with others in the community and nearly half described verbal abuse or physical attacks. Similarly, Campbell and Heginbotham (1991) found hostile action in employers' refusals of candidates who declared previous mental health problems. The stereotypical connection between violence and mental illness was confirmed in large US public surveys (Field Institute, 1984; DYG Corporation, 1990). The vote was split, though, indicating that public views are not universally hostile or prejudicial. The problem is that the negative position is sufficiently prevalent to have a discriminatory impact on people with mental health problems.

The third form of understanding of lay views comes from taking personal accounts of mental health (rather than mental illness) (Rogers and Pilgrim, 1997). In the Rogers and Pilgrim study, lay people found it extremely difficult to articulate a positive view of mental health and preferred to define it negatively by referring to the avoidance of mental illness. However, they did have views about how to avoid stress and how to positively parent children in order to encourage their wellbeing. They also believed that the source of mental health problems was mainly related to social stressors but that the solution to problems remained in the hands of the individual sufferer.

See also: *risks to and from people with mental health problems; social exclusion; stigma; the mental health service users' movement; the quality of mental health care.*

FURTHER READING

Kokanovic, R., Dowrick, C., Butler, E. et al. (2008) 'Lay accounts of depression amongst Anglo-Australian residents and East African refugees', *Social Science & Medicine*, 66 (2): 454–66.
Rose, D., Wykes, T., Leese, M., Bindman, J. and Fleischmann, P. (2004) 'Patients' perspective on electro-convulsive therapy: systematic review', *British Medical Journal*, 326: 1363–5.

REFERENCES

Barham, P. and Hayward, R. (1991) *From the Mental Patient to the Person*. London: Routledge.
Campbell, T. and Heginbotham, C. (1991) *Mental Illness: Prejudice, Discrimination and the Law*. Aldershot: Dartmouth.

key concepts in
mental health

Chamberlin, J. (1993) 'Psychiatric disabilities and the ADA: an advocate's perspective', in L.O. Gostin and H.A. Beyer (eds), *Implementing the Americans with Disability Act*. Baltimore, MD: Brookes.

Cochrane, R. (1983) *The Social Creation of Mental Illness*. London: Longman.

DYG Corporation (1990) *Public Attitudes Toward People with Chronic Mental Illness*. Elmsford, NY: DYG Corporation.

Field Institute (1984) *In Pursuit of Wellness: A Survey of California Adults*. Sacramento, CA: California Department of Mental Health.

Kokanovic, R., Dowrick, C., Butler, E. et al. (2008) 'Lay accounts of depression amongst Anglo-Australian residents and East African refugees', *Social Science & Medicine*, 66 (2): 454–66.

Read, J. and Baker, S. (1996) *Not Just Sticks and Stones: A Survey of the Stigma, Taboo and Discrimination Experienced by People with Mental Health Problems*. London: Mind Publications.

Rogers, A. and Pilgrim, D. (1997) 'The contribution of lay knowledge to the understanding and promotion of mental health', *Journal of Mental Health*, 6 (1): 23–35.

Rogers, A., Pilgrim, D. and Lacey, R. (1993) *Experiencing Psychiatry: Users' Views of Services*. Basingstoke: Mind/Macmillan.

Rose, D., Wykes, T., Leese, M., Bindman, J. and Fleischmann, P. (2004) 'Patients' perspective on electro-convulsive therapy: systematic review', *British Medical Journal*, 326: 1363–5.

Rosen, G. (1968) *Madness in Society*. New York: Harper.

Sayce, L. (2000) *From Psychiatric Patient to Citizen: Overcoming Discrimination and Social Exclusion*. Basingstoke: Macmillan.

The Biopsychosocial Model

DEFINITION

This model of ill health (especially mental ill health) emphasises the combined contributions of biological, psychological and social factors. Its focus is on their variable and contingent contributions to pathology, in both its objective aspects (of disease and impairment) and subjective aspects (of illness and disability).

KEY POINTS

- The model is described and the historical role of Adolf Meyer and George Engel is noted.
- The support offered by General Systems Theory is explained.
- Criticisms of the model are described.

The biopsychosocial (BPS) model, as its name indicates, is a *model* (a practical framework to account for and work with particular cases of disease and illness) and not a theory (a conceptual framework to explore pathology and the character of medical knowledge and its role in society more widely). Its popularity, in specific relation to 'mental illness', has arisen because of its claimed inclusiveness about aetiology (the original causes of illness) and pathogenesis (the mechanisms of how people become ill) and because it avoids the accusation of reductionism, especially biological reductionism.

It has been associated in particular with social psychiatry and the tradition developed originally by Adolf Meyer and his 'psychobiology' (Meyer, 1952). However, its roots can be traced back even further to Rudolph Virchow, the 'father' of social medicine, which for a while in the late 19th century was popular in the academy (Brown and Fee, 2006). Subsequently, the importance of social medicine was lost and a narrower biomedical approach came to predominate, in particular within the insecure medical specialty of psychiatry by the end of the 20th century.

THE IMPORTANCE OF GEORGE ENGEL

The BPS model was formally announced in the literature by a psychiatrist, George Engel, who had a primary interest in psychosomatics. He was critical of the bio-reductionist norm in medical training and practice. This had led to medical researchers becoming scientifically limited and clinicians becoming insensitive to the unique psychological features of their patients and their particular social contexts (Engel, 1980).

Disease and illness are embedded in a complex matrix of bodily, interpersonal and wider social influences in our lives and Engel wanted to highlight that complexity. He was not critical of the existence and societal role of the medical profession in principle; indeed, his work was about rescuing the authority of the latter by producing 'a new medical model [*sic*]' (Engel, 1977). There were writers far more critical of the whole medical enterprise at the time of his writing, for example Illich (1976). Thus, Engel was a reformist within his profession; he was not a general critic of modern medicine.

SUPPORT FROM GENERAL SYSTEMS THEORY

The BPS model came to be supported by health researchers committed to variants of General Systems Theory. The latter was developed by laboratory scientists who noted that living systems (including within them those events and processes attracting the attention of medicine) could not be understood by the limited logic of experimentalism (von Bertalanffy, 1969). The latter closed system reasoning (which, by *controlling* variables, controlled them *out* of the picture) needed to be replaced by open systems reasoning. This assumed that reality was in flux across time and place and multilayered in nature. Complexity was to be expected and prediction would be uncertain (Walby, 2007). Human systems are open systems and so have to be understood with these points about complexity and unpredictability borne in mind (Bateson, 1980).

Moreover, because human beings reflect on their experience and use language, the meaning of what happens to them (in this case when they are ill) is as important to understand as how their body works or any risks to health in their environment. Hence, this is why the 'psychological' is as important to understand as 'the biological' and 'the social'. This more holistic approach had proved useful in public health research and marks a return to a version of Virchow's 'social medicine' (Dahlgren and Whitehead, 1992).

CRITICISMS OF THE BPS MODEL

The merits of the BPS model have been assessed and some have found it lacking for not being humanistic enough (Ghaemi, 2009), not being biological enough (Guze, 1989), or even for being too biological (Read, 2005). In the latter regard, it is the case that medical research claiming to use the BPS model tends to privilege biological factors (e.g. Garcia-Toro and Auirre, 2007).

Bio-reductionism is very strong in those medically trained, even when they attempt to respect psychological and social factors. However, this tendency has not been accepted by others. For example, McClaren (2006) concedes that the BPS model has succeeded in resisting biological reductionism but it has not offered a scientific understanding much beyond common sense (about us living in a complex human world). (The counter-argument here is that models consistent with common sense might be both scientifically legitimate and acceptable and intelligible to non-experts.)

A final criticism is from those who endorse the model's good intentions but observe two limitations to its consistent application in practice (Álvarez et al., 2012). First, it would be politically costly to follow through the model fully and routinely (as it implicates sources of deprivation and threat beyond the identified patient, such as toxic environments and general material poverty). Second, Engel and other clinicians wanting to apply the model are humanistically inspired and motivated to interact cautiously and respectfully with patients, one by one. It is difficult to ensure that all clinicians are inspired and motivated in the same way. Having said this, the claim has been made in the past 20 years that doctors now are being trained to work in a person-centred way at all times with their patients, and protocols can be developed to ensure consistent clinical practice (Dolovich et al., 2016).

Unless the BPS model is rejected out of hand in favour of bio-reductionism, the contention about the model seems to be about its ability to deliver its apparent promise of holism. For example, it is challenging to constantly re-validate it in practice, case by case, especially when clinicians or researchers cannot access all potentially relevant data, past and present, all of the time (Schwartz, 1982). However, even if that is not achieved, the *attempt* to do so reminds clinicians to reason holistically about their patients.

To end with the starting point about this section, because it is a model and not a theory the BPS model has no reflective capacity about its own limitations.

The model is good at being inclusive about causes in individual cases but the task of truly theorising medical knowledge and its contested role in society is completely beyond its reach (Pilgrim, 2015). For example, the pre-empirical conceptual problems about psychiatric knowledge are ignored, as are the problems of medicalisation and the interests of the drug companies in creating new diseases to treat. These topics require a form of serious critical attention that is outside the scope of the BPS model.

See also: *public mental health; social models of mental health.*

FURTHER READING

Weiss, P.A. (1977) 'The system of nature and the nature of systems: empirical holism and practical reductionism harmonized', in K.E. Schaefer, H. Hensel and R. Brady (eds), *A New Image of Man in Medicine*, Vol. 1: *Towards a Man-Centered Medical Science*. New York: Futura.

Wolman, B.B. (1981) *Contemporary Theories and Systems in Psychology*. Amsterdam: Plenum.

REFERENCES

Álvarez, A.S., Pagani, M. and Meucci, P. (2012) 'The clinical application of the biopsychosocial model in mental health: a research critique', *American Journal of Physical Medicine & Rehabilitation/Association of Academic Psychiatrists*, 91 (Suppl. 1 13): S173–80.

Bateson, G. (1980) *Mind and Nature: A Necessary Unity*. New York: Bantam.

Brown, T.M. and Fee, E. (2006) 'Rudolf Carl Virchow', *American Journal of Public Health*, 96 (12): 2104–5.

Dahlgren, G. and Whitehead, M. (1992) *Policies and Strategies to Promote Equity in Health*. Stockholm: Institute of Futures Studies.

Dolovich, L., Oliver, D., Lamarche, L. et al. (2016) 'A protocol for a pragmatic randomized controlled trial using the Health Teams Advancing Patient Experience: Strengthening Quality (Health TAPESTRY) platform approach to promote person-focused primary healthcare for older adults', *Implementation Science*, 11 (5 April): 49.

Engel, G. (1977) 'The need for a new medical model: A challenge for biomedicine', *Science*, 196 (4286): 129–36.

Engel, G.L. (1980) 'The clinical application of the biopsychosocial model', *American Journal of Psychiatry*, 137: 535–44.

Garcia-Toro, M. and Auirre, I. (2007) 'Biopsychosocial model in depression', *Medical Hypotheses*, 68 (3): 683–91.

Ghaemi, N. (2009) 'The rise and fall of the biopsychosocial model', *British Journal of Psychiatry*, 195: 3–4.

Guze, S.B. (1989) 'Biological psychiatry: is there any other kind?', *Psychological Medicine*, 19: 315–23.

Illich, I. (1976) *Medical Nemesis*. London: Marion Boyars.

McClaren, N. (2006) 'The myth of the biopsychosocial model', Correspondence, *Australian and New Zealand Journal of Psychiatry*, 40 (3): 277–8.

Meyer, A. (1952) *The Collected Works of Adolf Meyer*. New York: Basic Books.

Pilgrim, D. (2015) 'The biopsychosocial model in health research: its strengths and limitations for critical realists', *Journal of Critical Realism*, 14 (2): 164–80.

Read, J. (2005) 'The bio-bio-bio model of madness', *The Psychologist*, 18 (40): 596–7.

Schwartz, G.E. (1982) 'Testing the biopsychosocial model: the ultimate challenge facing behavioral medicine?', *Journal of Consulting and Clinical Psychology*, 50 (6): 1040–53.

key concepts in
mental health

von Bertalanffy, L. (1969) *General System Theory: Foundations, Development, Applications*. New York: Braziller.

Walby, S. (2007) 'Complexity theory, systems theory and multiple intersecting social inequalities', *Philosophy of the Social Sciences*, 37 (4): 449–70.

Madness

DEFINITION

Madness is sustained unintelligible conduct and spoken thought. The person inhabits an idiosyncratic world, which does not make immediate sense to others.

KEY POINTS

- The relationship between lay and professional descriptions of madness is discussed.
- The merits of non-medical ways of framing madness are examined.

Madness has also officially been called 'lunacy' and 'insanity'. The latter is still used in our legal system but the former is now defunct. Since the 19th century, mental health professionals have also used 'mania', 'mopishness', 'melancholia', 'psychosis', 'dementia praecox', 'schizophrenia', 'manic depression', 'schizoaffective disorder' and 'bipolar disorder'. This emphasises the shifting ways in which the English language frames madness in the official world of politicians and clinicians.

Such is the fear or amusement that madness creates in the general population that we have quite a rich lexicon to describe it. Terms used in the English vernacular about madness have included 'crazy', 'crackers', 'deranged', 'bonkers', 'batty', 'bananas', 'psycho', 'potty', 'do-lally', 'away with the fairies', 'on another planet', 'spacey', 'loony', 'loopy', 'touched', 'wacky' or just 'mental'. The latter connotation has meant that those with learning disabilities (what were once called a '*mental* handicap') have also been stereotyped as being mad. Since the English language readily draws on foreign sources at times, we also have: to go 'loco' (from Spain); or 'berserk' (from Scandinavia); or to run 'amok' (from South Asia).

Many of the disparaging lay terms used above imply alienation (with the mad being under extra-planetary influence or being strangers to themselves or the rest of humanity). For many years, experts on madness were called 'alienists'. In the madhouses of the 17th and 18th centuries, the mad were seen as not really human and so they could be visited and viewed with horror or amusement by normal citizens, without any sense of guilt or remorse.

Although 'severe mental illness', 'psychosis', 'schizophrenia' or 'bipolar disorder' only began to exist with the emergence of the psychiatric profession, as its preferred codifications of madness, the latter has always existed. This point is made to emphasise that madness is not simply a slippery semantic construction. There does seem to have been a real and consistent pattern of description across the centuries. Since antiquity, records of various societies indicate that those who transgress social expectations, in ways that others cannot fathom, provoke some clear description of difference.

Two stereotypical and enduring descriptions of madness since ancient times have included violence and aimless wandering. Other features include mad people talking to themselves (outside an intelligible religious ritual or context of prayer) and expressing grandiose or ridiculous views, which the challenges of others do not modify. Madness has also invited emotional descriptions of being wild and exuberant or flat and dejected, in contexts in which these forms of expression were unexpected. In accord with the violent stereotype of madness, the word 'mad' also means furiously angry.

Before madness became medicalised in the 19th century, it was described and explained within moral and supernatural frameworks. The early asylum system was run by religious lay people who saw madness as evidence of demonic possession or influence, leading to corruption of the soul and the ensuing animalistic deterioration of the personality. For this reason, 'moral treatment' was the first systematic attempt to bring the insane back into the fold of normal society.

Although scientific medicine is critical of this outmoded view, it did locate madness in a moral context. To reframe it as mental illness (the current Western rational medical view) decontextualises mad conduct and attributes it to essential pathology within the individual. More strongly than this, it attributes it to some yet to be discovered disorder of the brain and pre-empts the possibility that madness might actually be meaningful, even if not in an immediate sense. By contrast, the older view meant that the mad person's actions were being evaluated within a moral and religious framework. Thus, the latter, not just the person, was open to interpretation or interrogation.

The clinical gaze of the psychiatric profession encourages us only to look at individuals as manifestations of mental illness and not the profession that claims expertise about them or those parties in society in whose interests it works. It is as if simply to describe symptoms of mental illness as pathology (and so meaningless communication) is all that is required in order to describe madness. This closes down rather than opens up an exploration of the mystery of madness and its regular negotiation by those who remain sane by common consent.

The religious framing of madness as negative or demonic has been far from unambiguous. Religious exuberance ('religiosity') has been seen as divine or inspired at times rather than devilish. Examples of this today can be found in some forms of ultra-orthodox Judaism. Similarly, religious madness was associated with positive Protestant revivalism in Northern Ireland during the mid-19th century. The capacity to 'talk in tongues' has been framed as a divine, not demonic, intervention in Pentecostal Christian sects. The Greek philosopher Socrates pointed out the equal value of sanity and madness, because good forms of the latter were supplied by the gods. He emphasised the positive aspects of mad rapture: prophesying (a 'manic art'); mystical initiations and rituals; poetic inspiration; and the 'madness' of mutual lovers. All of these points resonate in religious belief systems today. They are also a corrective to the negative view that madness is merely a comical, frightening or pitiful state.

In some cultures, some of the symptoms of madness (particularly the experience of hallucinations and thought insertion, where an idea comes to mind from an outside source) have been seen as a supernatural gift shown by shamans and religious leaders, rather than a defect or malady. Saints, prophets and pious hermits have also shown clear signs of madness, with their visions and claims of clairvoyance. Their claims of peculiar religious insights and their withdrawal from normal society would now readily invite a diagnosis of severe mental illness. Madness is defined by the attributions of others and the transgression of the fundamental rule in adult society of being able to render one's behaviour intelligible to others when required. This 'intelligibility rule' is a characteristic of societies, not individuals. Consequently, madness is a social judgement, not a medical scientific fact. Moreover, not only are exceptions tolerated to the intelligibility rule to various degrees in various societies, but also conformity to the rules of reason or rationality does not always produce healthy outcomes.

It is true that mad people are unintelligible to others and so lack credibility as citizens. However, it is also true that sane people may act reasonably and intelligibly but be highly destructive. The threats of warfare and ecological degradation to humanity as a whole, the pursuit of genocide and the building of concentration camps have been the collective outcome of sane people acting in a reasonable and intelligible way, according to the norms of their parent society.

In other words, the disvalue that is placed on the irrationality of individuals is only one way of attributing pathology. Descriptions of pathology ultimately are value judgements and health can be defined perversely as conformity to an unhealthy society. Rationality, transparency and efficiency (the ideal features of normal people in modern industrialised societies) taken to their ultimate conclusions can also be pathological. For this reason, many of those who are hostile to a naive mental illness view of madness have argued for concerted efforts to create productive conversations between normality and madness, with the assumption that advantages might accrue in both directions. Relevant examples here are of the works of Ronald Laing and Michel Foucault, who noted that in modern societies, the dialogue between reason and unreason has broken down. According to Laing's colleague, David Cooper, this broken dialogue now means that the opposite of madness is not sanity but normality.

See also: *anti-psychiatry; causes and consequences of mental health problems; creativity; psychiatric classification; spirituality; the myth of mental illness*.

madness

81

FURTHER READING

Bentall, R.P. (2003) *Madness Explained*. London: Penguin.
Cooper, D. (1968) *Psychiatry and Anti-Psychiatry*. London: Tavistock.

Coulter, J. (1973) *Approaches to Insanity*. New York: Wiley.

Foucault, M. (1965) *Madness and Civilisation*. New York: Random House.

Laing, R.D. (1967) *The Politics of Experience and the Bird of Paradise*. Harmondsworth: Penguin.

Le Francois, B., Menzies, R. and Reaume, G. (eds) (2013) *Mad Matters: A Critical Reader in Canadian Mad Studies*. Toronto: Canadian Scholars Press.

Porter, R. (1989) *A Social History of Madness*. London: Routledge.

Rosen, G. (1968) *Madness in Society*. New York: Harper.

Screech, M.A. (1985) 'Good madness in Christendom', in W.F. Bynum, R. Porter and M. Shepherd (eds), *The Anatomy of Madness*, Vol. 1. London: Tavistock.

Scull, A. (1979) *Museums of Madness: The Social Organization of Insanity in 19th Century England*. London: Allen Lane.

Wing, J. (1978) *Reasoning about Madness*. Oxford: Oxford University Press.

Attention Deficit Hyperactivity Disorder

key concepts in
mental health

DEFINITION

Attention Deficit Hyperactivity Disorder (ADHD) is a psychiatric description of children or adults, who have a persistent pattern of inattention, hyperactivity and impulsivity. According to DSM and ICD, these forms of conduct are assumed to interfere with the development and functioning of the person affected.

KEY POINTS

- This diagnosis is typically given in childhood and may be retained for those growing up, who then continue to manifest features of inattention, hyperactivity and impulsivity, despite long-term treatment. However, new cases are also diagnosed in adults, a trend which has increased in recent years.
- Both the diagnosis and its medicinal treatment have been the focus of controversy. Validity problems are noted in the former and iatrogenic impacts noted in the latter.
- We can reflect on the maintenance of a controversial diagnosis by attending to the interest work of various parties gaining from or querying its legitimacy.

This diagnosis has been controversial for three main reasons, which often interweave in their expression. First, its validity has been queried and the role of unreasonable medicalisation discussed. Second, the risks of the long-term treatment of those diagnosed with amphetamine-based drugs have been critiqued. Third, the interests of diagnosticians and the drug companies have been explored by critics.

THE VALIDITY PROBLEM

As with other functional psychiatric diagnoses, the one of ADHD is tautological:

Q: How do we know this child has ADHD?

A: Because they have persistent problems of poor concentration, distractibility and they find it very difficult to sit still at their school desk.

Q: Why do they behave in this way?

A: Because they are suffering from ADHD.

There are no biological markers to offer us an aetiological account of the diagnosed disorder. The diagnosis relies upon a medical consensus (within for now the *ICD* and *DSM* committee systems) about 'the fact' of ADHD.

Thus, we can separate three distinct questions. First, how does the diagnosis emerge? The answer is via the current norms of Western diagnostic medicine and the interests underpinning it (see later on interest work). Second, is the diagnosis valid according to our expectations of a good medical diagnosis? The answer is 'no'. Its aetiology cannot be specified and it relies on symptoms, not biological signs. Moreover, many of its component symptoms can be found in other diagnoses, thereby undermining its concept validity. Third, does the diagnosis encourage a full and open-minded biopsychosocial formulation of distractible impulsive behaviour in children and adults, case by case? The answer is 'no'. Instead, we find a form of 'hoped-for-reductionism' (Wolman, 1981), whereby those favouring the diagnosis insist that the conduct can be explained *already and fully* by a form of neuro-deficit inside diagnosed patients. Instead of case-by-case formulations, the diagnosis is a Procrustean bed constituted by this assumed biological substrate. Manifestations of hyperactivity are then reduced to the diagnosis in terms of its explanation and conceptualisation. People and their complex and particular context are reduced to a diagnosis.

That case-by-case context has a double significance. It might have a causal role to account for disruptive and distractible conduct in children exposed to poverty and abuse (the diagnosis is given disproportionately in these circumstances). Also, the social context provides the normative setting for how deviance is judged and then medicalised (Timimi and Leo, 2009). Bio-reductionism imposes social blinkers in both senses: we lose a sense of social causes and are oblivious to the normative expectations provided in different times and places.

As with all other functional diagnoses, that of ADHD is an epistemic fallacy, i.e. diagnosticians confuse what they *call* reality with reality itself. Such reductions of statements about reality to statements of knowledge are a feature of all functional psychiatric diagnoses and so this one is not peculiar. This particular epistemic fallacy means that social norms are excluded from analysis. In this case, it is assumed that ADHD is a condition existing inside individuals, independent of the context of the conduct being used to warrant the diagnosis (Conrad, 2006).

The shifting character of normativity is important in relation to this diagnosis (and many others). The particular forms of conduct that the diagnosis of ADHD subsumes are in themselves unremarkable or they might fall within the normal range in a time and place (Moncrieff and Timimi, 2011). (The very same criticism could be made of other forms of attributed mental disorder, such as shyness or sadness, when they become 'avoidant personality disorder' or 'depression'.) Some adults are impulsive and often mislay their car keys – so what? Some children are excitable and distractible at times – so what? The answers to these questions reside not in medical explanations and questionable biomedical treatments in response, but in our accul-turated social expectations. Apart from distractibility arising in children for such social or contextual reasons and the behavioural features of the diagnosis being present in normal functioning, it may also be present as a result of a range of other difficulties, such as anxiety, hearing impairments or mild learning difficulties.

IATROGENESIS

Psychostimulants used to treat ADHD have been associated with a range of iatro-genic effects, including sleep disruption, mood swings, nausea and reduced appetite, raised levels of reported anxiety, raised blood pressure, stunted growth and delayed puberty in boys (Poulton et al., 2013). Given that up to a third of children treated with psychostimulants for ADHD continue with their symptoms into adulthood, the long-term or permanent use of these drugs during the life span creates risks to the patient, some known and some not. While there is no correla-tion in the short term with their use on children's proneness to substance abuse, there is evidence that that risk increases in adult patients (Dalsgaard et al., 2014).

Concerns about the increasing use of psychostimulants in children in the USA began to appear in the paediatric literature during the 1990s. For example, one review at the time noted a 2.5 increase in the rate of prescribing in just the first five years of the decade (Safer et al., 1996). Today in the UK, the National Institute for Clinical Excellence recommends that psychological not pharmacological treatments should be prioritised, especially in very young children, but the former are more resource-intensive and so these recommendations are difficult to implement in practice. As a consequence, psychostimulant use in children has increased not decreased in recent years, even in a system of socialised medicine (the NHS in Britain). Between 2007 and 2012, there was a 60 per cent increase in their use. Between 1992 and 2001 in the UK, there was a 92-fold increase in the prescription of psychostimulants for children under the age of 6 (Hill and Turner, 2016). This means there was a 92-fold increase in iatrogenic risk to very young children whose nervous system was highly immature and who were not in a position to offer informed consent to exposure to that risk. Moreover, children of that age *ipso facto* are not socialised and so firm and clear judgements about the 'appropriateness' of their conduct by adults might be dubious and ill-judged. Accordingly, to label and medicate such young children is highly problematic and so invokes ethical and political objections.

INTEREST WORK

The unresolved debates about validity reflect protagonists with differing interests (professional, commercial, personal or ideological). No one is value neutral and there is no 'bird's eye' view that can be offered by analysts of the controversy. For example, the way I have framed this entry to the book reflects my position within that range. Child psychiatrists and child psychologists defending the diagnosis have a career interest in its perpetuation. The drug companies can spin out profits from a form of psychotropic medication (amphetamine) which in other contexts has lost its therapeutic credibility and has been re-cast now as a dubious recreational drug. Families of children with the diagnosis gain from individualising wider challenges in their social context. They also may gain extra educational resources by their child receiving the diagnosis. If a child is simply afflicted by a mental disorder, then few questions need to be asked about the personal responsibility of significant adults in their lives.

The gains for critics are political and usually reflect a wider intellectual critique from within psychology and psychiatry. This critique focuses on diagnosis as a mystification and diversion from the examination of the social context of both the process of diagnosis and the biographical uniqueness of each identified patient. The threat this poses to defenders of the diagnosis is then reflected in angry counter-attacks (e.g. https://aadduk.org/2018/01/23/letter-to-british-psychological-society-re-adhd-stigmatisation). The AADD-UK organisation is a group of adults with the diagnosis, who are offended by the post-diagnostic approach issued by the Division of Clinical Psychology, the 'Power Threat Meaning Framework' (Johnstone and Boyle et al., 2018). Those professionals expressing concerns about the over-diagnosis, or even the fundamental scientific legitimacy, of ADHD and its iatrogenic risks face campaigns of vilification from the conservative amalgam of professionals, families and drug companies favouring its use (LeFever Watson et al., 2013). All three of these groups contain people with a strong vested interest in retaining a diagnosis, which is both empirically contestable and ethically problematic. For their part, its critics are pursuing their own interests (which are ideological and sometimes disciplinary in nature).

To summarise, the controversy about ADHD centres on the validity of the diagnosis, the risks of biological reductionism (obscuring a needed assessment of psychological and social risks to children), the iatrogenic toll of treatment and the range of interests present in those supporting or critiquing the diagnosis.

See also: *challenging conduct in adults and children; the pharmaceutical industry.*

attention deficit hyperactivity disorder

85

FURTHER READING

Conrad, P. (2006) *Identifying Hyperactive Children: The Medicalization of Deviant Behavior.* Burlington, VT: Ashgate.

Timimi, S. and Leo, J. (eds) (2009) *Rethinking ADHD: From Brain to Culture.* Basingstoke: Palgrave Macmillan.

Conrad, P. (2006) *Identifying Hyperactive Children: The Medicalization of Deviant Behavior.* Burlington, VT: Ashgate.

Dalsgaard, S., Mortensen, P.B., Frydenberg, M. and Thomsen, P.H. (2014) 'ADHD, stimulant treatment in childhood and subsequent substance abuse in adulthood', *Addictive Behaviors*, 39 (1): 325–8.

Hill, V.C. and Turner, H. (2016) 'Educational psychologists' perspectives on the medicalisation of childhood behaviour: a focus on Attention Deficit Hyperactive Disorder (ADHD)', *Educational & Child Psychology*, 33 (2): 12–29.

Johnstone, L. and Boyle, M., with Cromby, J., Dillon, J., Harper, D., Kinderman, P., Longden, E., Pilgrim, D. and Read, J. (2018) *The Power Threat Meaning Framework: Towards the Identification of Patterns in Emotional Distress, Unusual Experiences and Troubled or Troubling Behaviour.* Leicester: British Psychological Society.

LeFever Watson, G., Arcona, A.P., Antonuccio, D.O. and Healy, D. (2013) 'Shooting the messenger: the case of ADHD', *Journal of Contemporary Psychotherapy*, 44 (1): 43–52.

Moncrieff, J. and Timimi, S. (2011) 'Critical analysis of the concept of adult attention hyperactivity disorder', *The Psychiatrist Online*, 35: 334–8.

Poulton, A.S., Melzer, P., Tait, P.R., Garnett, S.P., Cowell, C.T., Baur, L.A. and Clarke, S. (2013) 'Growth and pubertal development of adolescent boys on stimulant medication for attention deficit hyperactivity disorder', *Medical Journal of Australia*, 198 (1): 29–32.

Safer, D.J., Zito, J.M. and Fine, E.M. (1996) 'Increased methylphenidate usage for attention deficit disorder in the 1990s', *Pediatrics*, 98 (1): 1084–8.

Timimi, S. and Leo, J. (eds) (2009) *Rethinking ADHD: From Brain to Culture.* Basingstoke: Palgrave Macmillan.

Wolman, B.B. (1981) *Contemporary Theories and Systems in Psychology.* Amsterdam: Plenum.

Temporo-Spatial Aspects of Mental Abnormality

DEFINITION

Mental abnormality is defined by the norms of time and space but the latter also create the conditions of possibility for universal trends (particularly about the importance of distress and unintelligibility) as well as their situation-specific forms.

KEY POINTS

- Time and place provide particular norms about what is considered to be psychologically abnormal.

- Trends and fads about both naming that abnormality and responding to it are evident.
- A tension exists in the historical and cross-cultural literature about seeking to generalise across time and place, while conceding particular situated features of psychological abnormality.

Several entries in this book reflect a tension between two forms of description. The first refers to attempts to identify permanent features of psychological normality and abnormality across time and space. This assumes empirical invariance: mental disorders are depicted as being the same in character across time and place. The second refers to various rejections of this possibility in favour of descriptions that are situated or contextualised.

The first tendency is evident in both psychiatric and psychological positivism, which assume in advance that reality is fixed and has 'covering laws' which apply in all times and places. *ICD* and *DSM* reflect this tendency but even they have had to concede the occurrence of 'culturally specific syndromes' (see later in this entry). The second tendency can be found in a range of anti-positivist criticisms from 'critical psychiatry' rooted in postmodern ideas and objections from critical realists. These critics emphasise differing contexts which created a range of conditions of possibilities (or causes) as well as a range of social norms that make judgements about what is remarkable or unremarkable about psychological functioning in society.

The literature discussing these judgements includes that covering the history of psychiatry as well as cross-cultural psychiatry. As I have noted elsewhere in the entries relevant to these writings, no society on record has been indifferent to those who are manifestly distressed or unintelligible. However, their salience has varied from society to society, with madness tending to be the main social concern (whether or not it was subsequently framed in medical or religious terms). What today we might call 'the neuroses' and 'the psychoses' have been a long-term interest to those who have been sane by common consent because they disrupt the expectations of others in daily life. Modern psychiatry tends to then codify those concerns in diagnostic language but their origins are in the 'lay arena' of particular social contexts.

Other diagnoses, such as those of 'personality disorder' and 'substance misuse', have a much shorter medical history (since the 19th century). Prior to that, self-centred or self-indulgent incorrigibility in its various forms was described simply in moral terms. With these points in mind, I now shift to trends (or arguably 'fads') that have emerged since the development of modern psychiatry and psychology.

TRENDS IN DIAGNOSTIC AND TREATMENT RESPONSES IN MODERN WESTERN HEALTHCARE

Here I illustrate the point about more recent shifting trends by some brief case studies of diagnoses and preferred forms of treatment: neurasthenia and chronic fatigue syndrome; eating disorders; insulin coma therapy; cognitive-behavioural therapy; and mindfulness. These trends or fads in diagnostic and treatment emphasis are accounted for in different ways, as will be clear.

Neurasthenia and chronic fatigue sydrome

The diagnosis of neurasthenia was an orthodoxy in 19th-century Western medicine. Freud followed the lead of other doctors in assuming that the physical depletion of energy in the nervous system led to the behavioural outcome of lethargy and listlessness. Its associated symptoms were summarised by Beard (1869) as being malaise, debility, insomnia, poor appetite, headaches and feelings of chronic weakness. Today it remains a common diagnosis in China and is still included as a diagnostic category in *ICD*, although it has been dropped from *DSM*.

Chronic fatigue syndrome (CFS) has much in common symptomatically with neurasthenia, although its origins are claimed by its advocates to be in viral infections that create the long-term residual behavioural lethargy and experiental distress associated with it. After its naming during the 1980s by physicians, a tension arose between those claiming it unambiguously as a physical disease (i.e. a post-viral impact in all cases) and those arguing that psychosocial factors may be implicated in its emergence and maintenance (Wessely, 1995; cf. ME Association, 2016). Campaigning groups focus on its assumed physical basis by preferring the older diagnosis of 'myalgic encephalomyelitis' or 'ME'. The controversy about the diagnosis continues in the light of these differences of views and because it is a diagnosis of exclusion: fatigue is common in a number of conditions which are excluded before CFS is applied. It has no biological marker and its aetiology is contested. However, we can note that this is also the case with functional psychiatric diagnoses, such as schizophrenia and yet those diagnoses are applied confidently in medicine.

At the turn of this century, more specialist services were set up to treat those with the diagnosis, leading to reported symptomatic improvement in about a third of cases (Collin and Crawley, 2017). In the past ten years, the incidence has declined after peaking during the 1990s. The diagnosis of 'fybromyalgia' (generalised and persistent muscle pain) has been used more instead and changes have occurred in the demographic patterning (Collin et al., 2017).

Eating disorders

These are described in *DSM* and *ICD* and are only meaningful in cultures in which there is no food scarcity. The tendency to eat excessively and then vomit (bulimia), or to avoid and hide food (anorexia), occurs in cultures in which food is regularly available. Both bulimia and anorexia are more common in females and tend to emerge in adolescence. Bulimia typically emerges in late adolescence but anorexia has an earlier onset. (The incidence of eating disorders is very rare in young children and in older adults.) The typical anorexic girl fears weight gain and considers her body to be too large, even when she is demonstrably underweight. Some patients have alternating phases of binge eating and food avoidance, and may exhibit habits common to both (vomiting and laxative use) throughout. Some other activities, such as excessive exercise, also predict anorexia, although the direction of causality is not clear. (Do competitive runners, dancers and gymnasts need to keep their weight down to perform efficiently? Alternatively, are the excessive activity and the eating disorder both parts of a personal strategy to remain thin?)

Eating disorders can occur in isolation but they are often linked to other mental health problems, such as low mood and self-harming. Indeed, both anorexia and bulimia can themselves be framed as self-harming activities, as the patient is denying themselves sustenance to live or they are interfering with their body in an injurious way. Examples of the latter are vomiting, which inflames the oesophagus and rots the teeth, and starvation itself, which can lead to a range of health problems. The preponderance of eating disorders in girls has led to many feminist accounts (Malson, 1997). These emphasise both social norms (girls aspiring to an 'ideal' model figure) and the control of food and weight as political strategies. The latter may reflect the young girl's access to control, given the relative powerlessness of females in a patriarchal society. As the diagnosis became more established and services provided, the incidence remained stable but there was a continuing trend of girls rather than boys being diagnosed (van Hoeken et al., 2009).

Eating disorders throw into relief a number of features about food and its physical and symbolic relationship to human welfare. They indicate a global division between rich and poor. They are far more prevalent in conditions of dietary plenty for the bulk of the population. While it is true that poor diet and malnutrition are present in the poorest sectors of developed societies, even these may exhibit eating disorders, because food, of sorts, is regularly available. (The growth in food banks in developed societies since the global financial crisis of 2008 suggests a counter-trend, though.) In developing countries, mass starvation can be common. In these countries, the dominant problem is finding something to eat on a regular basis. Eating disorders can only meaningfully arise when the patient has a predictable source of food to regulate; hence they are a product of relative affluence (van Hoeken et al., 1998). For example, studies in Egypt, China and India suggest that anorexia nervosa is very rare in their young female populations (Tseng, 2003).

Insulin coma therapy

This was introduced by Sakel in 1927 and continued to be used extensively in Western psychiatry until the 1950s when it was superceded by the neuroleptic treatment of psychosis. Sakel noticed that a patient who had slipped into a coma recovered in a more lucid mental state. This triggered a biomedical enthusiasm for the technique, which was dangerous (errors of dose led to death). As with the later tolerance of iatrogenic risk to psychotic patients of the major tranquillisers, this acceptance of 'heroic' medical interventions in madness on behalf of those sane by common consent, signalled an indifference to the rights of patients with low social status and credibility.

Cognitive-behavioural therapy (CBT)

In recent times, mass media reports point to the use of cognitive-behavioural therapy (CBT) for all forms of mental disorder. Its popularity has emerged for a range of reasons. First, it has been promoted by psychologists and psychiatrists as a form of intervention that can be tested in randomised controlled trials (RCTs), in much the same way as a drug. Second, its brief form (claims of cure of mental illness in as few as six sessions) is attractive in cash-strapped healthcare systems like the British NHS. Third, it can be promoted as a form of scientific applied psychology (distinguishing it, for example, from the more dubious psychoanalytical forms of therapy). In the UK, these selling points for CBT were the successful basis for the lobbying of government by a labour economist, Richard Layard, and his psychiatric advisors. This lobbying led to the establishment in the UK of the Improving Access to Psychological Therapies initiative extant at the time of writing (Pilgrim, 2011).

Critics of the approach argue that it does not do justice to human complexity and that it legitimises uncritically the status of psychiatric categories (which themselves are scientifically dubious). Moreover, the empirical evidence from the RCT model noted above is undermined by a competing evidence base that suggests that the specific model of psychological therapy is not a predictor of client improvement. Instead, the latter arises largely from the quality of the relationship between clients and their therapists (the working relationship or treatment alliance). According to the latter argument, we improve in therapy because we like and trust our therapist, not because of the particular model they prefer or are trained in.

The trend to favour one model of psychological therapy over another reflects the cultural interests of dominant professional groups in a time and place. For now, in Western developed societies, this model is CBT.

Mindfulness

Mindfulness refers to the capacity to attend to our awareness of our inner and outer worlds at a particular moment in time. It is a concept derived from Buddhism and is used freely now in a range of contexts aspiring to improve mental health. It points to the role of inner processes as a source of personal change, thereby altering older behaviourist assumptions in psychology.

This psychological technique, which might be part of a psychotherapeutic programme learned as a separate ability for general use in life, has its origins in Buddhism. The latter (along with Stoicism) is an ancient tradition that has a continuing impact on modern psychological interventions, aimed at promoting mental health or treating mental health problems. Mindfulness is a necessary, but not sufficient, component of traditional forms of Buddhist meditation. In the confines of current mental health practice, it is largely a taught technique and as such does not necessitate either a knowledge of, or commitment to, Buddhism as a philosophical tradition. However, because it is taught and can be practised to improve its efficiency, it still retains an affinity with that meditative tradition. And in both cases, we vary in our natural (untutored) ability to be attentive to internal and external stimuli. This is analogous to psychoanalytic patients varying in their ability to free associate or report in a nuanced and honest way what comes to mind. It may be that such processes come easier to the quiet, watchful introvert than the garrulous and distractible extravert.

Its increasing recent importance as a psychological technology suggests the demise of behaviourism as a defining feature of scientific psychology. The growth of cognitivism in the wider discipline and the shift from behaviour therapy to cognitive behaviour therapy in the past 40 years within clinical psychology is an indication of that trend. This means that now clinical practice routinely engages with client subjectivity and agency. Mindfulness is one example of that engagement with the consciousness of the client.

Although it is now associated with being an adjunct to CBT or a general method to improve wellbeing and so has a mental health focus, its recent clinical origins were in relation to general health problems. However, despite enthusiasts encouraging mindfulness, to date its role in physical health problems has not proved to have any curative efficacy, though it can help in coping and living with chronic or terminal conditions.

CROSS-CULTURAL PSYCHIATRY

Cross-cultural (or 'transcultural') psychiatry can be explored in two ways. It can simply be read as a source of knowledge about mental disorder in different cultures. Alternatively, the contradictions it exposes about psychiatric knowledge are also noteworthy. In the first, a universal body of psychiatric knowledge is considered to be non-problematic. The main interest is then in the study of differences *within* this assumed universally legitimate body of knowledge. In the second, psychiatric knowledge is read sceptically, and cross-cultural differences are deemed to expose further the futility of claims of a unifying and valid body of psychiatric knowledge. This entry will consider both readings.

Cultural differences in mental disorder – the orthodox reading

Cross-cultural psychiatry starts with three assumptions. First, it is assumed that mental disorder, as defined and studied by Western psychiatry (developed in the 19th century mainly from German psychiatric diagnosis and classification – 'nosology'), is manifested universally. It is taken as read that the definitions of mental disorder set out by *DSM* and *ICD* are valid. Thus, say, 'depression' or 'schizophrenia' are considered to be valid diagnoses, with stable symptom profiles, that can be investigated internationally. The second assumption is that specific forms of mental disorder may be shaped in their expression, incidence and prevalence by cultural differences. One implication of this is that psychiatrists should be very careful to understand cultural meanings (especially semantic subtleties, non-verbal etiquette and folk belief systems) when making any diagnosis. Third, there is an assumption that sometimes there are expressions of mental abnormality which are culturally unique.

It is in this third area that cross-cultural psychiatry attracts most attention in Western readers because of the exotic connotations of what are called 'culturally related specific syndromes'. For example, in Malaysia, some men have a morbid fear that their penis is shrinking and that this is an indication of imminent death (*koro*). A female version of this is in relation to shrinking nipples. A similar genital fear is found in India, called the *dhat* syndrome. This is the belief that serious illness will be created by excessive loss of sperm (from nocturnal emission or masturbation). In another example, in China, there is a morbid fear of catching colds (frigophobia; *pa-len*; *wei-han*). This is in the context of the Chinese belief system about the balance between yin and yang. Those with a fear of colds predominating will over-dress in warm weather and avoid cold-inducing foods.

In Japan, with its particular sensitivity to the views of others, some adolescents develop *taijinkyofushio*. This entails the young person being excessively anxious about how they are viewed by others, especially classmates and those whom they must socially encounter who are not family members. A final example is Nigerian 'brain fag syndrome'. This is the anxious belief on the part of the patient that their intellectual and sensory capacities are impaired, accompanied by a burning sensation in the head and neck.

Cultural differences in mental disorder – the sceptical reading

The central problem for cross-cultural psychiatry is that if it introduces too much sensitivity to cultural differences (a form of relativism), then the core assumption about a universally stable body of knowledge is under threat. If, on the other hand, the latter is over-emphasised, then psychiatrists are accused of being culturally insensitive or of manifesting a form of Western cultural imperialism. The use of American society as a normative cultural base for *DSM* encourages this criticism. Those committed to cross-cultural psychiatry can either be accused of 'having it both ways', in their attitude towards the universal and the particular, or they are constantly struggling to advocate the correct or delicate balance between them.

In support of the universal hypothesis is the notion that some conditioned physiological processes (anxiety and the misery linked to 'learned helplessness') are demonstrably universal (see the entries on Sadness and Fear). Moreover, some broad generalisations can be made about these phenomena in other mammals, not just about all human beings. The problem comes when these expressions of distress are reified or codified using Western medical labels. Why should Western labels (specifically 19th-century Germanic ones) be deemed to be intrinsically valid or superior to ones preferred elsewhere? Also, why are these labels medical in nature? Why are medical codifications superior to religious or social ones or ordinary language descriptions?

These questions arise because of the centrality of language in human functioning. This allows us to rehearse alternative meanings for what we experience and what we see. This open-textured reflectiveness, for example, lets us view anxiety in ourselves or others as an illness or as an existential state (or both). Depression can be viewed as an illness or experienced as a religious experience invoked by sin.

Why is the first right and the second wrong? Who decides? When it comes to madness (see the entry on Madness), why is it mental illness rather than unrecognised creativity, religious insight or simply a mystery to be tolerated? These questions undermine our confidence in the universal applicability of psychiatric knowledge.

Despite these criticisms, invited by cross-cultural psychiatry, the latter provides an opportunity to discuss cultural relativism. It also encourages orthodox Western practitioners to be more sensitive to alternative belief systems and contextual reasoning. In doing so, it invites them to pay close attention to the particular meanings being expressed by an individual patient. Taken to its logical conclusion, this would then mean abandoning all diagnoses in favour of biopsychosocial formulations case by case. Genuine cross-cultural sensitivity may ensure that psychiatrists provide unique formulations when they encounter patients from alien cultures. Ironically, this habit is not encouraged by the application of standard diagnostic techniques, based on *DSM* or *ICD*, within a Western native culture.

See also: *biological interventions; fear; madness; race; psychological interventions; sadness.*

FURTHER READING

Abas, M., Broadhead, J.C., Mbape, P. and Khurnalo-Satakukwa, G. (1994) 'Defeating depression in the developing world', *British Journal of Psychiatry*, 164: 293–6.

Bruch, H. (1974) *Eating Disorders: Anorexia Nervosa and the Person Within*. London: Routledge.

Collins, P.Y., Patel, V., Joestl, S., March, D., Insel, T.R., Daar, A.S. et al. (2011) 'Grand challenges in global mental health', *Nature*, 475 (7354): 27–30.

Cox, N. and Webb, L. (2015) 'Poles apart: does the export of mental health expertise from the Global North to the Global South represent a neutral relocation of knowledge and practice?', *Sociology of Health & Illness*, 37 (5): 683–97.

Das, A. and Rao, M. (2012) 'Universal mental health: re-evaluating the call for global mental health', *Critical Public Health*, 22 (4): 383–9.

DelVechio Good, M.-J., Hyde, S., Pinto, S. and Good, B. (2008) *Post-Colonial Disorders*. Berkeley, CA: University of California Press.

Diala, C., Muntaner, C., Walrath, C., Nickerson, K.J., LaVeist, T.A. and Leaf, P.J. (2000) 'Racial differences in attitudes towards professional mental health care and in the use of services', *American Journal of Orthopsychiatry*, 70 (4): 455–64.

Kleinman, A. (1988) *Rethinking Psychiatry*. New York: Free Press.

Kokanovic, R. (2011) 'The diagnosis of depression in an international context', in D. Pilgrim, A. Rogers and B. Pescosolido (eds), *The SAGE Handbook of Mental Health and Illness*. London: Sage.

Krause, I.B. (1989) 'Sinking heart: a Punjabi communication of distress', *Social Science & Medicine*, 29 (4): 563–7.

Kuyken, W., Warren, F.C., Taylor, F.S. et al. (2016) 'Efficacy of mindfulness-based cognitive therapy in prevention of depressive relapse: an individual patient data meta-analysis from randomized trials', *JAMA Psychiatry*, 73 (6): 565–74.

Patel, N., Bennett, E., Dennis, M., Dosanjh, N., Miller, A., Mahtani, A. and Nadirshaw, Z. (eds) (2000) *Clinical Psychology, 'Race & Culture': A Training Manual*. Chichester: Blackwell.

Silove, D., Austin, P. and Steel, Z. (2007) 'No refuge from terror: the impact of detention on the mental health of trauma affected refugees seeking asylum in Australia', *Transcultural Psychiatry*, 44 (3): 359–94.

Summerfield, D. (2008) 'How scientifically valid is the knowledge base of global mental health?', *British Medical Journal*, 336: 992–4.

Watters, E. (2010) *Crazy Like Us: The Globalization of the American Psyche*. New York: Free Press.

REFERENCES

Beard, G. (1869) 'Neurasthenia, or nervous exhaustion', *Boston Medical and Surgical Journal*, 3: 217–21.

Collin, S.M. and Crawley, E. (2017) 'Specialist treatment of chronic fatigue syndrome/ME: a cohort study among adult patients in England', *BMC Health Services Research*, 17 (1): 488.

Collin, S.M., Bakken, I.J., Nazareth, I., Crawley, E. and White, P.D. (2017) 'Trends in the incidence of chronic fatigue syndrome and fibromyalgia in the UK, 2001–2013: a Clinical Practice Research Datalink study', *Journal of the Royal Society of Medicine*, 10 (6): 231–44.

Malson, H.M. (1997) 'Anorexic bodies and the discursive production of feminine excess', in J.M. Ussher (ed.), *Body Talk: The Material and Discursive Regulation of Sexuality, Madness and Reproduction*. London: Routledge.

ME Association (2016) *Liberating the NHS: No Decisions about Me, without Me*. London: The ME Association.

Pilgrim, D. (2011) 'The hegemony of cognitive behavioural therapy in modern mental health policy', *Health Sociology Review*, 20 (2): 120–32.

Tseng, W.-S. (2003) *Clinician's Guide to Cultural Psychiatry*. London: Academic Press.

van Hoeken, D., Bartelds, A., Hoek, H., van Son, G. and van Furth, E. (2009) 'Time trends in the incidence of eating disorders: a primary care study in the Netherlands', *Journal of Eating Disorders*, 43 (2): 130–8.

van Hoeken, D., Lucas, A.R. and Hoek, H.W. (1998) 'Epidemiology', in H.W. Hoek, J.L. Treasure and M.A. Katzman (eds), *Neurobiology in the Treatment of Eating Disorders*. Chichester: Wiley.

Wessely, S. (1995) 'The epidemiology of chronic fatigue syndrome', *Epidemiologic Reviews*, 17 (1): 139–51.

Challenging Conduct in Adults and Children

DEFINITION

Psychological difference brings with it a variety of forms of social non-conformity and discerning cause and effect is not easy. Some deviations from norms are subtle and barely noticed by others, but in some cases they constitute notable challenges within particular social contexts. In children, challenging conduct reflects value judgements about the identified individual failing to comply with 'age appropriate' norms.

> *The source of these deviations from expectations may be considered to be biological, psychological or social. In adults, such challenges might be acute or chronic and may be accounted for in a variety of ways. When learning disability and acute psychosis are excluded, chronic challenging conduct is often associated with diagnoses of personality disorder. The latter are defined by enduring disturbances of conduct that involve distress and/or recurrent interpersonal dysfunction in identified patients, which elicits offence or distress in others.*

KEY POINTS

- Challenging conduct in adults is linked to social non-conformity.
- The psychiatric classification of personality disorders is outlined.
- Criticisms of the personality disorder diagnosis are described.
- Particular considerations about challenging conduct in children are outlined.

Forms of non-conformity that pose challenges to third parties may or may not entail experienced distress on the part of the offending social actor. Also, psychological difference in any particular society may be highly valued (for example, extraordinary genius or benevolence). When and if it is disvalued, its causal source may be about attributed cognitive deficit (see the entry on Intellectual Disability) or acute irrationality (see the entry on Madness). Sometimes it attends the transgression of legal rules and this raises the question about whether criminality might be accounted for using psychological or psychiatric models. Within the latter, there has been an extensive and unresolved discussion about people who are incorrigibly challenging to others. This has culminated in the ambivalent inclusion of 'the personality disorders' within classification systems such as *ICD* and *DSM* (see the entry on Psychiatric Classification). Despite attempts by those developing *DSM* to argue that its remit is not about social non-comformity, all attributions of distress, unintellibility and incorrigibility inevitably refer to social norms. This point is at its most obvious when personality disorders are considered.

The origins of psychiatric interest in what are now described as personality disorders were limited to those who were deemed sane but also showed an absence of conscience and a lack of consideration for the rights of others. Today, this type of description would be limited only to what is called 'antisocial personality disorder' under *DSM-5* (American Psychiatric Association, 2013) and 'dissocial personality disorder' under *ICD-10* (World Health Organization, 1990).

Even this older antisocial focus (what was called 'moral insanity') does not find a ready current consensus. For example, the most extensive work in the area has been carried out by a psychologist, Robert Hare, who uses the term 'psychopathic disorder' to describe people with mixed features of antisocial, histrionic and narcissistic personality disorders (Hare, 1993). The term 'sociopathy' is used more in North America. However, there it may still be distinguished from 'psychopathy', with the latter being defined more by personal features than social (and especially criminal) consequences alone. Those labelled as psychopathic are also generally antisocial but they are not always detected as criminals: they may find successful roles in life but they distress those they manipulate and use for their own ends.

The following types of personality disorder can be found in *ICD-10*:

- Paranoid (suspicious, mistrustful, resentful, grudge-bearing, jealous, self-important).
- Schizoid (emotionally cold, detached, aloof, lacking enjoyment, introspective).
- Schizotypal (socially anxious, eccentric, oddities of thought and perception).
- Emotionally unstable (chronic feelings of emptiness and fear of abandonment, recurrently suicidal and self-harming, unstable mood states).
- Dissocial (callous to others, impulsive, lack of guilt and remorse, irresponsible, failure to take responsibility for actions).
- Anankastic (perfectionist, preoccupied by rules and details, over-conscientious, rigid and stubborn, pedantic, overly conventional).
- Histrionic (self-dramatising, shallow, attention-seeking, over-concern with physical attractiveness, suggestible).
- Anxious avoidant (fearful avoidance of others, fear of being criticised or humiliated).
- Dependent (compliant, lets others take responsibility, fear of being left to care for self, needs excessive help from others to make decisions).

When *DSM-5* was being drafted, experts in the field of personality disorders feared that it was going to be 'an unwieldy conglomeration of disparate models that cannot happily coexist and raises the likelihood that many clinicians will not have the patience and persistence to make use of it in their practices' (Shedler et al., 2010: 1026). Final adjustments to the text of *DSM* responded to this sort of critical feedback. Indeed, the personality disorders were so contentious that they were excluded from the main body of the document and placed in a separate section of *DSM-5*, signifying the need for 'further study'. *DSM-5* encourages clinicians to combine a consideration of six 'traits' (see below) with a focus on the patient's particular difficulties in 'personality functioning', although the latter is not precisely defined, so we assume that self-evident common sense is being encouraged. This 'hybrid' approach of trait assessment and current presenting problems retains a list similar to that in *DSM-IV* (American Psychiatric Association, 1994) and is reminiscent of that of *ICD-10* but with fewer disorders:

- Borderline Personality Disorder ('Emotionally unstable' in *ICD*).
- Obsessive-Compulsive Personality Disorder ('Anankastic' in *ICD*).
- Avoidant Personality Disorder.
- Schizotypal Personality Disorder.
- Antisocial Personality Disorder ('Dissocial' in *ICD*).
- Narcissistic Personality Disorder (not included in *ICD*, perhaps suggesting a North American cultural bias).

There are a number of criticisms that can be levelled at the concept of personality disorder and, by implication, any of its types (Blackburn, 1988; Dolan and Coid, 1993; Pilgrim, 2001). These criticisms can be explored using the following questions:

- *What is personality?* While most psychologists still use this term to describe a person's enduring or stable character, not all choose to embrace it. For example, the study of context-dependent identities has become more and more important for some psychologists. But for those who subscribe in principle to the concept of personality, there is a consensus, for now, that individuals can be described by the unique combination of points on five dimensions (openness to experience, conscientiousness, extraversion, agreeableness and neuroticism or emotional stability). These are often called the 'Big Five' in personality research (see Figure 2.1).

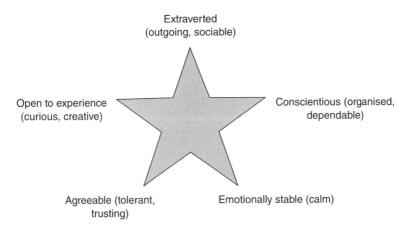

Figure 2.1   The Big Five personality traits

- *If, according to academic psychology, personality is a unique blend of points on five continua, is a categorical diagnosis of personality disorder logically possible?* This highlights a problem for any system of diagnosis which operates using the digital rule of present/absent or ordered/disordered. The compromise is to agree on a quantifiable cut-off on a dimension (an analogue decision). An example of this is the medical definition of hypertension being a persistent diastolic blood pressure of over 95 or 100. The total absence of measured blood pressure is a symptom of being dead and so blood pressure can only be described meaningfully for live subjects on a continuum rather than as a category. Similarly, personality is a description of live subjects and so has to be described in relative rather than categorical terms. If personality disorder were defined by personality characteristics from academic psychology, then a computation of five different scores on the personality dimensions would need to be measured. Currently, the diagnosis is not made using this method and no professional agreement exists on this method of case identification. It is important to note that in the field of psychopathy led by Hare (noted above), his psychological account insists that the disorder is not present or absent but exists on continua in different populations. For example, the general population contains about 1 per cent of people warranting the label but others have that tendency to some degree. (Note that most of us bunch up at the non-psychopathic end of the distribution, otherwise society would not function.) By contrast, in prison populations, the bunching is at the other end of the distribution (by definition, prisoners are a biased sample of antisocial people). However, even in those populations, Hare would argue that only about 15 per cent would warrant a label of extreme psychopathy but concedes that ultimately cut-offs on distributions are administrative and moral judgements.

- *Are psychologists and psychiatrists talking about personality 'traits' in the same way?* Under *DSM-5*, a discussion of six traits is present to guide diagnosis. These are: 'negative emotionality', including depression, anxiety, shame and guilt; 'introversion', which includes withdrawal from social interaction; 'antagonism', including an exaggerated sense of self-importance; 'disinhibition', which includes impulsivity; 'compulsivity', which includes perfectionism and rigidity; and 'schizotypy', which includes odd perceptions and beliefs. These reflect discussions of psychopathology scattered across psychiatric traditions and, with the exception of 'introversion' (the flip-side of 'extraversion'), they do not reflect the consensus about the 'Big Five' dimensions, agreed by orthodox personality theory in academic psychology and noted above. Thus, a clear epistemological gap seems to exist between psychiatric and psychological conceptualisations of personality.

- *Can personality disorder be distinguished from other forms of mental disorder?* For any diagnosis to be valid, it should be coherent and separate from other conditions. *ICD* explicitly distinguishes personality disorder from mental illness. However, earlier authorities on personality problems and insanity (Cleckley, 1941) saw an overlap between the two or a connecting continuum. Turning to neurosis, types such as 'anxious avoidant', 'dependent', 'histrionic' and 'obsessive-compulsive' personality disorder are basically descriptions of chronic neurotic symptom presentation. Not only are these types of personality disorder not distinguishable from neurosis, they are also fundamentally constituted by it.

- *Is the diagnosis of personality disorder used consistently?* This is known as the problem of reliability of diagnosis, which takes two forms. Inter-rater reliability is checking whether different professionals agree on the diagnosis of the same patient. Test–retest reliability is checking whether the patient is diagnosed consistently over time. This is more important in the diagnosis of personality disorder than of illness, because the latter may change with remission or recovery. Because personality disorder is about enduring personal qualities, we would therefore *expect* stability of scores. Reasonable test–retest reliability is found for antisocial, paranoid and borderline personality disorders but all of the other types have poor reliability.

- *Can personality disorder be readily differentiated from normality?* The problem this question highlights is that the qualities described as 'personality disordered' may lead to good social adjustment or significant success in some social contexts. The aggressive propensities of the psychopath may be expressed lucratively in a professional boxer or honourably in a soldier. The tedious, self-dramatising attention-seeking of a histrionic personality might find fame and fortune on the stage. An obsessive-compulsive personality might function very well and efficiently in an occupation which requires paying close and consistent attention to detail. A narcissist might find an esteemed career in political life or success in the leadership of a large organisation. Moreover, there are cultural and sub-cultural norms in which symptoms of personality disorder might blend. The passivity and dependency of some Asian and Arctic cultures may mirror many of the symptoms of dependent personality disorder. The dramatic and flamboyant norms of Mediterranean countries may mirror many of the symptoms of histrionic personality disorder.
- *Can the aetiology of personality disorder be specified?* This is easy to answer: 'No'. The validity of a medical diagnosis requires a clear aetiology. However, personality disorder shares this vulnerability with the diagnosis of functional mental illness. All functional diagnoses are defined in a circular way, rather than by aetiology. The diagnosis is made on the basis of symptoms and the symptoms are accounted for by the diagnosis:

Q: How do we know that this patient suffers from borderline personality disorder?

A: Because they are emotionally unstable, recurrently self-harm and are desperately concerned about being abandoned in intimate relationships.

Q: Why do they behave in this way?

A: Because they suffer from borderline personality disorder.

- *Can personality disorder be treated?* This awkward question persists. The short answer is that the consequences of the disorder *may* be mitigated but the underlying personality cannot. After all, can any of our personalities (rather than some of our particular attitudes and habits) be truly altered? And even when efforts have been made to change the social consequences of personality disorder, the results are not clear. Change in individual patients is often slow, faltering and difficult to demonstrate over long periods of time. Short-term gains are often demonstrated as grounds for warranting discharge or a loosening of surveillance and control and so they are biased by these factors. If a person's incorrigible conduct is deemed untreatable, then, arguably, they must remain outside psychiatric jurisdiction (a point that some psychiatrists often make to avoid responsibility for some patients). Treatment regimes for personality disorder either focus on mitigating the excesses of personal distress and dysfunction (as in the treatment of borderline personality disorder) or on reducing specific offending behaviours (as in the treatment of sex offenders, who might warrant a diagnosis of antisocial personality disorder). In other words, at best, some of the *symptoms or behavioural features* of personality disorder may be treatable but not the disorder itself.

A final point to make about personality disorder for emphasis is that it is basically a medical codification of people who recurrently act in a way that others disapprove of, condemn or find tiresome. The diagnosis is a way of expressing dislike, disgust or contempt for others. The term 'moral insanity' still has resonances today. The diagnosis of personality disorder is still about moral attributions.

CHALLENGING CONDUCT IN CHILDREN

As with adults, challenging conduct in children is always with reference to social norms. The difference is that adults are expected to have completed a process of 'primary socialisation' in which they have learned how to be citizens in their particular society and to comply with role–rule relationships. By contrast, children *ipso facto* are immature neurologically, psychologically and socially. They have not completed that process of socialisation (in our society, in their family and in the schooling system).

Accordingly, challenging conduct in children tends to refer to failed expectations about 'age appropriate' conduct. An example of this was given in the entry on ADHD, whereby children 'misbehave' in the family and at school in ways that reflect a lack of concentration and hyperactivity. The very notion of 'hyperactivity' is normative because it implies an optimal or expected form of 'activity'. In the other direction, a child who is intellectually slow and fails to learn bowel and bladder control by the age expected in their culture would be considered to have a learning disability. Other attributed causes might be neurological. For example, a brain-damaged child might be disinhibited if their frontal lobes are affected.

Another failed expectation relates to oppositional behaviour, which reflects the normative assumption that children should be obedient to parental directives or those used by teachers and others *in loco parentis*. 'Conduct disorder' in children brings in further normative expectations of emerging morality fitting for the social context involved. This disorder is described with reference to children lying, running away from home, vandalism, stealing and aggression to others. A vulnerability of this diagnostic approach is that such conduct could be accounted for by more fine-grain descriptions of the child's biography. A boy needy for social approval might conform to peer pressure to commit crime. A girl being sexually abused at home may run away, and so on.

With these cautions in mind, we can consider features of childhood that are separate from adulthood:

1. Children are not yet socialised so judgements about their conduct are more tentative and provisional, highlighting the risk of early labelling and potential stigmatisation.

2. Contextual explanations like the ones just given about the needy boy or the sexually abused girl are a clear caution about a reductionist diagnostic approach to deviant conduct.

3. In turn, early identification and treatment are politically ambiguous. Advocates of more resources for child and adolescent mental health services point out the gap between the incidence of mental health problems and the availability of treatments. However, the other side of the same coin is that identification brings stigma and treatment brings iatrogenesis. The moral justification for more mental health services has to be based on a child-centred and trauma-informed approach. An enlarged biomedical regime of 'diagnose-and-medicate' might create more problems than it solves. This caution is relevant given the increased use of anti-psychotic medication and mood stabilisers in young children in recent years.

4. Childhood brings with it a confluence of several forms of relational powerlessness, which makes considerations about their mental health particularly important. Rather than asking what is wrong with them (when their conduct is a cause for concern for adults), we might focus instead on what has happened to them. The infant with foetal alcohol syndrome is thrown into the world in an immediate state of biological vulnerability. The child brutalised by beatings is prone to repeating that brutality. The girl sexually abused will be prone to a life-time risk of distress, expressed potentially in a range of ways. Children lack the capacity to reflect on their situation and they lack the autonomy to take charge of risks to themselves. In the case noted above, about the abused girl who opts to run away from home, the central psychological and moral issue is not her attributed mental disorder but the crime committed against her. The first of these can obscure the second unless we offer formulations about why children behave in the way they do rather than categorising it as a form of pathology.

A final point is a reminder of one made earlier for emphasis: it is impossible to separate psychiatric diagnosis from descriptions of non-conformity. Under the *DSM* system, the American Psychiatric Association has traditionally argued that social non-conformity is not the same as mental disorder. Everything discussed in this entry suggests that the two are inevitably intertwined.

See also: *attention deficit hyperactivity disorder; creativity; fear; forensic mental health services; intellectual disability; psychiatric classification.*

FURTHER READING

Faulkner, A., Gillespie, S., Imlack, S., Dhillon, K. and Crawford, M. (2008) 'Learning the lessons together', *Mental Health Today*, February: 23–5.

Hare, R.D. and Neumann, C.S. (2008) 'Psychopathy as a clinical and empirical construct', *Annual Review of Clinical Psychology*, 4: 217–46.

Olfman, S. and Robbins, B.D. (2012) *Drugging Our Children: How Profiteers are Pushing Antipsychotics on Our Youngest, and What We Can Do to Stop It*. Santa Barbara, CA: Praeger.

challenging conduct in adults and children

Timimi, S. (2015) 'Children's mental health: time to stop using psychiatric diagnosis', *European Journal of Psychotherapy and Counselling*, 3: 342–58.

Tyrer, P., Coombs, N., Ibrahimi, F., Mathilakath, A., Bajaj, P., Ranger, M. et al. (2007) 'Critical developments in the assessment of personality disorder', *British Journal of Psychiatry*, 190: s51–9.

REFERENCES

American Psychiatric Association (APA) (1994) *Diagnostic and Statistical Manual of Mental Disorders* (4th edn) (*DSM-IV*). Washington, DC: APA.

American Psychiatric Association (APA) (2013) *Diagnostic and Statistical Manual of Mental Disorders* (5th edn) (*DSM-5*). Washington, DC: APA.

Blackburn, R. (1988) 'On moral judgements and personality disorders: the myth of psychopathic disorder re-visited', *British Journal of Psychiatry*, 153: 505–12.

Cleckley, H. (1941) *The Mask of Sanity*. St Louis, MS: C.V. Mossy.

Dolan, B. and Coid, J. (1993) *Psychopathic and Anti-social Personality Disorders: Treatment and Research Issues*. London: Gaskell.

Hare, R.D. (1993) *Without Conscience: The Disturbing World of the Psychopaths Amongst Us*. New York: Pocket.

Pilgrim, D. (2001) 'Disordered personalities and disordered concepts', *Journal of Mental Health*, 10 (3): 253–66.

Shedler, J., Beck, A., Fonagy, P. et al. (2010) 'Personality disorders in *DSM-5*', *American Journal of Psychiatry*, 167: 1026–8.

World Health Organization (WHO) (1990) *International Statistical Classification of Diseases, Injuries, and Causes of Death* (10th edn) (*ICD-10*). Geneva: WHO.

Self-harm

DEFINITION

Within medical services, self-harm tends to refer to self-injury that is neither life-threatening nor accidental. However, it can be thought of as a continuum between everyday obsessions with one's own body and completed suicide.

KEY POINTS

- Narrowly defined self-harm is outlined.
- The wider implications for human acts of aggression against the self are discussed.
- Questions for all of us to answer about these wider implications are posed.

The narrowly focused discourse about self-harm is about non-accidental self-injury which is not life-threatening. Examples here would be of people deliberately cutting or burning themselves or swallowing sharp objects. Non-fatal self-harm might also include drug overdose cases recorded in the casualty departments of hospitals.

Practitioners caring for self-harming patients typically distinguish it from intentional suicidal acts and from accidental self-harm. This 'pure form' of self-harm is typically linked to tension release in order to feel better about being alive rather than to suicidal intent. However, its perpetrators may still die accidentally from blood loss, self-poisoning or infection, and coroner's courts struggle at times to distinguish between 'suicide', 'death by misadventure' and 'accidental death'. Accidental self-harm might entail injury during an unrelated activity but linked to risk (for example, being injured in a car crash, when not wearing a seatbelt) or from ordinary daily tasks (such as cutting oneself while cooking or gardening). Thus, the question of patient intentionality is at the centre of professional deliberations about various manifestations of self-harm.

A range of views exists within this narrow focus about what should be done, from the coercive prevention of such acts to simple tolerance and the provision of hygienic first aid. In between lie various approaches to its treatment, including addressing the underlying reasons for the action. Self-harm is often seen by mental health professionals as a communication about, or a symptom of, other problems (such as diagnosed severe depression or personality disorder) or as indicative of a post-traumatic history.

While this narrow focus on non-fatal self-injury dominates the debates in mental health profession circles, a wider discussion can also be found. Obsessive behaviour about one's own body is commonplace. Examples of this would be scratching, knuckle cracking, nail biting, hair twisting and plucking, lip chewing, skin picking and teeth grinding. Their relationship to self-grooming can be ambiguous and they provide common examples of the tension release potential or function of paying any obsessive attention to one's own body. In many other species, scratching and self-grooming indicate 'displacement activity' in conditions of uncertainty or conflict, although as rule-following and acculturated language users it is unlikely that human activity, such as self-harm, could be reduced to this explanation alone.

There are various cultural forms of self-harm linked to time, place and tradition. A common recent example is the fashion for piercing and tattooing, both of which require painful insertions of sharp objects into healthy skin. Turning to tradition rather than fashion, religious observance and rituals involving painful self-harm can signal special piety. Examples here would be public self-flogging during some Islamic holy days and the painful spiked garter ('cilice') worn secretly by members of Opus Dei, the strict Catholic sect. In Christianity, 'mortification of the flesh' is justified in the scriptures by identification with the pain of Christ's crucifixion as a path to God and as a test of God's power to prevent death from injury. The latter testing out can be found in Appalachian sects in the USA, which handle venomous snakes in their rituals.

The less dramatic example in religious devotion is fasting, which deliberately invokes hunger pangs. All the major deistic faiths place a positive value on fasting. Self-harm in these circumstances can be expressed as a spiritually healthy alternative to self-indulgence. However, the difficult experiential distinction between pleasure and pain is highlighted by sadomasochism. The latter sexual 'perversion' or 'variation' entails the giving and receiving of pain, which at times leads to explicit injury in the process. This overall experience is positively enjoyed by its participants. Religious puritans might condemn the latter but proudly preserve their own noble traditions of self-harm.

Substance misuse entails routines of self-harm which are normalised in secular societies (especially alcohol use) but are met with ambivalence from religions. Sometimes substance use is frowned upon, but at other times it is woven into their rituals (for example, wine as the blood of Christ) or deployed to change consciousness (for example, the use of cannabis by Rastafarians). These various examples suggest an enduring confusion in religious and secular societies about the valued and disvalued expressions of self-procured pain and the risk of harm to the body.

In psychodynamic terms, all on the range, right up to and including deliberate suicide, indicate an intro-punitive stance towards the self (turning aggression inwards). However, it is also the case that extra-punitive action, such as fighting and other aggressive risk-taking more generally, typically culminate in a risk to the self, not just others. This ambiguity is highlighted by the recorded sex differences in self-harm (females have a fourfold incidence). However, risk to self in males may manifest itself more indirectly because of their greater proneness to substance use, fighting and fast driving.

To muddy the water further about the nature of self-harm, some of its perpetrators do not place an emphasis on aggression but on meaning. In particular, they focus on the way in which pain is a positive alternative to inner emptiness. In psychodynamic terms, this would be framed more as a schizoid rather than as a depressive phenomenon.

Also, whether motivated by aggression or meaning, there are victims other than those physically injured. Harm to the self can bring distress to others. A parent finding a teenager cutting themselves or the train driver who brakes frantically when a person appears on their track are predictably distressed secondary victims of self-harm. These prospective outcomes can evoke anger in those treating self-harming patients. This anger may compound, and help rationalise, the moral condemnation of self-harming patients, who are seen as diverting time and resources from those legitimately deserving medical treatment.

Self-harm, then, is open to contestation on a number of fronts. We might all have a view on the following implied questions about the topic:

- How extensive or narrow should be its definition?
- Can its rational and irrational aspects be readily distinguished?
- Are we all, to some degree, self-harming?
- Can turning against the self be readily distinguished from turning against others?

- Is self-harm about aggression or about meaning (or might it be about both)?
- If self-harm (like all behaviour) is also a communication, what does it mean and who is its target in particular cases and circumstances?
- Can self-harm make people feel more alive?
- What is the relationship between pain and pleasure?
- Is self-harm only a manifestation of mental distress or might it also be a fashion statement or a proud display of duty to God?

These questions take us well beyond the narrow group of medical and psychiatric patients introduced at the beginning of this entry.

See also: *spirituality; substance misuse; suicide.*

FURTHER READING

Brodsky, B.S., Cliotre, M. and Dulit, R.A. (1995) 'Relationship of dissociation to self-mutilation and childhood abuse in borderline personality disorder', *American Journal of Psychiatry*, 152: 1788–92.

Favazza, A.R. (1996) *Bodies under Siege: Self-Mutilation and Body Modification in Culture and Psychiatry* (2nd edn). Baltimore, MD: Johns Hopkins University Press.

Haines, J., Williams, C.L., Brain, K.L. and Wilson, G.V. (1995) 'The psychophysiology of self-mutilation', *Journal of Abnormal Psychology*, 104 (3): 471–89.

Redley, M. (2003) 'Towards a new perspective on deliberate self-harm in an area of multiple deprivation', *Sociology of Health and Illness*, 25 (4): 348–73.

Substance Misuse

DEFINITION

The use of a psychoactive substance in a way that causes harm to the self or others.

KEY POINTS

- Substance misuse is described, mainly using alcohol abuse as an example.
- The public health as well as individual consequences of substance misuse are discussed.

Psychiatrists consider substance misuse to be both a free-standing mental disorder and a common presenting problem in medicine, affecting health in a variety of ways. The diagnosis appears in both the *International Classification of Diseases*

(World Health Organization, 2016) and the *Diagnostic and Statistical Manual of Mental Disorders* (*DSM*) (American Psychiatric Association, 1994).

Because of the prevalent use of alcohol, it is considered to be a major public health problem and so will be the main exemplar provided in this entry. Excessive alcohol use has a demonstrable influence on both the health status of its users and on third parties affected by intoxicated behaviour. For example, excessive and prolonged alcohol consumption increases the chances of heart disease, neurological degeneration and some forms of cancer. It is specifically linked to premature death from cirrhosis of the liver. Suicidal behaviour and depressed mood, as well as job loss, are also linked to alcohol intoxication. At the same time, and arguably of greater importance because there may be multiple innocent victims, substance misuse increases the probability of road traffic accidents, domestic violence, child neglect, sexual offending and violent assaults on strangers.

The health effects related to the self and others of lesser-used drugs are more complicated. For example, the use of heroin and its prescribed medical substitute methadone increases the risk of road traffic accidents but do not seem to be linked strongly to violence against others. However, non-violent acquisitive crime and prostitution are linked to heroin use because of the drug's high financial cost to the user. By contrast, crack cocaine is strongly linked to violent action. In part, then, the criminal manifestations of illicit substance misuse are a function of the different physiological effects of the drugs involved.

The risk associated with the opioids (drugs synthesised to chemically mimic, or ones derived directly from, opium) is complicated by the way that these are used. The unsafe and illegal supply of heroin and its common intravenous method of administration create particular and often lethal hazards. These include accidental over-dosing, because drug purity in local supplies varies, and acquired infections, such as HIV and hepatitis. Intravenous use is preferred because of the 'rush' of euphoria it creates in the recipient. This is one reason why addicts are less keen on the oral use of methadone, which prevents distressing heroin withdrawal symptoms but provides no 'rush' prior to a comforting and prolonged heroin stupor ('nodding').

For those who consider substance misuse to be a diagnosable psychiatric condition rather than a bad habit, injurious to the self and others, then *ICD* and *DSM* are at hand. Both classificatory systems specify the following substances implicated in the diagnosis: alcohol, caffeine, cannabis, cocaine, hallucinogens, solvents (or inhalants), nicotine (or tobacco), opioids, and sedatives and hypnotics. Amphetamines and phencyclidine, an obsolete anaesthetic used as a recreational drug in the USA but rarely in the UK, are included in *DSM* but not in *ICD*.

The criteria used for the diagnosis in *DSM* are more elaborate than in *ICD*. The latter simply refers to 'a pattern of psychoactive substance use that is causing damage to health; the damage may be to physical or mental health'. The *DSM* list is longer and refers to one or more of the following 'clinically significant impairments' over a 12-month period, manifested in: failures in role obligations in work, school or home; substance use in situations of physical hazard; legal problems; and persistent interpersonal problems linked to the use. This stipulation of a 12-month defining period would exclude the public health implications of those who, when acutely intoxicated, episodically or on a one-off basis, might cause serious harm to others. Indeed, one important diversion of the chronicity of use and its effects is that we might ignore the more serious behavioural implications of acute intoxication in many who are not formally diagnosed. For example, the social consequences are far greater for the drunk driver who kills several people in one incident (but is not labelled as a substance misuser) than for the long-term heroin user who keeps out of trouble for years on end.

When it comes to defining dependency or dependence, both systems emphasise: a compulsion to use the drug; a tendency to increase dose levels because of tolerance; withdrawal effects; a persistent focus on the use of the drug to the detriment or exclusion of other activities; and a failure to control the habit, despite feedback about its consequences. It is clear that some of the substances listed in *DSM* and *ICD* are not dependency-forming but are very psychoactive (e.g. the hallucinogens). Others are very dependency-forming but barely psychoactive in the experience of the user, so only strong withdrawal effects are noted (e.g. caffeine and nicotine). The damage to users of nicotine is now well documented and so the imperceptible subjective gains make it a particularly pernicious drug. Sometimes 'dependence' is distinguished from 'addiction', with the presence of *physical* withdrawal effects indicating the latter and their absence suggesting the *psychological* nature of the former.

Estimates about the prevalence of substance misuse vary from place to place. North American studies of alcohol misuse indicate a one-year prevalence of 7–10 per cent, with a lifetime risk of 14–20 per cent (Regier et al., 1994). This compares with a one-year prevalence of 4.7 per cent in the UK (Meltzer et al., 1994). Some of this difference could be accounted for by different methods of data collection (the US studies included homeless populations but the UK one did not). When homeless populations are sampled, the prevalence rate of alcohol abuse rises to around 40 per cent in Britain (Gill et al., 1996).

Also, the demographic pattern of problem drinking changes over time as well as place. While cirrhosis levels have declined overall in recent years in Southern Europe, in Northern Europe excessive drinking has significantly increased in young females, indicating that women will increasingly become medical casualties of their habit with age. Given the recklessness linked to intoxication ('disinhibition'), this also means that female perpetrators of violence and other antisocial acts are tending to increase in number. Another indication of the social cost of alcohol consumption is its impact on hospital admission (in the UK, this is around 10 per cent in both psychiatric and general medical admissions). Young binge-drinking places a particular acute stress on both law enforcement and emergency medical services at weekends. It is also an important underlying factor in other health risks (such as self-harm, accidents and sexually transmitted diseases).

Because substance misuse occurs typically in people who are deemed to be sane, health professionals may hold an ambivalent attitude towards patients,

substance misuse

similar to that for those with a diagnosis of personality disorder. Indeed, sometimes persistent multiple drug use and its behavioural consequences are used to diagnose antisocial personality disorder. Because of the strong moral discourse surrounding drug use, a tension exists between traditional medical paternalism, in which the patient is treated sympathetically as the victim of an affliction, and the cultural norm (which health workers are embedded in and so reflect) of condemning the user and morally exhorting them to change for the better. This ambivalence also appears in the treatment programmes offered. These all require personal commitment and honesty from the user and so it is often difficult to separate medical descriptions of a cure or recovery from common-sense ones of moral reform.

A particular point about substance misuse is its role in the debate about violence and mental disorder. Psychotic patients who abuse substances are more dangerous than others in the general population. However, those who do not abuse substances are not more dangerous. Moreover, substance misuse *alone* leads to a significant increase in the risk of danger to the self or others. This is important because if substance misuse is formally within the jurisdiction of psychiatry, then users become psychiatric patients and raise the profile of violence in this particular population. It also skews our association of suicide with mental health problems. Suicidal behaviour is correlated with mental health problems but by no means limited to them.

If substance misuse were not framed as a psychiatric problem (but as, say, a social or moral one), then a sub-group of violent and suicidal intoxicated people would be removed from the 'dangerous to the self or others' component of psychiatric populations. This might then beg a question about whether the state should intervene to alter substance misuse and, if so, what alternative interventions and views of the problem would replace those associated with 'psychiatric treatment' and medical paternalism. A bridge between a psychiatric approach and that used within a lay view of morality is the widespread and sustained success of the organisation Alcoholics Anonymous (AA), which began in 1935 and continues to operate globally. It emphasises personal responsibility for recovery but starts with a confession that the person is powerless in the face of the drug and that life has become unmanageable.

AA has become a prototype self-help model for a range of addictive problems and so we now also see, for example, Narcotics Anonymous, Sex Addicts Anonymous, Gamblers Anonymous and Overeaters Anonymous. These self-help initiatives also point up the tendency for *any* compulsive habit (from cigarette smoking and shopping to sexual promiscuity and shoplifting) to be thought of as a psychiatric problem. Also, the ambiguous word 'compulsive' here indicates that some people are compelled to break rules (in the case of this section, rules of sobriety, moderation and decorum) and others are compelled to comply with them (in the case of the overly conformist 'obsessive-compulsive personality disorder'). The abstinence model of AA may suggest that people are exhorted and supported to move from one end to the other of a compulsive continuum.

The widespread contemporary societal preoccupation with a range of addictive behaviours throws into relief our modern struggle with the use and abuse of individual freedom. The wide inclusion of so many addictions reflects recent forms of social organisation based upon consumption, with the latter shaping identities and modern definitions of both normality and pathology (Reith, 2004).

An argument for retaining a medical view of substance misuse is the good evidence that it is a form of self-medication to reduce stress or to improve mood (even if these personal short-term strategies may be counterproductive in the long term). However, analysts of the role of substance use in the self-management of experienced stress point out that many do not progress to fulfil the criteria for a psychiatric disorder (Aneshensel, 1999). Put differently, beneath the lifetime risk of 14–20 per cent for alcohol misuse, noted earlier, lie a large number of people (probably most of the remaining 80 per cent plus) who use alcohol moderately, or excessively on occasions, to release tension or improve their mood. This point obviously applies less in those countries where alcohol use is illegal or is culturally constrained.

See also: *challenging conduct in adults and children; risks to and from people with mental health problems.*

FURTHER READING

Reith, G. (2004) 'Consumption and its discontents: addiction, identity and the problem of freedom', *British Journal of Sociology*, 55 (2): 283–98.

Royal College of Psychiatrists (2000) *Drugs: Dilemmas and Choices*. London: Gaskell.

REFERENCES

American Psychiatric Association (APA) (1994) *Diagnostic and Statistical Manual of Mental Disorders* (4th edn) (*DSM-IV*). Washington, DC: APA.

Aneshensel, C.S. (1999) 'Outcomes of the stress process', in A.V. Horwitz and T.L. Scheid (eds), *A Handbook for the Study of Mental Health*. Cambridge: Cambridge University Press.

Gill, B., Meltzer, H., Hinds, K. and Pettigrew, M. (1996) *Psychiatric Morbidity among Homeless People: OPCS Surveys of Psychiatric Morbidity in Great Britain*. London: HMSO.

Meltzer, H., Gill, B. and Pettigrew, M. (1994) *The Prevalence of Psychiatric Morbidity among Adults Aged 16–64 Living in Private Households: OPCS Surveys of Psychiatric Morbidity in Great Britain*. London: HMSO.

Regier, D.A., Narrow, W.E., Rae, D.S., Manderscheid, R.W., Locke, B.Z. and Goodwin, F.K. (1994) 'The *de facto* US mental and addictive disorders service', *Archives of General Psychiatry*, 50: 85–94.

Reith, G. (2004) 'Consumption and its discontents: addiction, identity and the problem of freedom', *British Journal of Sociology*, 55 (2): 283–98.

World Health Organization (WHO) (2016) *The ICD-10 Classification of Mental and Behavioural Disorders*. Geneva: WHO.

Intellectual Disability

DEFINITION

The term 'intellectual disability' is for now a preferred description, internationally, of people who from a young age show a developmental slowness, and then arrest, in relation to their intellectual, social and practical functioning. Generally, degrees of these deficits or impairments are described on a continuum from 'mild' through 'moderate' and 'severe' to 'profound'.

KEY POINTS

- The history of learning disability and its links to psychiatric services are described.
- The shift from a medical to a social model of learning disability is outlined.

Both the American Psychiatric Association and the World Health Organization now prefer the term 'intellectual disability' (ID). In Britain, the term 'learning disability' is still typically used in both legal and clinical contexts. The developmental focus has been a constant feature since the 19th century, despite a shifting terminological picture (or 'euphemism treadmill'). For this reason, the early appearance of ID distinguishes it, for example, from acquired brain damage or dementia emerging in adulthood.

If madness (and dementia) reflects a relative loss of reason, then ID reflects a failure in the development of reason (cognitive, social or practical). Accordingly, there has been a common assumption that ID reflects a collection of deficits of reason created by genetic defects. However, although some ID is, indeed, traceable to genetic causes (e.g. Down's Syndrome) or inter-uterine causes (e.g. foetal alcohol syndrome and Rubella), developmental impairments can also accrue at birth (e.g. due to oxygen deprivation) or be post-natal, when the brain is immature (e.g. from lead poisoning or malnutrition). However, for many people described as 'intellectually disabled', the cause of their problems is simply not known (especially those at the 'mild' and 'moderate' end of the spectrum).

At the turn of the 20th century in Britain, the separation of types of developmental slowness and arrest included 'imbeciles', 'idiots', 'feeble minded' and 'moral imbeciles'. The last of these did not necessarily reflect intellectual incompetence but its focus was on an absence of moral reasoning (later to be called 'psychopathy' or 'antisocial personality disorder'). Later terms used in the Anglophone world for what is now called ID included 'mental deficiency', 'mental retardation', 'mental subnormality', 'mental handicap' and 'learning difficulties'.

At the start of the 19th century, with the mass segregation of a range of deviant populations in hospitals, asylums, workhouses and 'colonies', those with learning disabilities and those with mental health problems could be found together. The Lunacy Act of 1845 stipulated that 'idiots, lunatics or persons of unsound mind' should be certified and detained in asylums (Saunders, 1985). A distinction was made by the end of the century between two forms of intellectual impairment: 'idiocy', manifest from infancy, and 'dementia', developing later in life. In Britain, as in the rest of Europe and North America, the gradual legislative division of 'idiocy' from 'lunacy' became apparent. For example, the 1890 Lunacy Act emerged separately from the 1886 Idiots Act. This separation was maintained in the subsequent 1913 Mental Deficiency Act and the 1930 Mental Treatment Act.

The prejudicial lay notion has long existed that mental health problems and ID are the same type of mental incapacity, disorder or disability. This amalgam prejudice cuts both ways. In ordinary language, all those with mental health problems might inaccurately be considered to be 'stupid' and those with learning problems might all wrongly be considered to be 'mad'. In English-speaking countries, both groups might be dismissed as being 'mental', in a pejorative or scoffing way, by others.

At the turn of the 20th century, this conflation of the two groups in the lay mentality was mirrored, to a degree, in the professional domain, as psychiatrists took over the jurisdiction of intellectual impairment in mental handicap hospitals, not just the management of madness in mental hospitals. A legacy of this today is that ID is a sub-speciality of psychiatry.

At times, professionals and relatives of patients have episodically made painstaking attempts to point out that the client's problems in each are quite different. However, this understandable attempt to put a conceptual distance between the two groups of patients is itself problematic. It may imply that someone with an ID is in some way immune from mental health problems. This is both logically and empirically untenable. People with a diagnosis of ID, like anyone else, can develop mental health problems. Also, on average, those with a diagnosis of schizophrenia have a lower intelligence than the measured norm (using the tradition of the tested intelligence quotient or IQ). They also usually manifest social impairments. Psychiatrists may see this as evidence of schizophrenia being a neurodevelopmental disorder. (However, the *upper range* of IQs in those with a diagnosis of schizophrenia is the same as the general population.)

In light of the above problems about overlapping psychological characteristics, attempts to keep the two types of patient groups separate may have had the perverse effect of disenfranchising ID patients, as their access to mental health provision is restricted. On the other hand, some psychotic patients may have unrecognised learning difficulties. Thus, those with both ID *and* mental health problems can 'fall between two stools' of service provision.

Because ID is defined by poor cognitive capacity, judged by the presence of both a low IQ and impaired social competence, then medical jurisdiction can be queried. ID patients overwhelmingly have training, educational and social, rather than medical, needs. However, for the time being, they and their families are largely cared for by the same occupational mix as those with mental health problems. The training of these psychiatrists, nurses and psychologists overlaps with, but is also different from, that of their colleagues working in mental health services. In the UK, while some ID services have now shifted from the NHS to social service jurisdiction, the professionals working in them are still predominantly trained in a health service context.

The retention of ID in medicalised settings can be justified partially by a large core group of patients with genetic abnormalities (such as Down's Syndrome) or a range of congenital metabolic abnormalities. Also, some post-natal acquired brain damage has an explicit neurological aetiology. The latter may include head injury, malnutrition, lead poisoning or brain infection. These inherited, congenital and post-natal medical histories can lead to ID emerging during early childhood and provide fair grounds for framing them as true medical neurology cases. Some of these infants have very short lives and so do not become adults with an ID diagnosis (for example, in those with Tay-Sachs Disease and Hurler's Syndrome).

This leaves an ambiguous or marginal role for psychiatry (rather than neurology or psychology). Even if there is a known biological cause for these patients, their behavioural problems require social and psychological responses. This is similar to the position of older people with dementia, where biological aetiology is proven or is likely but psychosocial interventions (especially with family members) are mainly implicated. As with much of the work of psychiatry, biological aetiology (known or assumed) does not always lead to appropriate, acceptable or effective biological treatments. For example, the use of major tranquillisers ('anti-psychotics') in ID treatment has been controversial. At the same time, the more appropriate use of psychological techniques, preferred by clinical psychologists, to deal with the violent or challenging behaviour of patients, is not without controversy (McDonnell and Sturmey, 1993).

Moves towards the de-medicalisation of ID and towards a social model of understanding and provision have come on three fronts. First, most of the old 'mental handicap' hospitals have now been closed down and their residents shifted to small community-based living facilities. Some of the challenging or dysfunctional problems of residents in large institutions were a result of social isolation and a lack of meaningful daily activity ('institutionalisation'). However, since patients have moved into the community, many of these problems are still reported, indicating that expectations about the benefits of simply resettling patients may have been over-optimistic.

Second, the demand for more human rights for ID patients arose in the 1970s, with the professionally driven 'normalisation' movement (Wolfensberger, 1972). Normalisation demands that devalued people have their right to a normal existence restored as much as possible. The campaign to educate children with learning disabilities in ordinary schools is a practical manifestation of this normalisation ideology.

Third, a new social movement of those with an ID diagnosis has campaigned for their increasing rights as citizens. This user-led but advocate-supported movement has reinforced the work on citizenship demands started by the normalisation movement. This parallels the emphasis on social inclusion demanded by people with mental health problems.

Returning to the development of mental health problems in those who are intellectually disabled, a paradox exists. On the one hand, the prevalence of some mental health problems is considered to be higher than in non-intellectually disabled populations. On the other hand, the ability to detect psychiatric disorders is confounded by communication difficulties. The higher rate of psychotic disorders in ID populations compared to the general population reinforces the psychiatric assumption that 'schizophrenia' is a neurodevelopmental disorder.

Mood disorders are diagnosed less often in people with an ID diagnosis. Estimates of diagnosable personality disorder in the latter within the community are as high as 30 per cent, with a further 20 per cent being described as having 'abnormalities of personality' (Khan et al., 1997). Also, anxiety may be expressed differently in this group of patients. The communication problems people with an ID diagnosis have when representing themselves to others suggest that an effective and helpful response to those who also have mental health problems requires particular professional skills and good interdisciplinary collaboration (Drotar and Sturm, 1996).

See also: *challenging conduct in adults and children; mental health; social exclusion; stigma.*

FURTHER READING

Goodey, C. (2011) *A History of Intelligence and 'Intellectual Disability'*. Farnham: Ashgate.
Thomson, M. (1998) *The Problem of Mental Deficiency*. Oxford: Oxford University Press.

REFERENCES

Drotar, D.D. and Sturm, L.A. (1996) 'Interdisciplinary collaboration in the practice of mental retardation', in J.W. Jacobson and J.A. Mullick (eds), *Manual of Diagnosis and Professional Practice in Mental Retardation*. Washington, DC: American Psychiatric Association.
Khan, A., Cowan, C. and Roy, A. (1997) 'Personality disorders in people with learning disabilities: a community survey', *Journal of Intellectual Disability Research*, 41: 324–30.
McDonnell, A.A. and Sturmey, P. (1993) 'Managing violent and aggressive behaviour: towards better practice', in R.S.P. Jones and C. Eayrs (eds), *Challenging Behaviours and People with*

intellectual disability

Learning Disabilities: A Psychological Perspective. Kidderminster: British Institute of Learning Disabilities.

Saunders, I. (1985) 'Quarantining the weak-minded: psychiatric definitions of degeneracy and the late Victorian asylum', in W.F. Bynum, R. Porter and M. Shepherd (eds), *The Anatomy of Madness*, Vol. 3. London: Tavistock.

Wolfensberger, W. (1972) *The Principle of Normalisation in Human Services.* Toronto: National Institute of Mental Retardation.

Causes and Consequences of Mental Health Problems

DEFINITION

The causes of mental health problems refer to those antecedent factors that may, or do, account for their existence. The consequences of mental health problems refer to their impact on the identified patient and other people.

KEY POINTS

- Consideration of the causal antecedents of mental health problems is separated from that of their consequences.
- It is concluded that while our social context provides one source of causal factors, our description and evaluation of mental health problems always take place in that context.

Previous entries have all referred to proven, assumed or contested causes of mental health problems. The question of causation has been fiercely debated for a number of reasons. First, a dominant form of causation (biodeterminism) has been associated with eugenics, with that political philosophy now being held in widespread suspicion within liberal democracies. Second, causation has been asserted rather than proved; it has been taken to be self-evident. This has been particularly the case within the biodeterminist tradition, although it was also the case that Freud rode two horses in this regard. He considered that ultimately a neuroscientific explanation of mental illness would accrue but also that, for now, psychological explanations were useful, plausible and necessary. Third, a commitment to causal assumptions has been closely entwined with professional interests and bids for legitimacy. As a branch of medicine, psychiatry has relied on biodeterminism in part to justify its authoritative role and power in the mental health industry. This point applies equally, though, to competing bids for legitimacy. For example, the credibility of clinical psychology as a profession has been bound up with the causal claims derived first from behaviourism and then cognitivism. These theories in the academy created confidence (or even arrogance) for applied psychologists, when they developed their rhetoric of professional justification. Fourth, the drug companies and politicians have also been communities of interest, which have favoured and promoted some models or assumptions about causation, and ignored or discounted others.

Thus, one implication of the substantial ambiguity of mental health problems ('functional psychiatric diagnoses') is that the very lack of certainty surrounding them allows a variety of claims to be asserted about their causation. And those claims are driven by ideology and economics, not dispassionate science, although the latter is selectively co-opted or invoked, in order to suit particular interests. For all parties, we can say when standing back from it all, and quite reasonably, 'Well, they would say that, wouldn't they?' about their favoured version of causal reasoning. When there is contestation, the most powerful voices tend to prevail. Science, as well as traditionally accepted cultural authority and money, are then drawn upon as linguistic and material resources in order to defend those voices. However, resistance is also provoked, with claim and counter-claim following, as evidenced by the recent *DSM-5* controversy.

Turning to consequences, these are quite a different matter. Before professional and commercial interests that shape some causal claims and seek to discredit others become evident, there is a ubiquity about what we would now broadly call 'mental health problems' or 'mental disorders'. Experiences of distress and dysfunction occur first in the lay arena. Some people feel distressed and it affects their confidence, self-esteem, social competence, quality of life, and even at times their willingness to carry on living. Fear and sadness are inherently distressing and debilitating. Some people will act in ways that others do not understand and that are perplexing and frightening. This has profound consequences for their credibility and trustworthiness in the eyes of those around them, who are sane by common consent. Some people are experienced by those around them as being incorrigibly egocentric. This leads to reactions of fear, distaste and exasperation in those around them, who in turn may act to reject or control the problematic conduct.

All of these experiences of the 'identified patient' and those around them become interpersonal events and social processes *whether or not there is professional intervention*. And when the latter is available and might be invoked at some contingent point, this is a consequence of someone expecting someone else to 'do something' about an unsatisfactory situation. And when professionals respond conveniently, that is when their claims of legitimacy about causation (discussed above) are invoked to justify their authority (and status and salaries). However, the most notable aspect of this authority, in the first instance and sometimes for a good while, is that they are offering to 'do something' about a situation that has become unmanageable in the lay arena. This can be done coercively or negotiated with the incipient patient. The distressed person may voluntarily and anxiously seek, and gratefully receive, these ministrations. A member of the public encountering madness in the street calls the police, who then negotiate a welcomed 'psychiatric disposal'. The despairing parent of an hallucinating and aggressive adolescent finds relief for a while when their child is involuntarily admitted to hospital. A similar respite is experienced by the 'significant others' who look forward with hope to a new therapist for a patient diagnosed with a 'personality disorder'.

Thus, the consequences of mental health problems are complex and implicate many others in both the lay and professional or 'service' arenas, with the latter term begging the question: 'Service for whom?' And just as there remains much ambiguity about causal factors (biological? psychological? social? past? present? an uncertain mixture of all of them?), ambiguity is also present about consequences. This is why overarching descriptions are found lacking. For example, in an attempt to avoid terms like 'mental illness' and 'mental disorder', the term 'distress' has been favoured at times. But who is distressed? Is it the patient? Is it others? Is it both?

The answers to these complex questions vary from one situation to another and so, for example, to replace the diagnosis of an 'eating disorder' wholesale with that of 'eating distress' marks a contestable switch. The distress of others seeing a loved one starving themselves to death is often an important aspect of decision-making. The distress of an 'anorexic patient' is typically about being asked to eat *rather than* being allowed to starve themselves into a life-threatening position. The distress of the 'treating professional' is about the prospect of mismanaging risk, when facing the consequences of a patient dying under their care. Therefore, the scenario of self-starvation is certainly distressing, but more than one party experiences the problem in their own particular way.

This example reminds us that while social factors are variably implicated in the causation of mental health problems, their consequences are *always evaluated* in a social context. This is because mental health problems are always about normativity. They are about a lack, or loss, of reason and the attendant rule transgressions and role failures that they contingently bring into being. Thus, when we come to consider consequences, we must deal with the social processes that contingently *constitute* the problem in the first place. It is not sufficient simply to consider the 'impact' of 'mental disorder' or its 'burden'. 'Mental disorder' is an attribution about one or more social scenarios, with different parties seeking to pursue their interests, their understanding of causation and their need to live their life in this way rather than another. Psychiatric crises are social crises and so the matter of consequences requires a social, not a medical, frame of understanding.

Finally, and to reinforce this point about socially contingent reasoning, some symptoms of 'mental disorder' might – in certain social settings – be connoted positively (the madness of poets, prophesy and lovers of antiquity). The witchdoctor is expected to have supernatural visions. The restrictions of distressing obsessionality for one person might be the job description of another, such as the efficient accountant. Catatonia might have a functional advantage for the artist's model. Manic exuberance might be required to succeed in some competitive arenas of life, such as show business or academia. We can never escape the need to consider social context when thinking about the consequences of mental health problems and, indeed, whether they are seen as being problematic at all.

See also: *madness; neuroscience; psychiatric classification; subjective and objective aspects of mental health.*

FURTHER READING

Bentall, R.P. (2003) *Understanding Madness: Psychosis and Human Nature*. London: Penguin.

Cosgrove, L. and Krimsky, S. (2012) 'A comparison of *DSM-IV* and *DSM-5* panel members' financial associations with industry: a pernicious problem persists', *PLoS Medicine*, 9 (3): e1001190.

Healy, D. (2004) 'Psychopathology at the interface between the market and the new biology', in D. Rees and S. Rose (eds), *The New Brain Sciences: Perils and Prospects*. Cambridge: Cambridge University Press.

Kingdon, D. and Young, A.H. (2007) 'Research into putative biological mechanisms of mental disorders has been of no value to clinical psychiatry', *British Journal of Psychiatry*, 191: 285–90.

Lillehet, E. (2002) 'Progress and power: exploring the disciplinary connection between moral treatment and psychiatric rehabilitation', *Philosophy, Psychiatry and Psychology*, 9 (2): 167–82.

Moncrieff, J. (2008) *The Myth of the Chemical Cure*. Basingstoke: Palgrave Macmillan.

Pilgrim, D. and Tomasini, F. (2012) 'On being unreasonable in modern society: are mental health problems special?', *Disability and Society*, 27 (5): 631–46.

Pols, J. (2001) 'Enforcing patients' rights or improving care: the interference of two modes of doing good in mental health care', *Sociology of Health and Illness*, 25 (4): 325–47.

Sedgwick, P. (1982) *PsychoPolitics*. London: Pluto Press.

Summerfield, D. (2008) 'How scientifically valid is the knowledge base of global mental health?', *British Medical Journal*, 336: 992–4.

Szasz, T.S. (1963) *Law, Liberty and Psychiatry*. New York: Macmillan.

Trauma

DEFINITION

Trauma is an emotional response to a terrible event like an accident, rape or natural disaster. Immediately after the event, shock and denial are typical. Longer-term reactions include unpredictable emotions, flashbacks, strained relationships and even physical symptoms like headaches or nausea. While these feelings are normal, some people have difficulty moving on with their lives.

KEY POINTS

- Trauma describes both an objective set of events suddenly and detrimentally affecting an individual and its subjective impact and legacy.
- There are both psychological and legal aspects to trauma.
- Traumatised individuals constitute the bulk of those acquiring a diagnosis of post-traumatic stress disorder, the only functional psychiatric diagnosis that retains a clear aetiological source.

The above definition of trauma is offered to us by the American Psychological Association (APA) and indicates our contemporary tendency to use the word in its psychological sense. However, in the older general medical sense, the term 'trauma' referred to our bodily health being compromised by a sudden injury, whether or not the impact was life-threatening. Note that the APA definition at the outset emphasises that trauma is an *internal* state (similarly, today, the word 'stress' ambiguously alludes to both outer events and a subjective state). The older medical definition focused more on detrimental *external* forces on the normally functioning bodily system. However, this is a point of balance and emphasis, as both versions of trauma do consider both outer events and their personal consequences.

The above definition also signals the blurred line, at times, between physical and mental health. The expression 'you scared me to death' signifies the extent of a personal shock metaphorically. However, as an example of the interplay between physical and mental health, those with a cardiovascular vulnerability could really be killed by a shocking event in their life (from a stress-induced stroke or heart attack). And in the other direction, physical trauma can have psychological consequences. A life-threatening injury means that the near-death experience could lead to a continuing distress after the event. A woman raped outside her home may suffer consequential sexual dysfunction, become agoraphobic and develop chronic physical health problems. The man driving a train that killed a suicidal jumper on the track may be unable to work again, which then has an impact on both his physical and mental health.

LEGAL AND PSYCHOLOGICAL ASPECTS OF TRAUMA

The idea of psychological trauma has been part of a legal discourse, with the notion of 'nervous shock'. The latter, though, is focused upon the duty of others, rather than a wider one of random shocking events, such as seeing a person die when struck by lightning. With 'nervous shock', in British and Australian law, another party is deemed to have *caused* the psychological injury by their action (recklessness) or inaction (negligence). This introduces a potential contention about the trustworthiness of a reported experience of psychological trauma (because it might be claimed insincerely in order to gain financial compensation). Given this dilemma, expertise in discerning true from false cases is often sought from mental health professionals. In North America, the term 'nervous shock' is not used but criteria for emotional distress are applied likewise in legal claims of psychiatric injury.

Psychological trauma has an unusual status within psychiatric diagnosis, especially in recent iterations of *ICD* and *DSM* (World Health Organization, 1990;

American Psychiatric Association, 2013). The reported experienced symptoms are part of the only functional psychiatric diagnosis, for now at least, in which the distressed or dysfunctional state is tied to a very clear antecedent. (In other functional diagnoses, the aetiology of the disorder by definition is not known, that is why they are called 'functional'.) This is important because much of the reasoning about functional disorders is that they reflect in whole or part the learned or inherited personal or *internal* vulnerability of the incipient patient. In the case of post-traumatic stress disorder (PTSD), the emphasis is clearly on an *external* and serious shock to the person who otherwise would probably be, or was seen previously to be, psychologically normal.

PTSD AND ITS HISTORY

PTSD is now typically diagnosed in certain recurring scenarios of warfare, torture and genocide, road traffic or industrial accidents, sexual and non-sexual violent assaults and being affected by natural disasters, such as earthquakes or sudden floods. The coherence of the diagnosis is contested because a range of symptoms of anxiety and depression can occur in various permutations, although a unique aspect of PTSD is a focus on re-experiencing the trauma. The latter in various ways can preoccupy the affected person in their waking life and while asleep in recurrent nightmares. In the former case, the person may also experience intrusive 'flashbacks' to the event. Experiences such as emotional numbing and hyperarousal are used to distinguish PTSD from other disorders implying types of distress, when the diagnosis is applied. The most important criterion though is proven exposure to an acute and extreme stressor. Thus, unlike other functional disorders, PTSD has an explicit and definable external referent.

PTSD emerged under *DSM-III* (American Psychiatric Association, 1980) but, subsequent to the First World War, other terms were well rehearsed in relation to traumatised combatants, such as 'shell shock' and 'war neurosis' (Salmon, 1929). The term 'shell shock' was introduced in the midst of the war by Myers (1915), and connoted the assumption that the condition arose from the brain being jolted against the inner scull, when the incipient patient was near to an explosion.

The context of warfare now is different from that of the early 20th century, when those affected were overwhelmingly military personnel. Today, numerically, it is defenceless civilians who are more likely to be traumatised. Their displacement as refugees means that loss, not just trauma, are typically experienced concurrently, which undermines the idea of trauma as an isolated and discrete event. The same ambiguity applies to those traumatised during periods of childhood adversity (see below) because they experience other relevant sources of distress (such as the loss of trust in caregivers).

The shifting notion of PTSD is noteworthy. Initially, under *DSM-III* the main focus was on acute anxiety symptoms but latterly (under *DSM-5*) other 'dysphoric' symptoms have been added to the mix (i.e. sad feelings and negative thoughts). Also, reckless acting out is now attributed to some with the diagnosis (substance misuse and aggression). In the latter case, violent criminal acts by ex-combatants have been linked to their traumatisation during active service (Beckham et al., 1997).

A problem with circumscribing a seemingly neat category called 'PTSD' is that its constituent parts overlap with, or 'bleed into', many other diagnosed disorders, especially with symptoms related to acute anxiety, depression, sleep disturbances, impulse control and substance misuse (Kilpatrick et al., 2003). Another problem is that the prospect of claiming a truly objective definition of the disorder relates to the identified traumatic source, which is culturally and generally deemed to be extreme or 'catastrophic'.

Designating an external shocking event offers the promise of an objective starting point. However, as with all functional psychiatric diagnoses, the nuanced and idiosyncratic meanings attributed by a person diagnosed are not considered (i.e. the *a priori* criteria used by the *clinician* define the problem). Community surveys suggest that lay people have a very wide range of experiences they may define as traumatic in their lives (Taylor and Weems, 2009). By contrast, clinicians tend to incorporate and replay their own current social norms. Accordingly, if they consider that the patient's mixed symptoms, which broadly look like PTSD, are out of sync with, or proportion to, the stress that induced them, they may opt instead for a different diagnosis (such as 'adjustment disorder') (Horwitz, 1997).

THE TRAUMAGENIC MODEL OF MENTAL HEALTH PROBLEMS

As well as the literature on PTSD, some mental health professionals have developed a theory of adult mental health which focuses on the role of early trauma. Whereas the PTSD literature has focused on exposure to a traumatic event in adult life, the traumagenic neurodevelopmental model is about what happens to people in childhood, and subsequently how they adapt to those events. In particular, survivors of emotional, physical or sexual abuse in childhood are now thought to be at increased risk of manifesting a range of subsequent disturbances in how they trust the world and people around them. For example, children who are sexually abused are at significant risk of attracting a diagnosis of borderline personality disorder later in life. They are also more likely to abuse substances, with all the material and personal disruption that creates for them and their significant others.

And these adverse psychological manifestations may include psychotic symptoms. Read and colleagues (2014) reviewed the evidence that childhood adversities are risk factors for psychosis. This aspect is important because the previous biological explanations for vulnerability to psychosis have tended to emphasise *genetic* factors. A neurodevelopmental approach instead reminds us that 'the biological' can also be a product of events after birth and not about inherited vulnerability. The relational context emphasised in this model also reminds us that the narrow assumption of PTSD being about a discrete event is problematic. Children traumatised by the corruption of care, at the hands of adults, rarely experience one isolated event. Typically, the trauma is protracted and repeated and includes permutations of physical and emotional neglect or abuse.

See also: *causes and consequences of mental health problems; corruption of care; warfare.*

FURTHER READING

Herman, J.L. (1997) *Trauma and Recovery*. New York: Basic Books.

Read, J., Fosse, R., Moskowitz, A. and Perry, B. (2014) 'The traumagenic neurodevelopmental model of psychosis revisited', *Neuropsychiatry*, 4 (1): 64–79.

REFERENCES

American Psychiatric Association (APA) (1980) *Diagnostic and Statistical Manual of Mental Disorders* (3rd edn) (*DSM-III*). Washington, DC: APA.

American Psychiatric Association (APA) (2013) *Diagnostic and Statistical Manual of Mental Disorders* (5th edn) (*DSM-5*). Washington, DC: APA.

Beckham, J.C., Feldman, M.E., Kirby, A.C., Herzberg, M.A. and Moore, S.D. (1997) 'Interpersonal violence and its correlates in Vietnam veterans with chronic posttraumatic stress disorder', *Journal of Clinical Psychology*, 53 (8): 859–69.

Horwitz, M.J. (1997) *Stress Response Syndromes: PTSD, Grief, and Adjustment Disorders*. Lanham, MD: Jason Aronson.

Kilpatrick, D.G., Ruggiero, K.J., Acierno, R., Saunders, B.E. and Resnick, H.S. (2003) 'Violence and risk of PTSD, major depression, substance abuse/dependence, and comorbidity: results from the National Survey of Adolescents', *Journal of Consulting and Clinical Psychology*, 71 (4): 692–700.

Myers, C.S. (1915) 'Contribution to the study of shellshock', *The Lancet*, 16 (1): 316–30.

Read, J., Fosse, R., Moskowitz, A. and Perry, B. (2014) 'The traumagenic neurodevelopmental model of psychosis revisited', *Neuropsychiatry*, 4 (1): 64–79.

Salmon, T.W. (1929) 'Care and treatment of mental diseases and war neurosis ("shell shock") in the British Army', in T.W. Salmon and N. Fenton (eds), *The Medical Department of the United States Army in the World War, Vol. 10: Neuropsychiatry*. Washington, DC: US Government Printing Office.

Taylor, L.K. and Weems, C.F. (2009) 'What do youth report as a traumatic event? Toward a developmentally informed classification of traumatic stressors', *Psychological Trauma: Theory, Research, Practice, and Policy*, 1 (2): 91–106.

World Health Organization (WHO) (1990) *International Statistical Classification of Diseases, Injuries, and Causes of Death* (10th edn) (*ICD-10*). Geneva: WHO.

Psychological Formulations

DEFINITION

Psychological formulations are biographically unique descriptions of human experience and behaviour, which may or may not include explanatory reasoning. They are applied to patients in mental health settings but also appear in all 'idiographic' accounts within human psychology.

- The implications of the above definition are expanded and explored.
- Psychological formulations in mental health settings have emerged to augment or challenge psychiatric diagnosis.
- Their diverse forms are an indication of contestation in human science.

Psychological formulations represent the outcome of individual case studies and are not limited to people with mental health problems. This reflects an 'idiographic approach' within psychology generally, which is about in-depth or intensive individual case studies of human subjects. Note here that psychologists study non-human species as well, but an idiographic approach can only be established with human subjects because they are language users and therefore meaning givers. Case study investigations are thus a form of psychological *research*, in which the data are co-produced by the psychologist and the subject about the latter and their context. Case studies are used in a similar fashion by sociologists and anthropologists, except their interest is less intrinsically about the person and more about using them to understand aspects of the subject's context.

Psychological formulations are important for the mental health industry for both epistemological reasons (they offer a different knowledge base to diagnostic psychiatry) and political reasons (at times, they are used by psychologists and others to oppose that biomedical knowledge base). As the above definition indicates, they may, and often do, include explanatory aspects but, at their most basic, they are descriptive. Factors included can refer to the past, present and future. Moreover, they generally combine descriptions of events (agreed ontological claims about occurrences in a person's life) and the person's experience of these events. That experience is an important, albeit fallible window into events and thus a critical resource for discussion and potential beneficial change during forms of psychological therapy. Case studies from the latter are both accounts of personal change or stasis *and* a form of the idiographic psychological research noted above. Whereas a psychiatric diagnosis certainly is arrived at during a professionally centred form of conversation, the dialogue during the production of formulations is different in three main ways.

First, the client's perspective is given much more credence than in diagnosis. In the diagnostic interview, personal accounts are used only in a limited sense, as symptoms to be identified by the clinician. This means that elaboration outside this process by the patient is ignored or discarded for its lack of diagnostic relevance. Diagnosis is a convergent form of conversation, whereas a formulation relies on dialogical elaboration.

Second, a formulation is an elaborate, but always provisional, statement *about the person and their context*. By contrast, a diagnosis is a focused description at a point in time of what is *wrong with the person*, according to a given and medically agreed set of criteria. In line with the idiographic approach noted earlier, a formulation may or may not be about pathology, whereas a diagnosis is only about pathology being present or absent.

Third, the model used in diagnosis assumes *a priori* that the patient will be an embodied example of a general and naturally occurring disease structure and process (such as, say, 'schizophrenia' or 'depression'). The aim of diagnosis is to establish that this is, or is not, the particular case by 'eliciting symptoms' during the professional's assessment of the patient. By contrast, psychological models vary in their *a priori* assumptions (see below). If no symptoms are elicited, then the diagnosis of a particular mental disorder is left uncertain or the person is not deemed to be a patient at all. (This contention has arisen at times when psychiatry has been accused of being used in a politically abusive way.)

Thus, although psychological formulations are less crude and are more person-centred than psychiatric diagnoses, ultimately, they still reflect expert bodies of knowledge. The least professionally inflected formulations would come from the phenomenological and narrative traditions of psychological therapy and the most from the psychoanalytical tradition. The latter has been a strong lobby in the American Psychiatric Association to retain a developmental approach to aetiology, while also retaining a form of diagnosis. Moreover, psychoanalysis utilises diagnostic language to signal that developmental and dynamic approach to formulation. For example, it uses terms such as 'manic defences', 'narcissistic disturbance', the 'paranoid position' and the 'schizoid position', thus blurring the boundaries between psychiatric diagnosis and presumed psychological (in this case 'psychodynamic') processes and structures.

Notwithstanding this linguistic blurring between diagnostic psychiatry and psychoanalysis, generally formulations are more sophisticated because they are sensitive to, and flexibly open about, the particular biographical context and personal meanings ascribed to their experience by the patient. Moreover, a space for the legitimacy of formulations has been created by the proven shortcomings of functional psychiatric diagnoses. The latter have poor conceptual validity (two patients with the same label may have little in common), poor predictive validity (future outcomes or prognosis are not clear for particular patients), poor aetiological specificity (we do not know the cause of the problem), poor understanding of pathogenesis (we do not understand the mechanisms leading to particular symptoms) and poor treatment specificity (common treatments are used across diagnostic boundaries).

However, for psychological formulations to establish a mandate from society in general, or the people they are applied to in particular, they must offer clear advantages to the summary labelling of diagnostic psychiatry. And this is where arguments about logic, evidence and values begin to interweave from different communities of interest in different ways. For example, the logic of diagnosis is different from formulation, as has just been indicated. However, the logic of different models of psychological formulations also varies. A formulation about client X will be different if offered by a psychoanalyst rather than by a cognitive-behavioural therapist. Both would take the client's experience and meaning attributions seriously, but they would describe their preferred formulation using differing concepts and terminology. They also will have different explanatory paradigms when articulating their formulation verbally to the client or, say, in writing to a third party, such as a referrer.

When we compare diagnosis to formulation, two eventualities emerge. The first is that the latter is used as an elaboration of the former: diagnosis is accepted as a *broad starting point*, which is then fleshed out with a tailored biographically specific formulation. The second is that formulations are articulated as a *clear and preferred alternative* to diagnosis in all cases. In the second group are those who reject diagnosis in principle and who consider that psychological formulations are more respectful of the client's view. Intuitively, we would expect the latter advantage of formulation to always trump that of diagnosis for patients. Generally, this is true (for example, diagnosis has been a topic of complaint and resistance from disaffected service users), but there are some patients who actually prefer a diagnosis to a formulation. The former can be a comforting certainty or a damning form of professional stigma, depending on the label and the person involved.

See also: *causes and consequences of mental health problems; philosophical aspects of mental health; psychiatric classification; subjective and objective aspects of mental health; the biopsychosocial model; the myth of mental illness.*

FURTHER READING

Bracken, P. and Thomas, P. (2006) *Postpsychiatry: Mental Health in a Postmodern World*. Oxford: Oxford University Press.

British Psychological Society (2011) *Response to the American Psychiatric Association: DSM-5 Development*. Available at http://apps.bps.org.uk/_publicationfiles/consultationresponses/DSM-5%202011%20-%20BPS%20response.pdf

Cromby, J., Harper, D. and Reavey, P. (2013) *Psychology, Mental Health and Distress*. Basingstoke: Palgrave Macmillan.

Davis, M. (1996) *Disorders of Personality: DSM-IV and Beyond*. New York: Wiley.

Goldstein, B. and Rosselli, F. (2003) 'Etiological paradigms of depression: the relationship between perceived causes, empowerment, treatment preferences and stigma', *Journal of Mental Health*, 12 (4): 551–64.

Johnstone, L. and Dallos, R. (2013) *Formulation in Psychology and Psychotherapy: Making Sense of People's Problems*. London: Routledge.

Johnstone, L., Whomsley, S., Cole, S. and Oliver, N. (2011) *Good Practice Guidelines for the Use of Psychological Formulation*. Leicester: British Psychological Society.

McWilliams, N. (1994) *Psychoanalytic Diagnosis: Understanding Personality Structure in the Clinical Process*. New York: Guildford Press.

Meyer, A. (1952) *The Collected Works of Adolf Meyer*. New York: Basic Books.

Pilgrim, D. (2007) 'The survival of psychiatric diagnosis', *Social Science & Medicine*, 65 (3): 536–44.

Szasz, T.S. (1961) 'The use of naming and the origin of the myth of mental illness', *American Psychologist*, 16: 59–65.

Thomas, P. and Longden, E. (2013) 'Madness, childhood adversity and narrative psychiatry: caring and the moral imagination', *Journal of Medical Humanities*, 10 June (online), doi:10.1136/medhum-2012.

The Myth of
Mental Illness

DEFINITION

The term 'myth of mental illness' indicates that minds, like economies, can be sick only in a metaphorical sense. People may be frightened, sad, incorrigible or incomprehensible, but unless a bodily disease can be proved to underpin these forms of conduct, they are not an indication of true illness.

KEY POINTS

- The logic of the 'myth of mental illness' is explained.
- Critical responses to the notion are outlined.

This term was introduced by the American psychiatrist and psychoanalyst Thomas Szasz in the early 1960s (Szasz, 1961). He argued that mental illness is a myth because it does not fulfil the criteria, required by scientific medicine, to describe true pathology. Originally, he used the terms 'illness' and 'disease' interchangeably. More recently, in both medicine and medical sociology, the term 'disease' tends to refer to formal professional descriptions of pathology. 'Illness', more typically, refers now to an individual patient's *experience* of being unwell.

Szasz argues that mental illness is a metaphor, rather than a valid description of reality, which is conveniently used by a number of parties. The profession of psychiatry accrues the status of a proper medical specialty by claiming jurisdiction over illness. The state gains from the notion of mental illness because it can delegate lawful powers to medicine for the social control of disruptive psychological deviance. Those who do not attract the label of mental illness also gain from the concept because their troublesome fellow citizens can be dealt with by medical paternalism and removed from sight and mind. Occasionally, some patients gain advantages from the label (although this is less common than it being a disadvantage to them).

Thus, Szasz starts with a rather pedantic conceptual point (about the nature of true illnesses), but he quickly moves into a bold form of social and ethical analysis about the role of psychiatry in society, particularly as an agent of social control. He also discusses the history of societal reactions to non-conformity. He concludes that the modern mental patient occupies the same devalued, oppressed and stigmatised role as witches did in the Middle Ages.

Szasz begins with a traditional medical assumption that diseases require that *both* signs and symptoms must be present in an individual to warrant any confident diagnosis. Because psychiatry in its description of functional mental illness *only uses* symptoms (what people say and do) and lacks clear evidence of signs (evidence of bodily abnormality), it is on very weak or even fraudulent grounds as a medical speciality.

The very fact that the medical speciality of psychiatry restricts its own description to mental *illness* (not disease) tends to support Szasz's point that psychiatric diagnosis is based primarily on the patient's experience and conduct.

Szasz argues that diseases of the brain, which lead to marked changes in thinking and behaviour (for example, tertiary syphilis or alcoholic psychosis), are just that – diseases of the brain with psychological consequences. These, he says, should be called proper neurological diseases.

By contrast, where a diagnosis starts and finishes *only* with examples of thoughts and action, which others do not understand or do not approve of, then unless a biological cause can be unequivocally demonstrated in the person, they are not really ill. Hence, to call a person 'mentally ill' is to deploy a metaphor dressed up as a fact. Szasz argues that a mind can only be sick in a metaphorical sense – like an economy or a society.

For Szasz, psychiatry's codification of non-conformity as 'mental illness' is thus a logical error. The error then leads to and justifies, for its users and sympathisers, a political scandal and a moral outrage: the coercive control of madness under the guise of medical beneficence and paternalism.

By describing mental illness as a 'myth', Szasz does not imply that people are not sad, mad or frightened. His point is that these are ways of being, or 'problems in living', not symptoms of illness. By keeping an open mind about their nature, we may find different ways of making sense of them. Alternatively, sometimes they may simply remain mysterious. Szasz expresses a preference to interpret 'problems in living' as games or communications, with particular situated meanings for a person in their interpersonal context and life as a whole. (The term 'problems in living' was picked up by Szasz from another psychiatrist and psychoanalyst, Harry Stack Sullivan.)

One implication of Szasz's argument is that if a clear set of biological signs of, say, 'schizophrenia' was ever found, it should then be classified as a true biological disease or illness. Until then, according to Szasz, all functional psychiatric diagnoses, like 'schizophrenia', 'bipolar disorder', 'depression' and so on, should be deemed unscientific and invalid. Psychiatry makes sporadic claims that brain abnormalities can indeed be demonstrated in those with functional diagnoses. However, these claims have been varied, inconsistent and even contradictory. Moreover, cause and effect have never been proven. For example, a detected change in brain biochemistry in a patient could be a *cause* of psychotic symptoms or it could be a *consequence* of stress or the patient's drug treatment.

This provocative position taken by Szasz has attracted both enthusiastic supporters and indignant critics. Despite being a professor of psychiatry, he has repeatedly attacked modern psychiatric theory and practice, and reactions from his colleagues have varied from fury to exasperation. Many simply ignore him and place him beyond the pale. For example, many standard texts in psychiatry significantly omit allusions to his work (e.g. Nicholi, 1999) and it is silent denial that characterises these texts. Other texts (wrongly) depict the position about the 'myth of mental illness' as being external to the profession, as a form of 'anti-psychiatric' *sociological* attack (e.g. Gelder et al., 2001). This may seek to move the problem of psychiatric knowledge to an envious or hostile enemy without.

Some psychiatrists listen to the attack but still come to the conclusion that the symptom presentation of patients indicates that they are 'obviously mentally ill'. Others argue that while psychiatry may be over-reliant on symptoms, this is also true of physical medicine at times. For example, some conditions, such as multiple sclerosis, are difficult to diagnose. Some diagnoses of reported bodily symptoms have unknown or questionable bodily signs. A reported headache (a symptom) might be a result of muscle tension, a brain tumour or temporary dehydration. In other words, an over-reliance on functional symptoms does not neatly mark off psychiatry from other medical specialities.

Another academic reaction to the work of Szasz has been the argument that *all* illness represents a form of deviance, as it is associated with rule-breaking or role failure (Sedgwick, 1980). This sociological reframing of illness as deviance from norms *is* conceded in Szasz's original article, but he still argues that we can come to a stable, democratic and scientific consensus about bodily norms. By contrast, social norms shift over time and place, and policies about their violation are subject to the whims of the powerful in society. As a result, Szasz argues that we would be wise to treat psychiatry and its activity in a different way from the rest of medicine.

His case is supported by the fact that mental illness is treated in a uniquely coercive manner in most modern societies. It is very rare for people *with* physical illnesses to be controlled coercively by medicine on behalf of the state and society. By contrast, it is common for mentally ill patients to have their liberty taken from them without trial and for their bodies to be forcibly interfered with. While detained, patients may also be subject to solitary confinement at the discretion of staff ('seclusion'). These daily realities in mental health services give substance to Szasz's original concern about the peculiar character of psychiatric diagnosis and the nature of the treatments the profession typically prescribes.

Those, like Sedgwick, who agreed with Szasz about mental illness as deviance, disagreed with him on two fundamental matters. First, all illness, not just mental illness, is a form of deviance (Pilgrim, 1984). Second, Szasz set up a crude binary between determinism and moralism, with us being *afflicted* by physical illness but being *fully responsible* for what is called 'mental illness'. This moral absolutism about one part of the division is problematic. For example, maybe some of the time those with a psychiatric diagnosis really are impaired in their capacity to be full moral agents. In the other direction, we might be physically ill because of our moral judgements, for example when indulging in smoking or unprotected sex. If we are both determined and determining beings, then that assumption should apply to both physical and mental illness.

A final point to note about the gauntlet thrown down by Szasz is that it has probably contributed to more recent demands and criticisms from mental health service users about terminology. The use of 'mental distress', as a preferred alternative to 'mental illness', is an example here of this point. Even the more cautious tendency of writers about (rather than within) psychiatry to talk of 'people with a *diagnosis* of mental illness' (rather than 'people with mental illness') probably reflects the legacy of Szasz and his claim about the 'myth of mental illness'. It suggests that we can be confident that psychiatric diagnosis regularly occurs but not necessarily that it is legitimate, meaningful or valid.

See also: *neuroscience; psychiatric classification.*

FURTHER READING

Sedgwick, P. (1980) *PsychoPolitics*. London: Pluto Press.

Szasz, T.S. (1961) *The Myth of Mental Illness: Foundation of a Theory of Personal Conduct*. New York: Harper & Row.

REFERENCES

Gelder, M., Mayou, R. and Cowen, P. (2001) *Shorter Oxford Textbook of Psychiatry*. Oxford: Oxford University Press.

Nicholi, A.M. (ed.) (1999) *The Harvard Guide to Psychiatry*. Cambridge, MA: Belknap.

Pilgrim, D. (1984) 'Some implications for psychology of formulating all illness as deviancy', *British Journal of Medical Psychology*, 57: 227–33.

Sedgwick, P. (1980) *PsychoPolitics*. London: Pluto Press.

Szasz, T.S. (1961) *The Myth of Mental Illness: Foundation of a Theory of Personal Conduct*. New York: Harper & Row.

Part III

Mental Health Services

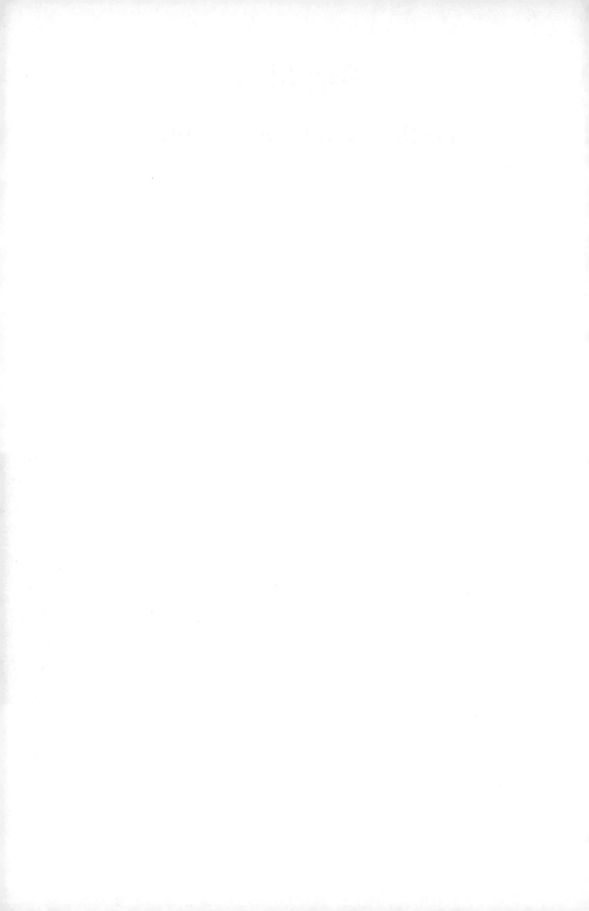

Primary Care

DEFINITION

Primary care refers to the first point of contact patients have with a health service. Staffed by general medical practitioners and other healthcare workers, it provides an initial diagnosis and treatment and it may be the start of a referral pathway to other services.

KEY POINTS

- The importance of primary care for people with mental health problems is discussed.
- Problems associated with the medicalisation of psychosocial problems in primary care are outlined.

Primary care is important for people with mental health problems for three main reasons. First, over 90 per cent of them will be in contact with their general practitioner (GP) or other primary healthcare worker during a year (Goldberg and Huxley, 1980). Second, only a small minority (about 10 per cent) of such patients are then referred on to specialist mental health services. Consequently, most people with mental health problems only receive a primary care response and the bulk of these would be described as having 'common mental health problems' (Chew-Graham, 2011). Third, in the wake of large hospital closures, most people with a history of psychosis are now living in the community, for most of their lives. Whether or not they return occasionally to acute service inpatient stays, for the most part, primary care will be their point of contact with the health service.

There are international differences in the salience of primary care and the above is a summary of the relevance of the current British NHS to people with mental health problems. For example, both the USA and the former Eastern European Communist bloc countries have seen shifts in recent years towards a greater primary care emphasis. Previously in the USA, specialist facilities predominated. In the case of the Eastern bloc, there were community-based polyclinics.

An implication of a primary *medical* response to mental health problems is that what are essentially psychosocial problems are framed from the outset as medical diagnoses (Chew-Graham et al., 2008). This is particularly the case with so-called 'mild to moderate' mental health problems, which GPs codify as anxiety states and depression. Psychiatric epidemiologists estimate that about 25 per cent of a typical GP caseload involves those with a mental health problem, the bulk of which is diagnosed as anxiety or depression (Ustun and Sartorius, 1995). About a fifth of these patients have persistent symptoms and so consult regularly in primary care (Goldberg et al., 2000). This medical framing is important because it has led to a predominance of biomedical interventions (psychotropic drugs). As a result, the drug companies target GPs for psychotropic drug marketing (Lyons, 1996).

This biomedical emphasis in primary care has resulted in two credibility problems for this service response. First, the availability of psychological interventions has lagged behind drug treatments (though there are several indications that this is being recognised and changed). Second, social problems are individualised (as medically diagnosed conditions). Moreover, psychiatrists have reinforced this individualising process by complaining that GPs do not accurately diagnose and that they under-diagnose mental illness (Freeling et al., 1985; Littlejohns et al., 1999). This discourse suggests that psychosocial problems are not medicalised *enough*. Thus, from a psychiatric perspective, the problem with primary care is its medical inefficiency. By contrast, critics of medicalisation complain of the mystification that a diagnosis of, say, 'depression' brings (Pilgrim and Bentall, 1999).

In the recent British mental health policy context, primary care has been charged with improving services to people with mental health problems in two ways. First, primary care practitioners are now expected to ensure consistent advice and help to people with mental health problems (including patients with a history of psychosis or 'severe mental illness'). Second, all patients should have their mental health needs assessed. Treatment should then be provided directly or by referral to specialist mental health services. In recent years, a number of government initiatives have been evident to boost primary mental health care. These include the introduction of psychology graduates to act as primary care mental health workers, an increased number of GPs with a special interest in mental health, and a policy to improve access to psychological therapies.

These policy changes, triggered by the *National Service Framework for Mental Health* (Department of Health, 1999), provide primary care workers with clear aims and objectives when responding to mental health problems. However, GPs find it much easier to implement other National Service Frameworks that have harder biomedical targets to achieve. For example, a study comparing the National Service Framework for coronary heart disease with the one on mental health showed that the former is implemented much more readily than the latter in primary care (Rogers et al., 2002).

Thus, primary care is a site of many contradictions. It deals with psychosocial problems but they are processed and recorded as medical problems. Although mental health problems are diagnosed as illnesses, they are not addressed within a medical framework as convincingly as bodily conditions like heart disease. GPs are criticised for their lack of medical knowledge (by psychiatrists) and yet they are responsible for most people with mental health problems. This point now applies to psychotic patients who previously would have lived most of their lives in large institutions. Primary care is the gateway to specialist services but, because of limited capacity in the latter, non-specialist staff are often left to manage complex cases.

Primary mental health care is also racialised and gendered. For example, Afro-Caribbean people do not access primary care as often as whites for mental health consultations. Women attend primary care services more than men in general (not just about mental health problems). This pattern alters the types of intervention offered to those who attend compared to non-attenders and also skews the population being both diagnosed and referred on to specialist services. (More is said about these implications in the entries for Race and Gender/Sex.)

Primary mental health care has come into focus because it both deals with 'common mental health problems' that rarely are referred on to specialists and it deals with people who have been in the latter but now live at home. Also, primary care manages people with long-term physical conditions, which often trigger depressive symptoms because of the pain and demoralisation associated with them. This very broad responsibility for a mixed caseload is reflected in the emphasis that primary care innovators are now placing on mental health. For example, the paramount obligation of primary care workers to be person-centred and mindful of the particular stressors impinging on patients is reflected in progressive primary care literature (e.g. Dowrick, 2018).

In light of this mixed caseload picture in primary care, the World Organisation of Family Doctors (WONCA) has issued an evidence-based consensus statement on core competencies required in good primary mental health care. These competencies refer to: values; being person-centred; sensitive case management; ensured collaborative practice; and reflective practice. This implies that all family doctors (GPs and community physicians) should: value mental health work; demonstrate good communication skills; be competent assessors of mental health problems; attend to the needs of those patients who are anxious or depressed (or both), as well as provide good physical healthcare for psychiatric patients on their list; coordinate care across disciplines and agencies; and be aware of their own health and wellbeing (www.globalfamilydoctor.com/Mental/Health/Core/competencies/20January2018).

This shift of focus to support and treatment in primary care settings has thrown into relief the extent to which conveyer-belt biomedical routines (diagnose-a-mental-illness-and-treat-it-medicinally) are any longer tenable. An implication of the core competency approach is that primary mental health care should focus on psychosocial aspects of the lives of patients, while recognising the importance of good general medical care for all (including the recognition of the iatrogenic impact of psychotropic medication). At present, innovations in primary mental health care include consultations offered by specialist services, and that alignment or embeddedness of specialists in generalist settings can now be tested against the six core competencies noted above. This broad aspiration about person-centredness and collaboration implies a service philosophy, which genuinely and routinely delivers a biopsychosocial approach to patient care.

See also: *acute mental health services; fear; gender/sex; madness; race; sadness; the biopsychosocial model.*

primary care

FURTHER READING

Chew-Graham, C.A., Mullin, S., May, C.R., Hedley, S. and Cole, H. (2008) 'Managing depression in primary care: another example of the inverse care law?', *Family Practice*, 9: 632–7.

Goldberg, D., Mann, A. and Tylee, A. (2000) 'Psychiatry in primary care', in M.G. Gelder, J.J. Lopez-Ibor and N.C. Andreasen (eds), *The New Oxford Textbook of Psychiatry*. Oxford: Oxford University Press.

REFERENCES

Chew-Graham, C. (2011) 'Common mental health problems: primary care and health inequalities in the UK', in D. Pilgrim, A. Rogers and B. Pescosolido (eds), *The SAGE Handbook of Mental Health and Illness*. London: Sage.

Chew-Graham, C.A., Mullin, S., May, C.R., Hedley, S. and Cole, H. (2008) 'Managing depression in primary care: another example of the inverse care law?', *Family Practice, 9*: 632–7.

Department of Health (DH) (1999) *A National Service Framework for Mental Health*. London: Department of Health.

Dowrick, C. (2018) *Person-Centred Primary Care: Searching for the Self*. London: Routledge.

Freeling, P., Rao, B.M., Paykel, E.S., Sireling, L.I. and Burton, R.H. (1985) 'Unrecognized depression in general practice', *British Medical Journal, 290*: 1180–3.

Goldberg, D. and Huxley, P. (1980) *Mental Illness in the Community*. London: Tavistock.

Goldberg, D., Mann, A. and Tylee, A. (2000) 'Psychiatry in primary care', in M.G. Gelder, J.J. Lopez-Ibor and N.C. Andreasen (eds), *The New Oxford Textbook of Psychiatry*. Oxford: Oxford University Press.

Littlejohns, P., Cluzeaut, F., Bale, R., Grimshaw, J., Feder, G. and Moran, S. (1999) 'The quantity and quality of clinical practice guidelines for the management of depression in primary care in the UK', *British Journal of General Practice, 49*: 205–10.

Lyons, M. (1996) 'C. Wright Mills meets Prozac: the relevance of "social emotion" to the sociology of health and illness', in V. James and J. Gabe (eds), *Health and the Sociology of Emotions: Sociology of Health and Illness Monograph*. Oxford: Blackwell.

Pilgrim, D. and Bentall, R.P. (1999) 'The medicalization of misery: a critical realist analysis of the concept of depression', *Journal of Mental Health, 8* (3): 261–74.

Rogers, A., Campbell, S., Gask, L., Marshall, M., Halliwell, S. and Pickard, S. (2002) 'Some national frameworks are more equal than others: implementing clinical governance for mental health in primary care groups and trusts', *Journal of Mental Health, 11* (2): 199–212.

Ustun, T.B. and Sartorius, N. (1995) *Mental Illness in General Health Care: An International Study*. Chichester: Wiley.

Secondary Prevention

DEFINITION

Secondary prevention strategies in relation to both physical and mental health refer to 'nipping problems in the bud'. Accordingly, this implies the accurate early identification of risks to health as well as effective policy intervention to eliminate or reduce those risks.

KEY POINTS

- Mental health promotion implies prevention in three senses, which are described.
- Dealing with the early indications of mental health problems implies an accurate identification of them before they deteriorate and become chronic as well as a recognition of the context generating these difficulties. Thus, the importance of recognising the particular vulnerabilities of individuals is implied during their interaction with stressors in their lives.

Primary prevention refers to the elimination of the original causes of mental health problems. Tertiary prevention refers to the reduction in relapse in already established problems and overlaps substantially with treatment. Secondary prevention sits in between these two health policy positions and focuses on 'nipping problems in the bud'.

The early identification of vulnerable individuals itself implies two indicators. The first is the valid observation of early symptom formation (for example, bedwetting in children or stress-related sick leave in adult workers). This is a recognition of differential vulnerability in the population; some of us are more resilient to stress than others for a range of reasons. A limited or lopsided interest in early case identification runs the risk of biological or psychological reductionism, creating a policy drift towards the pathologisation of sub-populations. However, this can be balanced by giving due weight (and, where appropriate, even prioritising) to scrutinising the role of stressors in the population, which themselves are unevenly distributed. Both of these are important: this is not an either/or policy consideration.

Before considering both vulnerability and stressors, a caution can be introduced about a policy enthusiasm for secondary prevention, when and if it is dominated by a screening and early diagnosis approach. This runs the risk of introducing stigmatising psychiatric labelling and iatrogenic medicinal treatments in early life. This caution needs to be borne in mind as we consider vulnerability.

VULNERABILITY

This was dealt with in the entries on Mental Health Promotion and Public Mental Health. Biological, psychological and social vulnerability are not random in the population. This is one reason why campaigning figures that refer to, say, one in four people having a mental health problem are fairly meaningless, because it is not *any* one in four. Our vulnerability is non-random and inflected by a range of biological, psychological and social causes.

Biological vulnerability includes congenital risks, such as foetal exposure to maternal substance misuse as well as older people with a family history of cardiovascular problems putting them more at risk of vascular dementia. Another example of biological vulnerability to mental health problems is in relation to the

secondary prevention

135

adverse effects of drug use (prescribed or recreational). Physical conditions such as diabetes can affect mood and chronic physical pain is demoralising.

Psychological vulnerability is relevant in children from abusive or neglectful family systems or where they are expected to take on a premature caring role for their own parents. Social vulnerability is most evident in relation to children living in poverty or in war zones. More generally, both children and adults living in congested urban areas are more at risk of developing symptoms of anxiety, depression and even psychosis.

Vulnerability, then, has both synchronic aspects (a moment in time) and diachronic aspects (across time). What has happened to people in the past may leave a legacy of vulnerability but new stressors emerge in our lives and they might trigger mental health problems in any one. These considerations bring us inevitably to the contingencies of external stressors.

EXTERNAL STRESSORS

These reflect extrinsic pressures on our wellbeing and our sense of personal security. An individualised approach focusing only on vulnerability will not do justice to this matter, because it is prone in its logic to biological and psychological reductionism. Commercially and politically, the vulnerability focus might be more convenient and so represents a conservative bias in policy formation. For example, treating children for ADHD (and its assumptions of biodeterminism) will divert attention from the context of disruptive conduct and provides an opportunity for profits for the drug companies (see the entry on Attention Deficit Hyperactivity Disorder).

By contrast, an external stressor perspective has enormous implications for public policy. Individualisation can enable politicians to focus on 'services' for vulnerable people without addressing political responsibility for the social causes of mental health problems (see the entry on Neuroscience). For example, poverty reduction would impact on primary, secondary and tertiary prevention but is politically fraught. After the 2008 crisis in international capitalism, the British government implemented a series of austerity measures which impacted disproportionately on those already poor.

Thus, policies that amplify rather than reduce poverty will have a deleterious impact on mental (and physical) health and undermine well-intended prevention policies. For those in work (some of whom will also be poor), the goal of profit efficiency places a pressure on employees to work quicker and more efficiently, which is stressful. A failure to meet production targets or time deadlines encourages surveillance, performance management and bullying in the workplace. Conditions of low status and weak task control by the worker exert a double stress upon them (Marmot et al., 1991). For some, that stress is added to being in insecure employment, with short-term contracts and now 'zero hours' contracts (Ferrie et al., 1995).

Workplace policies to reduce stress (see the entry on Economic Aspects of Mental Health) therefore occur in a context of opposing forces driven by matters of profit in the private sector and targets in the public sector. The workplace, then, is a contradictory space, with psychosocial processes evident that *both* threaten *and* improve mental health.

Apart from poverty reduction, an obvious list of external pressures, if corrected, would improve secondary prevention. These measures include successful anti-bullying policies in schools and the workplace (now including cyber-bullying), the reduction of exposure of children to abuse and neglect in their families, the assured provision of benign quiet spaces in urban environments and improved opportunities for social connections in order to increase social capital (Brimblecombe et al., 2018; Williford et al., 2013; Takizawa et al., 2014; Lindert, 2017; McDaid et al., 2018). An elephant in the room about this topic is living in a peaceful society: living in a war zone is fundamentally incompatible with the good mental health of non-combatants (see the entry on Warfare).

THE STRESS PROCESS MODEL

The discussion of stressors has led to their further differentiation within a broad stress process that impacts on us in different ways in different contexts over time. Stressors are threats or demands upon us, which limit our opportunities. This general process increases physiological arousal (creating anxiety) and may be inescapable (entrapment is depressing). Examples implied above would be children trapped in abusive or neglectful families or employees trapped in work that is high on demand and low on task control. Insecure employment creates ontological insecurity (a subjective experience) but also limits financial security to ensure routine household payments (an objective outcome).

Roxburgh (2011) notes that research in this area has separated the stress process into three components which can coexist in variable ratios over time and place for individuals: life events, chronic strains and daily hassles. Again, these have subjective and objective aspects and so it is not possible to standardise a measurement of them. For example, a life event such as a bereavement or divorce may be experienced as a distressing loss or a welcomed relief. Another example of this would be the vulnerability of students leaving home to go to university. This might be a point of mental health crisis for some and a sense of enjoyment and liberation for others (Holm-Hadulla and Koutsoukou-Argyraki, 2015).

Thus, the meanings we attach to what happens to us, not just the latter, inflect the probability of symptom formation (Johnstone and Boyle, 2018). Also, personal control varies between people within what appears to be a similar life event (Dohrenwend, 2006). Chronic strains in our lives are not random but are structured by our class position and educational level (with poverty dominating this picture) and they are influenced by social group membership (sex, race and age) (Wheaton, 1983; Pearlin, 1989). Racial discrimination and micro-insults experienced by black and ethnic minority people are sources of chronic strain that white people may be oblivious to. The same is true of sexism and homophobia.

The notion of 'daily hassles' is important but less clear to describe and measure than life events and chronic strains. Nevertheless, their cumulative effects are obvious stressors in our lives, which, if we are vulnerable to mental health problems, may generate a tipping point for symptom formation (Kanner et al., 1981; Wheaton, 1999; Almeida et al., 2002).

The interaction of these sources of stress is important. For example, a person under chronic strain may encounter a point of daily hassles (for example, transport failures on a day coinciding with conflict with their boss at work). If the person then takes time off work with a stress reaction, they may then experience social isolation that depresses them further. If their depression is chronic, eventually they may lose their job, creating financial pressures. Social defeat then amplifies their depression. If they cannot pay their mortgage, they may become homeless. We can see here a jumble of interacting factors creating a vicious circle for a person's mental health. Social context provides both structural biases in this non-random pattern and the ecological particularities impacting on people across time and place.

To conclude, secondary prevention policies need to take into account the non-random vulnerability of people to symptom formation and stressors (life events, chronic strains and daily hassles). Political strategies to mitigate the impact of the interaction between these domains are possible to imagine and examples were given above in relation to family and work settings. Virtually every part of public policy is a potential point of influence to reduce the probability of a mental health problem being triggered and to acknowledge the impact of those triggers by offering compassionate early support to those affected detrimentally. That range includes but is not limited to: optimal child protection policies; anti-bullying policies in school and work; good medical treatment for all in order to mitigate the psychological impact of pain and disability; noise and crime reduction in urban areas; the provision of dedicated support for bereaved people; poverty reduction; efficient uncrowded public transport; quiet green spaces for all; and routine access to meaningful social activities.

See also: *causes and consequences of mental health problems; economic aspects of mental health; mental health promotion; physical health; public mental health; the biopsychosocial model; warfare.*

FURTHER READING

Commonwealth of Australia (2000) *National Action Plan for Promotion, Prevention and Early Intervention for Mental Health 2000.* Canberra: Commonwealth Department of Health and Aged Care.

https://mhfa.com.au/sites/default/files/GUIDELINES-for-workplace-prevention-of-mental-health-problems.pdf

Johnstone, L. and Boyle, M., with Cromby, J., Dillon, J., Harper, D., Kinderman, P., Longden, E., Pilgrim, D. and Read, J. (2018) *The Power Threat Meaning Framework: Towards the Identification of Patterns in Emotional Distress, Unusual Experiences and Troubled or Troubling Behaviour.* Leicester: British Psychological Society.

Patton, G.C., Sawyer, S.M., Santelli, J.S., Ross, D.A., Afifi, R., Allen, N.B., Arora, M., Azzopardi, P., Baldwin, W., Bonell, C., Kakuma, R., Kennedy, E., Mahon, J., McGovern, T., Mokdad, A.H. and Patel, V. (2016) 'Our future: a Lancet commission on adolescent health and wellbeing', *Lancet*, 387: 2423–78.

Sarkar, C., Webster, C. and Gallacher, J. (2018) 'Residential greenness and prevalence of major depressive disorders: a cross-sectional, observational, associational study of 94, 879 adult UK Biobank participants', *Lancet Planet Health*, 2: e162–e73.

Singham, T., Viding, E., Schoeler, T., Arseneault, L., Ronald, A., et al. (2017) 'Concurrent and longitudinal contribution of exposure to bullying in childhood to mental health: the role of vulnerability and resilience', *JAMA Psychiatry*, 74: 1112–19.

REFERENCES

Almeida, D.M., Wethington, E. and Kessler, R.C. (2002) 'The Daily Inventory of Stressful Events (DISE): an investigatory approach for measuring daily stressors', *Assessment*, 9: 41–55.

Brimblecombe, N., Evans-Lacko, S., Knapp, M., King, D., Takizawa, R., et al. (2018) 'Long term economic impact associated with childhood bullying victimisation', *Social Science & Medicine*, 208: 134–41.

Dohrenwend, B.P. (2006) 'Inventorying stressful life events as risk factors for psychopathology', *Psychological Bulletin*, 132 (3): 477–95.

Ferrie, J.E., Shipley, M.J., Marmot, M.G., Stansfeld, S. and Davey Smith, G. (1995) 'Heath effects of anticipation of job change and non-employment: longitudinal data from the Whitehall II study', *British Medical Journal*, 311: 1264–9.

Holm-Hadulla, R.M. and Koutsoukou-Argyraki, A. (2015) 'Mental health of students in a globalized world: prevalence of complaints and disorders, methods and effectivity of counseling, structure of mental health services for students', *Mental Health & Prevention*, 3 (2): 1–4.

Johnstone, L. and Boyle, M., with Cromby, J., Dillon, J., Harper, D., Kinderman, P., Longden, E., Pilgrim, D. and Read, J. (2018) *The Power Threat Meaning Framework: Towards the Identification of Patterns in Emotional Distress, Unusual Experiences and Troubled or Troubling Behaviour.* Leicester: British Psychological Society.

Kanner, A.D., Coyne, J.C., Schaefer, C. and Lazarus, R.S. (1981) 'Comparisons of two models of stress measurement: daily hassles and uplifts versus life events', *Journal of Behavior Medicine*, 4: 1–39.

Lindert, J. (2017) 'Cyber-bullying and its impact on mental health', *European Journal of Public Health*, 27 (3): 1. https://doi.org/10.1093/eurpub/ckx187.581

Marmot, M.G., Smith, G.D., Stansfeld, S., Patel, C., North, F., Head, J., White, I., Brunner, E. and Feeney, A. (1991) 'Health inequalities among British civil servants: the Whitehall II study', *Lancet*, 337: 1387–93.

McDaid, D., Park, A.-L. and Wahlbeck, K. (2018) 'The economic case for the prevention of mental illness', *Annual Review of Public Health*, 40 (1): 373–89.

Pearlin, L.I. (1989) 'The sociological study of stress', *Journal of Health and Social Behavior*, 30: 241–56.

Roxburgh, S. (2011) 'Stressors and experienced stress', in D. Pilgrim, A. Rogers and B. Pescosolido (eds), *The SAGE Handbook of Mental Health and Illness*. London: Sage.

Takizawa, R., Maughan, B. and Arseneault, L. (2014) 'Adult health outcomes of childhood bullying victimization: evidence from a five-decade longitudinal British birth cohort', *American Journal of Psychiatry*, 171: 777–84.

Wheaton, B. (1983) 'Stress, personal coping resources and psychiatric symptoms: an investigation of interactive models', *Journal of Health and Social Behavior*, 24: 208–29.

Wheaton, B. (1999) 'The nature of stressors', in A.V. Horwitz and T.L. Scheid (eds), *A Handbook for the Study of Mental Health*. New York: Cambridge University Press.

Williford, A., Elledge, L.C., Boulton, A.J., DePaolis, K.J., Little, T.D. and Salmivalli, C. (2013) 'Effects of the KiVa antibullying program on cyberbullying and cybervictimization frequency among Finnish youth', *Journal of Clinical Child and Adolescent Psychology*, 42: 820–33.

Acute Mental Health Services

DEFINITION

Acute mental health services are accessed by, or imposed upon, people who are deemed to be in immediate need of containment to assess their needs, or to intervene when they are acting in a very distressed, disturbing or perplexing way.

KEY POINTS

- The history of acute mental health care is outlined along with its professional advantages to psychiatry.
- Problems on these units are discussed in relation to their social control function.
- Alternatives to inpatient care are considered.

The 1890 Lunacy Act required that all people entering asylums were detained compulsorily and a certificate of insanity issued. They were 'certified' – a term that is still used in jest in the vernacular today. The 1930 Mental Treatment Act introduced the notion of 'community care' and allowed for 'voluntary boarders'. After the Second World War, the first moves became evident to reduce the size of, or even to abolish, the old large Victorian asylums. However, it was not until the late 1980s that this programme of hospital closures became a reality in most localities.

In the run-up to this, during the 1970s, more and more acute psychiatric care was being sited in District General Hospitals. The psychiatric profession advocated this shift in order to raise its status and align itself with other medical specialities, already present in general hospitals (Baruch and Treacher, 1978). The dominance of medical forms of treatment in psychiatry by this period (drugs and electroconvulsive therapy) meant that siting a 'department of psychiatry' in a general hospital was in line with a biomedical environment of beds, blood tests and drug trolleys. It gave the appearance of scientific medicine coming of age in relation to mental illness.

For a while, the coexistence of these new general hospital facilities, alongside the yet-to-be-closed large asylums, meant that the majority of people being admitted to either type of facility were voluntary patients. For example, by the mid-1980s, only 8 per cent of admissions were classified as being 'formal' (i.e. involuntary). Even for this period, this figure was probably an underestimate of the amount of coercion required, as patients reported that they were told to agree to admission as an alternative to compulsion being used. In other words, for as long as the threat of compulsion exists, some patients will be under duress to go to hospital voluntarily. These are 'pseudo-voluntary patients' (Rogers, 1993). Indeed, as long as lawful compulsory powers exist to admit patients to a facility, then it is impossible to provide an accurate estimate of those who might be genuinely voluntary.

By the time that the large Victorian asylums had been closed in the 1990s, the pressure on the small units in general hospitals had increased for a number of reasons. First, the availability of beds was dramatically reduced, as the 'backstop' of the asylum acute admission ward disappeared. Second, some (but not all) patients, who had been long-term residents in the old hospitals and had moved to community residences, episodically went on to develop crises. Previously, these crises had been contained in the long-term hospital. Third, the increasing prevalence of substance misuse, in the poor localities in which many patients with long-term mental health problems had been settled, led to more and more 'dual diagnosis' patients being managed in acute units. Substance misuse increases the chances of chaotic and violent behaviour in psychotic patients.

As a result of these aggregating pressures, the ratio of officially recorded voluntary to involuntary admissions was reversed. By the mid-1990s, the great majority of patients entering acute units did so under a formal section of the civil part of the 1983 Mental Health Act (hence the expression 'sectioned patient'). This altered the prospects for these acute units. In the early 1970s, their advocates in the psychiatric profession aspired to offer medicalised treatment centres for people in acute mental health crises. Thirty years later, at the turn of the century, these had become holding containers for coercively admitted patients who might be intoxicated, chaotic or dangerous. Assaults against staff increased and the units became a site for illicit drug dealing. Risks from patients themselves were joined by others from the local impoverished culture. The function of acute units had been reduced to one of crisis containment. A census of activity in these units in the late 1990s concluded that they were 'non-therapeutic' (Sainsbury Centre for Mental Health, 1998).

However, this scenario had always been likely. The biomedical ethos and its attendant confidence in the 1970s were never evidence-based. They were driven instead by professional rhetoric. The preferred biomedical reliance on drug treatment brought in its wake adverse effects ('side-effects') that were life-diminishing and sometimes life-threatening. Moreover, the titles of these drugs are misleading. 'Anti-psychotic' medication does not cure madness and 'antidepressants' do not cure sadness (although they alter some symptoms, some of the time, in some people). The psychiatric profession's belief in, and triumphant claim about, a 'pharmacological revolution' has been misplaced. The burgeoning range of drugs produced after the 1950s was not the reason why the large hospitals were closed. The latter occurred for a mixture of financial and ideological reasons. The large hospitals had become too costly for the state to run and many parties objected to the wholesale segregation of devalued people (Busfield, 1986).

In the past 20 years, many critical professionals and disaffected users have pointed out that removing a person from the social context in which their mental health crisis had appeared – and then returning them to the same situation – was not a helpful response. The point was made many years earlier in a classic critique of the mental hospital (Goffman, 1961). Goffman noted that tinkering with problems and using hospitals as a garage for human breakdowns was not a form of service that was likely to be effective. People are not automobiles and so their problems cannot be rectified mechanistically in an isolated setting. Indeed, the notion of 'service' is inherently problematic, if and when compulsion is used – a 'service' to or for whom? Can a 'service' be imposed on a client?

Many involved with acute care are now more than aware of the problems they face, whether or not the above brief analysis of their nature is conceded. A number of points could be made about these challenges. First, staff could accept realistically that the acute services they provide are not likely to create mental health gains in patients, although they might temporarily give some respite to them and their significant others. Second, acute mental health problems might be better understood and managed by offering crisis intervention services in the community, rather than insisting that patients go into hospital. Third, where acute units are being used for purposes of coercive social control (as they are now in the majority of cases), it might be wise to admit to this function and not mystify it with the claim that acute services are simply providing 'treatment under the Mental Health Act'.

See also: *coercion; mental health policy; substance misuse; the quality of mental health care.*

FURTHER READING

Clearly, M. (2004) 'The realities of mental health nursing in acute inpatient environments', *International Journal of Mental Health Nursing*, 14: 134–41.

Deacon, M., Warne, T. and McAndrews, S. (2006) 'Closeness, chaos and crisis: the attractions of working in acute mental health care', *Journal of Psychiatric and Mental Health Nursing*, 13: 750–7.

REFERENCES

Baruch, G. and Treacher, A. (1978) *Psychiatry Observed*. London: Routledge.

Busfield, J. (1986) *Managing Madness*. London: Hutchinson.

Goffman, E. (1961) *Asylums*. Harmondsworth: Penguin.

Rogers, A. (1993) 'Coercion and voluntary admission: an examination of psychiatric patients' views', *Behavioural Sciences and the Law*, 11: 259–67.

Sainsbury Centre for Mental Health (1998) *Acute Problems: A Survey of the Quality of Care in Acute Psychiatric Wards*. London: Sainsbury Centre for Mental Health.

Forensic Mental Health Services

DEFINITION

Forensic mental health services detain or treat mentally disordered offenders.

KEY POINTS

- Secure mental health facilities are described.
- Problems associated with these facilities are outlined.

Most of the work of forensic mental health services involves the detention and treatment of offender-patients. In addition, they provide some community support and treatment for mentally disordered offenders released from prison or discharged from hospital facilities. In Britain, inpatient facilities for mentally disordered offenders are overwhelmingly in the NHS, although some prisons, or units within them, focus on work with those with a diagnosis of personality disorder. Conditions in prison for psychotic patients are extremely poor.

The NHS facilities are layered by security level. There are three high-security hospitals in England (Ashworth, Broadmoor and Rampton) and one in Scotland (Carstairs). Northern Ireland and Wales have no maximum-security facilities. Smaller medium-secure facilities can be found regionally. Many open facilities have locked wards (for example, dealing with dementing patients). These are usually described as 'low-secure' environments. Some low-secure environments may be rehabilitation services for long-stay offender-patients attached to medium-secure units.

In the UK, mentally disordered offenders can be found in prisons but they may be referred by the courts at trial or transferred from prison later to a range of secure mental health care facilities (largely in the NHS but also in the private sector). The physical security levels of these hospitals and units are such that escapes are very rare. The high-security hospitals (until recently called the 'Special Hospital' system) have been controversial in the last 30 years, with official inquiries about care standards and their physical condition being evident in all three. Some of these inquiries have been triggered by 'whistle-blowing staff' and media exposés of mistreatment or corruption. Two of the official inquiry reports in the 1990s (Blom-Cooper, 1992; Fallon et al., 1999) recommended the closure of Special Hospitals.

By and large, the treatment regimes in secure facilities are similar to acute inpatient units for those with a diagnosis of mental illness, combining containment with biological and psychological interventions. However, for those with a diagnosis of personality disorder, treatment regimes have been developed which are peculiar to secure settings and in which psychological interventions predominate.

Forensic mental health facilities are permitted to detain patients indefinitely and the average length of stay tends to be at least as long as would be expected had the offender gone to prison for a defined sentence (although this broad correlation contains individual variability). Thus, any advantage afforded to offenders going to hospital rather than prison is mainly about the living environment rather than about loss of liberty. Judgements about discharge from secure hospitals are based upon both evidence of improvement in symptoms of mental disorder and reduced risk to others. Because the prediction of reoffending is not perfect, staff making discharge decisions will tend to err in favour of 'false positives' to pre-empt criticism.

As a consequence, many patients feel aggrieved that their stay in hospital has been unduly long.

High-security mental health facilities are gendered – they are mainly used to contain male offender patients. A small number of female patients are detained at Rampton Hospital and others are dispersed in medium-secure facilities. At the same time, prevalence rates of mental disorder in female prisons are higher than in male prisons (but high in both). Male offender-patients are much more likely to be sex offenders. Also, male offenders are more likely to acquire the label of anti-social personality disorder or psychopathic disorder, whereas women are more likely to be labelled as 'borderline personality disorder'. The offending profile of women is more likely to include infanticide and arson. Substance misuse is prevalent in both groups, as is a history of maltreatment in childhood.

The following controversies have attended secure mental health services:

- *Risk management* This has been double-sided. On the one hand, overly liberal risk management can lead to dangerous patients being released who seriously reoffend. On the other hand, the authoritarian culture common in any high-security environment can tilt into negligence and harm to patients (possibly resulting in death). Also, the tendency towards 'false positive' decision-making was noted above. Thus, a conflict exists in secure environments between efforts to cultivate patient-centred care and third-party interests, which ensure the security of others (potential victims in open society). The latter emphasis inevitably encourages a distrustful attitude to detained patients, which can undermine the mutual trust required to create therapeutic optimism.

- *Isolation and institutionalisation* Secure facilities have been frequently characterised by professional, organisational and physical isolation. These factors together can lead to what the policy analyst John Martin described as a 'corruption of care' and the mistreatment of patients (Martin, 1984). At times, organisational isolation can also lead to the risky behaviour of patients going undetected. (For example, at Ashworth Hospital, a child was brought in as a visitor to be abused by sex offenders.) Those who have argued for the abolition of the large Special Hospitals have recognised that the varied psychological problems of people in them still require a response involving containment and not just treatment. The issue in this debate has been about size – the larger the number of beds in a residential facility, the greater the risk of isolation and institutionalisation. While these problems were widespread in 'mental illness' and 'mental handicap' hospitals in the 1960s and 1970s, they rapidly diminished with hospital run-down and closure. Because high-security hospitals are a remnant of an older network of large institutions, they remain vulnerable to old organisational problems.

- *Problems of indefinite detention* Whatever the mental state of detainees at the outset, indefinite detention brings with it particular forms of demoralisation, anger and dysfunctional conduct. This point applies to those in prison as well as in hospital. If an offender faces no prospect of liberty, then this affects their mental health. Also, it affects their motivation to collaborate with treatment. They may refuse treatment or they may comply with it disingenuously in order to negotiate their discharge. This poses a particular problem for risk assessors. The risk of offending can be tested ultimately and properly only in open settings. Dealing with long-stay patients is also potentially demoralising for staff and can make a contribution to the 'corruption of care' noted earlier.

- *The medicalisation of criminality* This controversy is mainly in relation to those with a label of antisocial personality disorder or psychopathic disorder. Placing rapists, paedophiles and murderers in a medical setting signals to them that they are not responsible for their actions and this can form a substantial barrier to treatment. (They 'patiently' wait for the medical problem they 'suffer' from to be 'treated'.) All agree that changes in antisocial behaviour rely overwhelmingly on the agency of the offender: they must be responsible for their actions, past, present and future. For this reason, many argue that those with a diagnosis of personality disorder should only be rehabilitated in prisons. This debate has been fuelled further by the question of whether personality disorder is 'treatable' at all. In strict terms, it is not (because, by definition, personality characteristics are stable). However, there is evidence that *offending behaviour* can be altered by psychological interventions even in those with a diagnosis of personality disorder.

Despite the above controversies, a couple of points can be made about secure mental health facilities which suggest that, in some respects, they are *less* problematic than those services dealing with non-offenders. The latter may be detained in acute mental health facilities without committing an offence. By contrast, offender-patients would warrant detention as prisoners and they would have the protection of due legal process and careful government inspection once detained. Consequently, their detention is consistent with natural justice. By contrast, 'civil' patients (i.e. those detained under 'civil' sections of the Mental Health Act rather than as 'mentally disordered offenders') are detained without trial. Another point in favour of mentally disordered offenders is that more is spent on them compared to those in contact with open mental health services. However, this financial advantage to mentally disordered offenders applies only to hospital, not prison, placements.

See also: *acute mental health services; biological interventions; challenging conduct in adults and children; intellectual disability; psychological interventions; risks to and from people with mental health problems.*

forensic mental
health services

FURTHER READING

Blom-Cooper, L. (1992) *Report of the Committee of Inquiry into Complaints about Ashworth Hospital*. London: HMSO.

Fallon, P., Bluglass, R., Edwards, B. and Daniels, G. (1999) *Report of the Committee of Inquiry into the Personality Disorder Unit, Ashworth Special Hospital*. London: HMSO.

Freckleton, I. and Keyzer, P. (2010) 'Indefinite detention of sex offenders and human rights: the intervention of the human rights committee of the United Nations', *Psychology, Psychiatry and Law*, 17 (3): 345–54.

Gostin, L. (ed.) (1985) *Secure Provision: A Review of Special Services for the Mentally Ill and Mentally Handicapped in England and Wales*. London: Tavistock.

Howerton, A., Byng, R., Campbell, J., Hess, D., Owens, C. and Aitken, P. (2007) 'Understanding help seeking behaviour among male offenders: qualitative interview study', *British Medical Journal*, 334 (7588): 303–6.

Kaye, C. and Franey, A. (eds) (1998) *Managing High Security Psychiatric Care*. London: Jessica Kingsley.

Martin, J.P. (1984) *Hospitals in Trouble*. Oxford: Basil Blackwell.

Marzano, L., Hawton, K., Rivlin, A. and Fazel, S. (2011) 'Psychosocial influences on prisoner suicide: a case-control study of near lethal self-harm in women prisoners', *Social Science & Medicine*, 72 (6): 874–83.

McGuire, J. (ed.) (1995) *What Works: Reducing Reoffending*. London: Wiley.

Pollack, S. and Kendall, K. (2005) 'Taming the shrew: regulating prisoners through women-centered mental health programming', *Critical Criminology*, 13 (1): 71–87.

Taylor, P.J. (1985) 'Motives for offending among violent psychotic men', *British Journal of Psychiatry*, 147: 491–8.

Thomas, S., McCrone, P. and Fahy, T. (2009) 'How do psychiatric patients in prison healthcare centres differ from inpatients in secure psychiatric inpatient units?', *Psychology, Crime and Law*, 15 (8): 729–42.

REFERENCES

Blom-Cooper, L. (1992) *Report of the Committee of Inquiry into Complaints about Ashworth Hospital*. London: HMSO.

Fallon, P., Bluglass, R., Edwards, B. and Daniels, G. (1999) *Report of the Committee of Inquiry into the Personality Disorder Unit, Ashworth Special Hospital*. London: HMSO.

Martin, J.P. (1984) *Hospitals in Trouble*. Oxford: Basil Blackwell.

The Mental Health Service Users' Movement

DEFINITION

The mental health service users' movement is an international network of people with mental health problems who are critical of orthodox psychiatric theory and practice and who demand full rights of citizenship.

KEY POINTS

- Different ways of understanding the role of psychiatric patients are discussed.
- One of these (the 'survivor') is elaborated in relation to new social movements.

- The concerns and demands of the mental health service users' movement are described.

Those studying the accounts of psychiatric patients living in the community have found that they have a number of daily concerns about social exclusion and their ability to cope in poor conditions of support (Barham and Hayward, 1991). Patients who are in contact with specialist mental health services are also critical of the way professionals frame their problems, the use of coercion and the narrow range of treatment responses offered (Rogers et al., 1993).

Rogers and Pilgrim (2014) point out that mental health service users can be thought of in four ways: as patients, as consumers, as survivors, or as providers. Literature about the third use of the term user, 'survivor', emphasises the collective oppression of psychiatric patients by mental health services and their wider host society. The term 'survivor' is itself ambiguous. It can indicate that a person has survived their mental health problem and it can refer to surviving the ordeal of mental health service contact. The term 'mental health service users' movement' is used here, but it is not universal. In the USA, where the term 'user' strongly connotes substance misuse, the term 'ex-patient' tends to be preferred. Even in the UK, as well as 'users' movement', the term 'survivors' movement' can also be found.

Dutch literature alludes to an 'opposition movement'. The latter is useful because it points up an important bias in the movement. Although they make demands about citizenship, much of the anger and debates of disaffected patients focus on disappointments or frustrations about the psychiatric profession and mental health services. This antagonistic link to psychiatry is exemplified in *Shrink Resistant: The Struggle Against Psychiatry in Canada* by Bonnie Burstow and Don Weitz (1988). Given this disaffection with psychiatry and mental health services, the term 'user' is problematic because patients do not always see services as being 'of use', nor is the contact always voluntary. Whether this contact means that they 'use a service' is a moot point. It suggests that third parties, benefiting from patients' removal from society, might be the real users of services.

The reactions of psychiatry to these attacks have been mixed. Sometimes they are dismissed as the collective and unreliable accounts of people who, by definition, have lost their reason (they are mentally ill). At other times, though, the criticisms have been taken seriously, particularly by that group of critical psychiatrists forming the 'post-psychiatry' movement. The focus on the failings of psychiatry also links the mental health service users' movement to 'anti-psychiatry', with the latter being built on and endorsed favourably by movement members.

The mental health service users' movement grew in the 1970s in the USA and mainland Europe, and in the mid-1980s in the UK (Rogers and Pilgrim, 1991; Campbell, 1996). It can be thought of as one example of a new social movement. The latter is a group containing people with a common identity who seek to promote their interests in opposition to dominant forms of power and organisation preferred by the state (Toch, 1965). The obvious examples of this are the women's movement, the black consciousness movement, the disability movement and the ecology movement. These can be distinguished from older social movements, such as versions of the labour or workers' movement, which focus on formal bureaucratic forms of organisation and on economic and political demands. By contrast, new social movements are less bureaucratic and they tend to make wider demands about personal liberation and citizenship or, in the case of ecology, the prevention of a global disaster. They emphasise civil, not just political, demands and they establish new agendas outside the normal democratic processes of the state bureaucracy (Habermas, 1981).

If they can be characterised in traditional political terms at all, the new social movements tend to have a mixture of liberal, left-libertarian and anarchist values. These generalisations need to be tentative, though. For example, some parts of the black consciousness movement show marked authoritarian and patriarchal tendencies. Sometimes the term 'identity politics' is also used to capture the nature of new social movements. However, the ecology movement does not neatly fit this definition.

Turning to the content of the mental health service users' movement, a number of themes can be identified:

- *The opposition to coercion* The focus here is on the way in which mental health problems are forcibly segregated from society.
- *The opposition to compulsory treatment* As well as the issue of compulsory detention, compulsory treatment is also opposed. Indeed, the notion of medical treatment is inherently problematic if it is imposed. Assaults on resistant bodies are cast as 'treatment' because the state delegates lawful powers to professionals. Similarly, what is solitary confinement in prison becomes 'seclusion' in mental health services. The users' movement seeks to expose the mystification of these oppressive practices carried out under the cloak of medical paternalism.
- *The opposition to psychiatric diagnosis* This varies in its salience in the movement but many patients resent the application of a medical diagnosis to a problem they prefer to frame in biographical, social or spiritual terms.
- *The demand for greater treatment choice* This relates to the dominant use of physical treatments in psychiatry. Users demand a greater choice of treatment responses than are on offer. Common demands are for psychosurgery and electroconvulsive therapy to be outlawed and for psychological therapies to be more available.
- *The demand for greater citizenship* This feature is shared with the physical disability movement. It is the one area of demand that lies outside complaints about psychiatry and specialist services, although the latter may still be criticised for not promoting social inclusion.

Earlier, the notion of user-as-consumer was noted. This has had the effect of diverting time and energy from the new social movement of psychiatric patients. The consumer emphasis is associated with 'user involvement' in mental health services (Pilgrim and Waldron, 1998). This draws users into the narrower agenda of the state's reforms of its pre-existing forms of organisation – professionally dominated mental health services.

See also: *anti-psychiatry; mental health; service-user involvement; the myth of mental illness*.

FURTHER READING

Campbell, P. and Rose, D. (2011) 'Action for change in the UK: thirty years of the user/survivor movement', in D. Pilgrim, A. Rogers and B. Pescosolido (eds), *The SAGE Handbook of Mental Health and Illness*. London: Sage.
Crossley, N. (2006) *Contesting Psychiatry: Social Movements in Mental Health*. London: Routledge.

REFERENCES

Barham, P. and Hayward, R. (1991) *From the Mental Patient to the Person*. London: Routledge.
Burstow, B. and Weitz, D. (eds) (1988) *Shrink Resistant: The Struggle Against Psychiatry in Canada*. Vancouver: New Star.
Campbell, P. (1996) 'The history of the user movement in the United Kingdom', in T. Heller, J. Reynolds, R. Gomm, R. Muston and S. Pattison (eds), *Mental Health Matters*. Basingstoke: Macmillan.
Habermas, J. (1981) 'New social movements', *Telos, 48*: 33–7.
Pilgrim, D. and Waldron, L. (1998) 'User involvement in mental health service development: how far can it go?', *Journal of Mental Health, 7* (1): 95–104.
Rogers, A. and Pilgrim, D. (1991) '"Pulling down churches": accounting for the mental health users' movement', *Sociology of Health and Illness, 13* (2): 129–48.
Rogers, A. and Pilgrim, D. (2014) *A Sociology of Mental Health and Illness* (5th edn). Maidenhead: Open University Press.
Rogers, A., Pilgrim, D. and Lacey, R. (1993) *Experiencing Psychiatry: Users' Views of Services*. Basingstoke: Mind/Macmillan.
Toch, H. (1965) *The Social Psychology of Social Movements*. New York: Bobbs Merrill.

Service-user Involvement

149

DEFINITION

User involvement is part of a wider political consensus that those who use public services should have a say in how these are organised and planned. When applied to users of mental health services, it reflects a range of initiatives to include users in: their individual care plans; staff recruitment and training; and service quality.

- A brief background to service-user involvement policy in Britain is given.
- Constraints on its development are discussed and estimates of its success are presented.

In Britain, mental health service-user involvement is now a well-rehearsed and endorsed position from service managers and politicians. With regard to the latter, it reflects both a Thatcherite legacy and a Blairite policy of consumerism in public services. As will be noted again later, it is particularly difficult to reconcile consumerism (with all of its assumptions about voluntary choice) with forms of service provision that have coercion at their centre. The notion of user-as-consumer is only one connotation: Rogers and Pilgrim (2001) note that users also appear in the literature as patients, as survivors and as providers.

This official central consumerist emphasis is important to note because user involvement can be justified in other ways or demanded for other reasons. For example, it can be seen as a human right. Alternatively, it can be used as a Trojan horse by the mental health service users' movement to insinuate oppositional arguments, when disaffected patients are angry with their treatment (in its widest sense), at the hands of services and service professionals.

When user involvement was mooted in the late 1980s, some of those involved in the service users' movement expressed the concern that it might deflect scarce time and energy. This suggested that user involvement was viewed by some more radical users as a form of diversionary co-option (Campbell, 1996; Campbell and Rose, 2011).

Another opening clarification is about relatives of users. In the separate entry on Carers, it is noted that sometimes the consumerist position leads to an amalgam discourse from service managers, who will sometimes refer to 'users and carers' in the same phrase. A version of this is 'user and carer involvement'.

As Diamond and colleagues (2003) note, the term 'user involvement' is ambiguous. The most conservative use of the term is in relation to eliciting consumer feedback (Bhui et al., 1998). This is analogous to the consumerist process of, say, hotels asking guests to fill in a satisfaction survey. It involves no direct negotiation between provider and recipient and the former can use their discretion about data utilisation. The progressive limits of user involvement are defined by projects which encourage users to be directly involved in service planning or in service improvement (Barnes and Shardlow, 1997; Pilgrim and Waldron, 1998). The conservative aspiration is the easiest to achieve. It is not labour-intensive. It requires little or no new financial or workforce resources. It can be acted upon or ignored. It can be cherry-picked and selectively attended to. By contrast, the more radical scenario is harder to achieve but, if successful, its impact on changing services would be greater.

Constraints on the progress of service-user involvement can thus be summarised as follows:

- *The current status of the factors prompting user involvement* It was noted in the introduction that consumerism was the main driver that started user involvement and has been retained. Two other triggering factors were present in the 1980s. The first was the eventual implementation of desegregation (hospital run-down and closure). The second was the problem of psychiatric knowledge, which was attacked first by 'anti-psychiatry' and then by the mental health service users' movement. These two triggers are still present but their influence may be less than in the past. For example, although the large hospitals were closed, we have also witnessed both trans-institutionalisation (the greater presence in prisons of people with mental health problems) and re-institutionalisation (the movement of long-stay patients into private hospitals and other smaller residential units). In other words, part of the hoped-for success of user involvement was that it would entail partnerships to collaborate on ensuring quality of life in the community. In practice, the community as a central site of user satisfaction is hedged around now by older forms of residential containment. To confirm this, more money is currently spent on inpatient facilities than on service changes to make them more community orientated (see the entry on Economic Aspects of Mental Health). More on the second factor will be noted in the next point.

- *The resilience of the biomedical approach to care* Since user involvement emerged as a policy in the 1980s, there has been no evidence that a more holistic approach to care has become an established norm in most localities. The balance between biological and psychological interventions remains skewed towards the former for most people in contact with specialist services. While all psychotic patients receive medication (new or old 'anti-psychotics'), only a minority receive psychosocial interventions. This is important because a recurring message from user consultations is that the balance should shift from medication to talking treatments.

- *The lack of money to support user involvement* Central government provides no ring-fenced money to guarantee user involvement. This is left to the discretion of local providers. Pressures on funding in services are such that user involvement can be given a low priority.

- *The ultimate constraint of coercion* As with the retention of biomedical interventions, this is also an important factor: 'What users recurrently demand is more options and greater voluntarism in their service contact. Pressures on inpatient beds in the last 20 years, since hospital run-down, have made acute units into unambiguous sites of coercive social control, with the majority of patients being involuntary and the remaining minority having a questionable voluntary status' (Rogers, 1993: 260).

- *Consumerism based on the assumption that service recipients can take or leave what is offered* Clearly, this is not the case with mental health services, where involuntary detention is ever present. In what sense can the logic of voluntary partnerships, suggested by the notion of user involvement, have any genuine meaning in the context of this coercive service character? Put differently, the more that coercion dominates a service site, the less meaning user involvement can have. This may be why those aspects of the service that are voluntary, psychologically orientated and community-based tend to receive a stronger endorsement from users (Diamond et al., 2003).

Given the above list of constraints, estimates of the success of user involvement have been variable in recent years. Pilgrim and Waldron (1998) reported minor successes in relation to local changes to day centre provision, advocacy services and improved communications with local mental health service professionals. Bowl (1996), in a social service setting, found that staff did not manage to successfully share power or build partnerships with users and that there were insufficient financial resources to sustain user involvement. Bowl also found staff resistance to involving users in staff selection. (This can be contrasted with many NHS mental health services that now include users on staff selection panels.)

The study by Diamond and colleagues (2003) was more optimistic. They found that success had been achieved in relation to the presence of regular service-user meetings and in user involvement in staff recruitment and in organising and planning services. There was weaker success reported in relation to involvement in staff training and in contacts with advocacy services. Given these ambiguous results in relation to the early days of user involvement, perhaps more time is needed to provide a clear research picture of its success or failure as a policy.

See also: *carers; economic aspects of mental health; mental health policy; segregation; the mental health service users' movement.*

FURTHER READING

Campbell, P. and Rose, D. (2011) 'Action for change in the UK: thirty years of the user/survivor movement', in D. Pilgrim, A. Rogers and B. Pescosolido (eds), *The SAGE Handbook of Mental Health and Illness*. London: Sage.

Faulkner, A. and Layzell, S. (2000) *Strategies for Living: A Report of User-led Research into People's Strategies for Living with Mental Distress*. London: Mental Health Foundation.

REFERENCES

Barnes, M. and Shardlow, P. (1997) 'From passive recipient to active citizen: participation in mental health user groups', *Journal of Mental Health*, 6: 289–300.

Bhui, K., Aubin, A. and Strathdee, G. (1998) 'Making a reality of user involvement in community mental health services', *Psychiatric Bulletin*, 22: 8–11.

Bowl, R. (1996) 'Involving service users in mental health services: social services departments and the NHS and Community Care Act 1990', *Journal of Mental Health*, 5 (3): 287–303.

Campbell, P. (1996) 'The history of the user movement in the United Kingdom', in T. Heller (ed.), *Mental Health Matters*. Basingstoke: Macmillan.

Campbell, P. and Rose, D. (2011) 'Action for change in the UK: thirty years of the user/survivor movement', in D. Pilgrim, A. Rogers and B. Pescosolido (eds), *The SAGE Handbook of Mental Health and Illness*. London: Sage.

Diamond, B., Parkin, G., Morris, K., Bettinis, J. and Bettesworth, C. (2003) 'User involvement: substance or spin?', *Journal of Mental Health*, 12 (6): 613–26.

Pilgrim, D. and Waldron, L. (1998) 'User involvement in mental health services: how far can it go?', *Journal of Mental Health*, 7 (1): 95–104.

Rogers, A. (1993) 'Coercion and voluntary admissions: an examination of psychiatric patients' views', *Behavioural Sciences and the Law*, *11*: 259–68.

Rogers, A. and Pilgrim, D. (2001) 'Users and their advocates', in C. Thornicroft and G. Szmukler (eds), *Textbook of Community Psychiatry*. Oxford: Oxford University Press.

Carers

DEFINITION

This term is currently used by politicians and health and social care managers to describe the relatives of service users or their significant others.

KEY POINTS

- Problems with the term 'carer' are described.
- Aspects of the relationships between people with mental health problems and their relatives are outlined.

It is now common in policy documents about both mental illness and physical disability to see the term 'carers'. It is sometimes used in an amalgam way (as in 'users-and-carers') (Department of Health, 1999, 2002). Both the single and amalgam terms are problematic for a variety of reasons. When people with mental health problems and their significant others are asked, they do not always feel comfortable with the term 'carer' (Henderson, 2004). The problem is that the convenient social administrative category of 'carer' does not accurately convey the day-to-day complexity of intimate relationships. Dependency in intimate relationships is typically mutual rather than one way, even when one party is sick, impaired or disabled. The highly restricted and one-way connotation of 'carer' and 'cared for' does not do justice to this complexity. Also, the term 'cared for' implies passivity. For this reason, Forbat (2002) has argued that the term 'caree' would be more accurate, as it provides a notion of personal agency on the part of the person who is the identified patient or client.

Given that terms such as 'health care' and 'social care' are administrative descriptions of health and welfare bureaucracies, we also have 'health care' and 'social care' professionals. In the case of those paid to care, the more restricted notion of one-way dependency is more applicable. Generally, this is associated with much clearer personal boundaries and role descriptions. The paid carer is not expected to have their personal, social or sexual needs satisfied by those they care for. Indeed, when and if this occurs, the paid carer is usually deemed to be acting

carers

153

in an unprofessional, unethical or abusive way. By contrast, this moral and legal discourse does not apply to unpaid care. In the latter case, need satisfaction is a two-way process. In the case of paid caring, need satisfaction must be suppressed or managed. It is not merely that one group is paid and the other is not – the way that those cared for are helped or supported is governed by different rules.

With these ambiguities and distinctions in mind, some further points can be made about the notion of 'carer'. Within the broad literature on informal caring in relation to physically disabled people, two features predominate. First, there is a strong feminist critique, which emphasises that women, more than men, absorb the pressures of unpaid care (e.g. Finch and Groves, 1983). Second, there is an emphasis on 'tending' – the physical support and procedures needed to respond to a physically disabled or sick person.

Neither of these points can be wholly applied in the case of those with mental health problems. In 'mental health care', the need for tending is largely absent in the case of functional problems but extensive in the case of dementia care (see the entry on Economic Aspects of Mental Health). Given that living with a person with a diagnosis of functional mental disorder is about coping with a range of tensions in the family, both male and female relatives are drawn into these interpersonal demands and dramas. Thus, when we turn to the peculiarities involved in applying an informal notion of care to mental health, the following points can be made (Rogers and Pilgrim, 2014):

- *Families and aetiology* Some of the professional literature has located intimate family life as the causal source of madness (e.g. Laing and Esterson, 1964). This 'anti-psychiatric' position fell out of favour after the 1970s (Howells and Guirgis, 1985). More recently, there has been a return to this aetiological theory to an extent (Bentall, 2003).
- *Families and relapse* While the family causation model has been controversial, a consistent professional orthodoxy is that the emotional climate of a family can affect relapse rates in psychotic patients (Jenkins and Karno, 1992; cf. Johnstone, 1993).
- *Relatives as risk assessors* The efficiency of risk assessment and prediction (in terms of relapse and risk to self and others) is significantly improved if significant others are included in discussions with staff (Klassen and O'Connor, 1988). However, this can create a role tension for relatives – are they an extension of the mental health system or is their first loyalty to the identified patient? In other words, the policy emphasis upon co-opting the views of relatives now extends to them working on behalf of mental health professionals (Forbat and Henderson, 2003).
- *Relatives as perpetrators and victims of abuse* This links back to the first point about aetiology. Families can be sites of two-way victimisation. Relatives of people with mental health problems may sometimes be abusive. Early childhood abuse is a good predictor of a range of mental health problems in adulthood (Briere and Runtz, 1987). In the other direction, the parents of psychiatric patients can be victims of intra-familial violence at times (Estroff and Zimmer, 1994).

- *Relatives as a lobby group* As relatives of those with mental health problems do not work together to advance their own personal liberation, they cannot be described as a full new social movement (see the entry on the Mental Health Service Users' Movement). However, they are an organised mental health policy lobby (Manthorpe, 1984). Organisations such as SANE and Rethink (previously the National Schizophrenia Fellowship) in the UK and the National Alliance for the Mentally Ill in the USA are dominated by relatives of patients. Many of their demands about service improvements are similar to those of the mental health service users' movement. However, they are more likely to prefer a biomedical model of causation and they place more of an emphasis on the provision of inpatient care and the need for greater coercive control of madness. Despite the tendency to use the amalgam term 'users-and-carers' (noted in the introduction earlier), it is important to note that while both groups have overlapping needs and priorities, these are not identical.

See also: *economic aspects of mental health; risks to and from people with mental health problems; the mental health service users' movement.*

FURTHER READING

Forbat, L. and Henderson, J. (2003) 'The professionalization of informal carers', in C. Davies (ed.), *The Future of the Health Workforce*. Basingstoke: Palgrave Macmillan.

Manthorpe, J. (1984) 'The family and informal care', in N. Maim (ed.), *Implementing Community Care*. Buckingham: Open University Press.

REFERENCES

Bentall, R.P. (2003) *Madness Explained: Psychosis and Human Nature*. London: Penguin.

Briere, J. and Runtz, M. (1987) 'Post-sexual abuse trauma: data implications for clinical practice', *Journal of Interpersonal Violence*, 2: 367–79.

Department of Health (DH) (1999) *National Service Framework for Mental Health*. London: DH.

Department of Health (DH) (2002) *Developing Services for Carers and Families of People with Mental Illness*. London: DH.

Estroff, S. and Zimmer, C. (1994) 'Social networks, social support and violence among persons with severe and persistent mental illness', in J. Monahan and H. Steadman (eds), *Violence and Mental Disorder: Developments in Risk Assessments*. Chicago, IL: University of Chicago Press.

Finch, J. and Groves, D. (1983) *A Labour of Love: Women, Work and Caring*. London: Routledge.

Forbat, L. (2002) '"Tinged with bitterness": re-presenting stress in family care', *Disability and Society*, 17 (7): 759–68.

Forbat, L. and Henderson, J. (2003) 'The professionalization of informal carers', in C. Davies (ed.), *The Future of the Health Workforce*. Basingstoke: Palgrave Macmillan.

Henderson, J. (2004) 'Constructions, meanings and experiences of "care" in mental health', PhD thesis, Open University, Milton Keynes.

Howells, J.G. and Guirgis, W.R. (1985) *The Family and Schizophrenia*. New York: International Universities Press.

Jenkins, J.H. and Karno, M. (1992) 'The meaning of expressed emotion: theoretical issues raised by cross-national research', *American Journal of Psychiatry*, 149: 9–21.

Johnstone, L. (1993) 'Family management in "schizophrenia": its assumptions and contradictions', *Journal of Mental Health*, 2: 255–69.

Klassen, D. and O'Connor, W. (1988) 'A prospective study of predictors of violence in adult mental health admissions', *Law and Human Behaviour, 12*: 143–58.

Laing, R.D. and Esterson, A. (1964) *Sanity, Madness and the Family*. Harmondsworth: Penguin.

Manthorpe, J. (1984) 'The family and informal care', in N. Maim (ed.), *Implementing Community Care*. Buckingham: Open University Press.

Rogers, A. and Pilgrim, D. (2014) *A Sociology of Mental Health and Illness* (5th edn). Maidenhead: Open University Press.

Mental Health Professionals

DEFINITION

The term 'mental health professionals' refers to those who work with people with mental health problems. A variety of occupational groups specialise in the field, notably psychiatrists, clinical psychologists, mental health nurses, mental health occupational therapists and mental health social workers. Other groups to be found are counselling psychologists, forensic psychologists, counsellors, psychotherapists and some pharmacists who specialise in mental health work.

KEY POINTS

- The occupational backgrounds of those working with people with mental health problems are outlined.
- The relationship between these occupational groups is discussed.

Mental health work is constituted by a range of professionals. The term 'psy complex' is used at times to capture this complexity but is more general, as it also denotes other professional activities informed by psychological approaches (such as teaching and advertising).

Historically, mental health services were politically dominated by the medical specialism of psychiatry though latterly this dominance is less clear, given the competition evident from other professions. For example, the general management of mental health services is commonly dominated now by mental health nurses. The management of certain client groups (those with a diagnosis of personality disorder or learning disability) is often led by clinical psychologists.

A legal reflection of this shift is the recently proposed English mental health legislation, which replaces the older notion of 'Responsible Medical Officer' with one of 'Clinical Supervisor', which could be held by a 'Consultant Psychologist'. This role is responsible for the admission and discharge of formally detained patients and as such highlights the peculiarity of a form of health work, which at times involves coercion and captive clients.

The range of occupational groups mentioned in the definition above is associated with a variety of academic disciplines. Only psychologists have a single academic discipline underpinning their work (psychology). Postgraduate training then transforms and separates this core academic discipline into different applied wings. Clinical psychologists work in a variety of health settings, including but not limited to mental health work, whereas counselling psychologists, a smaller group, mainly do mental health work. Forensic psychologists mainly work in prisons and, less commonly, in health services.

The disciplinary background of the other mental health professions, including medicine, is mixed. For example, medical and nurse training includes inputs from sociology, psychology, pharmacology and neurology. A complication, when discussing the mental health professions, is that the term 'discipline' is used in mental health services to indicate occupational background (as in 'multidisciplinary team' or 'interdisciplinary collaboration'). By contrast, in higher education, the term 'discipline' tends to refer to a core body of knowledge (such as mathematics, philosophy, sociology, geology, anatomy, physiology and so on).

As all mental health professionals are now graduates (until quite recently, this was not the case for mental health nurses), one way of examining the field of mental health is to explore its diverse knowledge base. The term 'profession' indicates a form of occupation which is different from that of 'worker'. Professionals are defined by the possession of more credentials and their focus on working with people rather than goods. However, in mental health services, at different times, the words 'worker', 'practitioner', 'professional', 'discipline' or 'occupation' can all be used to connote the same notion.

The history of the professions suggests a different bias towards one or other of these meanings. For example, male asylum attendants in the 19th century prefigured psychiatric nursing. They were employed to manhandle and restrain disturbed lunatics. This working-class and trade-unionised emergent wing of a profession was rejected by mainstream nursing. The latter, under the guidance of Florence Nightingale, was wholly female and middle class. From the outset, these genteel Victorian spinsters saw themselves as professionals, not workers. The reverse was the case in what was to become mental health nursing.

The different educational backgrounds of the mental health professionals shape their character. For example, psychiatrists, being trained in medicine, generally work diagnostically and use physical treatments, such as drugs and electroconvulsive therapy. Psychologists, being trained in psychology, are more likely to use formulations about a patient's problems and offer some form of psychological intervention. Nurses vary in between these positions. The lesser professional confidence of mental health nurses is indicated by the continued use of the term 'psychiatric nurse', reflecting the subordinate relationship between medicine and nursing.

These are only general trends of work being described, which typically characterise each occupational group. Exceptions can also be found and are not uncommon. For example, some psychiatrists train as medical psychotherapists and do not prescribe drugs. Some clinical psychologists use diagnostic terms when assessing patients' problems. Thus, approaches to mental health work overlap across the occupational groups.

A consequence of this overlap of roles and approaches across the mental health workforce is that sometimes the identity of a practitioner is defined more by their treatment orientation than by their occupational origins. For example, psychoanalytical psychotherapists from different occupational backgrounds might share a common identity. As a result, an individual practitioner with this orientation may lose their sense of belonging to the occupational group that originally provided them with the legitimate credentials to do mental health work.

As well as the blurring of roles between groups within mental health work, some mainly trained in the field can be found working outside specialist mental health services. For example, both clinical psychologists and psychiatrists work with people with physical health problems and those with learning disabilities.

Some forms of treatment for mental health problems imply a traditional division of labour centred on medicine. For example, drug therapy flows from a medical diagnosis and prescribed treatment controlled by psychiatrists. Nurses are responsible for accurately administering medication on a daily basis (or via less frequent injections) and then monitoring the positive or negative effects of the treatment.

At other times, treatments are controlled autonomously by professionals from different backgrounds, who carry and regulate their own caseloads with the support of a personally negotiated supervisor. For example, forms of psychological therapy might be deployed autonomously by nurse therapists, psychologists (of different types), medical psychotherapists, social workers or occupational therapists.

Outside specialist mental health services, a greater number of counsellors and psychotherapists can be found in the private sector. The credentials and regulation of these groups are less consistent than in mainstream health service work with people with mental health problems. In order to work in statutory mental health services in Britain, then, all professionals must come within the framework of health legislation. They must also demonstrate their competence through specific credentials presented on the occasion of their appointment and they must demonstrate regular knowledge updates ('continued professional development'). In the private sector, these legal requirements are absent, although to stay registered with a particular parent training body, practitioners must still subscribe to a code of conduct and give a personal commitment to continued professional development.

Finally, the definition of mental health professionals given at the outset focuses on those most closely associated, on a regular basis, with specialist mental health services. However, two other occupational groups are important in regulating access to the latter. First, police officers are involved with mental health crises in the community and their resolution or in securing a specialist referral. Second, GPs are an important gatekeeper into specialist services. They are also involved in the assessment and treatment of the majority of people with 'mild to moderate' mental health problems. GPs are taught that there will be a psychological dimension to around a third of all the patient presentations they see on a daily basis. Therefore, it might be argued that because of the volume of patients they see, GPs are a type of mental health worker.

See also: *causes and consequences of mental health problems; coercion; intellectual disability; primary care; psychological interventions*.

FURTHER READING

Cheshire, K. and Pilgrim, D. (2004) *A Short Introduction to Clinical Psychology*. London: Sage.

Colombo, A., Bendelow, G., Fulford, B. and Williams, S. (2003) 'Evaluating the influence of implicit models of mental disorder on processes of shared decision making within community-based multi-disciplinary teams', *Social Science and Medicine*, 56 (7): 1557–70.

Craddock, N., Antebi, D., Attenburrow, M.-J. et al. (2008) 'Wake-up call for British psychiatry', *British Journal of Psychiatry*, 193: 6–9.

Gask, L. (2004) *A Short Introduction to Psychiatry*. London: Sage.

Goldie, N. (1978) 'The division of labour amongst mental health professions – a negotiated or an imposed order?', in M. Stacey and M. Reid (eds), *Health and the Division of Labour*. London: Croom Helm.

Onyett, S., Pillinger, T. and Muijen, M. (1997) 'Job satisfaction and burnout among members of community mental health teams', *Journal of Mental Health*, 6 (1): 55–66.

Pilgrim, D. and Rogers, A. (2009) 'Survival and its discontents: the case of British psychiatry', *Sociology of Health and Illness*, 31 (7): 947–61.

Priebe, S., Burns, T. and Craig, T. (2013) 'The future of academic psychiatry may be social', *British Journal of Psychiatry*, 202: 319–20.

Saks, M. and Allsop, J. (eds) (2003) *The Regulation of the Health Professions*. London: Sage.

Biological Interventions

DEFINITION

Biological interventions for mental health problems include medication, electro-convulsive therapy (ECT) and psychosurgery.

KEY POINTS

- Biological interventions are the mainstay of psychiatric treatment, although they are sometimes used in combination with psychological interventions.

- Biological interventions are described and criticisms of them summarised.

Biological interventions are the mainstay response to mental health problems. These interventions may be offered or imposed alone or in combination with psychological interventions (Olfson and Pincus, 1999).

The following points summarise biological interventions and the controversies surrounding them:

- *The most prevalent form of intervention is medication* Psychiatric (or psychotropic) drugs are used in the treatment of all forms of mental disorder and there is an evidence base to support their appropriate use (Baldessarini, 1999). For this reason, it is virtually unheard of for a person with a mental health problem to be unmedicated. This statement is particularly true for those in contact with a specialist mental health service. The psychiatric profession has tended to describe these drugs in relation to their impact on a diagnosed mental disorder (e.g. 'antidepressants', 'anti-psychotics'). However, before the Second World War, this was not the case – drugs were seen only as an adjunct to psychiatric treatment, to suppress or manage symptoms. They were called 'sedatives' or 'tranquillisers'. After the 1950s, the so-called 'pharmacological revolution' brought with it a curative rhetoric, encouraged by the pharmaceutical industry (even though the newer drugs still only suppress symptoms).

- *Drugs have been associated with recurrent criticism from their recipients* Because psychotropic drugs, by definition, have powerful effects on the central nervous system, they have been associated with a range of negative or adverse effects. (These are sometimes called 'side-effects', which is misleading, as they are not secondary or marginal in the experience of patients.) These effects are often life-diminishing and sometimes they can be life-threatening (Kellam, 1987; Waddington et al., 1998). As well as individual drugs having effects, which may both reduce symptoms and create problems, the psychiatric profession has been criticised for using cocktails of drugs ('polypharmacy'). Another criticism has been that of therapeutic over-dosing ('megadosing'). Both polypharmacy and megadosing have been linked to the death of recipients (Breggin, 1993). Two high-profile critiques have been associated with the minor and major tranquillisers (Fisher and Greenberg, 1997). The first of these refers to the benzodiazepines, used as anxiolytics (to reduce anxiety symptoms) and hypnotics (to aid sleep). These widely prescribed drugs in primary care were addictive and ineffective after a few weeks. The second group refers to the older anti-psychotic drugs called 'neuroleptics'. These have been associated with three disabling and disfiguring adverse effects: Parkinsonism, tardive dystonias (painful muscle cramps) and tardive dyskinesia (involuntary muscle movements, grimacing, eye rolling and tongue flicking). These problems accumulated over the decades after the 1950s, as the average prescribed dose level kept rising (Segal et al., 1992).

- *The lack of political concern about some adverse drug effects reflects the low social status of psychiatric patients* In the 1950s, when the major tranquillisers were introduced, they were used in low doses. As the years progressed and dose levels were raised and cumulative chronic treatment had its effect, more and more patients complained of disabling effects, particularly in relation to tardive dyskinesia. Brown and Funk (1986) note that the 'pandemic' of these drug-induced symptoms was only tolerated by society because of the passivity and low social status of chronic psychotic patients. To confirm this, when the National Association for Mental Health (Mind) launched a publicity campaign about the use of major tranquillisers in the 1970s, in conjunction with the popular TV programme *That's Life*, little public concern was forthcoming. However, the programme was overwhelmed by responses about *minor* tranquillisers and the latter became the focus of the campaign thereafter.

- *The use of ECT is less common than medication but it remains a controversial intervention* Although medication dominates the lives of psychiatric patients, electroconvulsive therapy is hardly a rare event. In their study of 1,000 long-term psychiatric patients, Rogers and colleagues (1993) found that nearly half had received it at some point in their lives. More recent official data suggest that in excess of 11,000 patients receive it annually and a fifth of these under conditions of compulsion (Department of Health, 1999). ECT has always been a controversial treatment, especially in its early days when patients were shocked without anaesthesia or muscle relaxants (backs were broken from the induced fit). In more recent times, the modifications in the procedure have not diminished the hostility from its critics (Breggin, 1993). Critics argue that it is frightening to its recipients and that it leads to long-term cognitive deficits (Rose et al., 2003). By contrast, professionals convinced of the treatment's efficacy dismiss user concerns as being unfounded and in the minority (Wheeldon et al., 1999).

- *The use of psychosurgery is rare but highly controversial* This procedure involves cutting or destroying specific parts of the brain in order to treat resistant psychiatric conditions. Its use is now restricted to depressed or obsessive-compulsive patients who are unaffected by all other forms of intervention. Its use diminished after the 1950s when there was clear cumulative evidence of permanent adverse effects, including apathy, epilepsy and intellectual impairment. The ethical concerns about the procedure are threefold: first, by their nature, randomised controlled trials cannot be conducted and evidence has to rely on case follow-up; second, the intervention is irreversible; and third, the adverse effects can be very serious (Merskey, 1999).

A point of particular controversy has been that biological treatments reflect an enmeshment between the medical profession and the pharmaceutical industry. This has led to accusations that the psychiatric profession is in the pay of the drug companies in various ways from payments for educational events, to marketing inducements and research sponsorship (Healy, 2004; Tsai et al., 2011). Also, this enmeshment is part of a process of medicalisation in which more and more variations in physical and psychological functioning are being subjected to medical authority and products. Drugs which claim to improve mood or sexual or socio-economic performance have thus become contentious. The early advocates of the SSRIs (Selective Serotonin Reuptake Inhibitors), such as Peter Kramer in his well-known *Listening to Prozac,* suggested that their utility went beyond the treatment of depressants: they could be extended to enhancing the quality of life of the non-symptomatic mentally healthy (Kramer, 1993).

Attacks on pharmaco-consumerism, then, reactively have a part in this picture of contention. For example, Breggin and Breggin (1994) emphasised in their retort to Kramer that the scale of psychotropic drug consumption in the USA was not warranted, given the recorded evidence on poor efficacy and extensive iatrogenesis. In *Talking Back to Prozac,* they demonstrated the scale of the problem by alluding to government drug audits. By the turn of this century, about 25 million patient visits in the USA were made for 'depression', with 69 per cent of these resulting in prescriptions for SSRIs. By 2004, one in ten American women were taking an SSRI, and by 2007, antidepressants were the most prescribed among all classes of drugs, with a total of 227.3 million prescriptions in the USA. With a total revenue of $13.5 billion for Big Pharma, the SSRIs were the third best-selling drugs in the USA that year. Other critics of this emphasis on drug company marketing have linked it to the diagnostic expansionism evident in *DSM-5* (Frances, 2010; American Psychiatric Association, 2013). (This discussion is extended in the entry on The Pharmaceutical Industry.)

See also: *anti-psychiatry; psychiatric classification; psychological interventions; the mental health service users' movement; the pharmaceutical industry.*

FURTHER READING

Guze, S.B. (1989) 'Biological psychiatry: is there any other kind?', *Psychological Medicine,* 19: 315–23.
Healy, D. (2002) *From Psychopharmacology to Neuropsychopharmacology.* Budapest: Animula.
Kingdon, D. and Young, A.H. (2007) 'Research into putative biological mechanisms of mental disorders has been of no value to clinical psychiatry', *British Journal of Psychiatry,* 191: 285–90.

REFERENCES

American Psychiatric Association (APA) (2013) *Diagnostic and Statistical Manual of Mental Disorders* (5th edn) (*DSM-5*). Washington, DC: APA.
Baldessarini, R.J. (1999) 'Psychopharmacology', in A.M. Nicholi (ed.), *The Harvard Guide to Psychiatry.* London and Cambridge, MA: Harvard University Press.
Breggin, P. (1993) *Toxic Psychiatry.* London: Fontana.
Breggin, P.R. and Breggin, G.R. (1994) *Talking Back to Prozac.* New York: St Martin's Press.
Brown, P. and Funk, S.C. (1986) 'Tardive dyskinesia: barriers to the professional recognition of iatrogenic disease', *Journal of Health and Social Behavior,* 27: 116–32.
Department of Health (DH) (1999) 'Electroconvulsive therapy: survey covering the period January 1999 to March 1999', *Statistical Bulletin,* 22. London: DH.
Fisher, S. and Greenberg, R.P. (eds) (1997) *From Placebo to Panacea: Putting Psychiatric Drugs to the Test.* New York: Wiley.
Frances, A. (2010) 'Opening Pandora's Box: the 19 worst suggestions for *DSM-5*', *Psychiatric Times,* 11 February.
Healy, D. (2004) 'Psychopathology at the interface between the market and the new biology', in D. Rees and S. Rose (eds), *The New Brain Sciences: Perils and Prospects.* Cambridge: Cambridge University Press.

Kellam, A.M.P. (1987) 'The neuroleptic syndrome so called: a review of the literature', *British Journal of Psychiatry, 150*: 752–9.

Kramer, P. (1993) *Listening to Prozac.* New York: Viking.

Merskey, H. (1999) 'Ethical aspects of physical manipulation of the brain', in S. Bloch, P. Chodoff and S.A. Green (eds), *Ethical Aspects of Drug Treatment.* Oxford: Oxford University Press.

Olfson, M. and Pincus, H.A. (1999) 'Outpatient psychotherapy in the United States: the National Medical Expenditure Survey', in N.E. Miller and K.M. Magruder (eds), *Cost Effectiveness of Psychotherapy.* New York: Oxford University Press.

Rogers, A., Pilgrim, D. and Lacey, R. (1993) *Experiencing Psychiatry: Users' Views of Services.* Basingstoke: Mind/Macmillan.

Rose, D., Wykes, T., Leese, M., Bindman, J. and Fleischmann, P. (2003) 'Patients' perspective on electro-convulsive therapy: systematic review', *British Medical Journal, 326*: 1363–5.

Segal, S.P., Cohen, D. and Marder, S.P. (1992) 'Neuroleptic medication and prescription practices with sheltered care residents – a 12-year perspective', *American Journal of Public Health, 82* (6): 846–52.

Tsai, A.C., Rosenlicht, N.Z., Jureidini, J.N., Parry, P.I., Spielmans, G.I. et al. (2011) 'Aripiprazole in the maintenance treatment of bipolar disorder: a critical review of the evidence and its dissemination into the scientific literature', *PLoS Medicine, 8* (5): e1000434.

Waddington, J.L., Yuseff, H.A. and Kinsella, A. (1998) 'Mortality in schizophrenia: anti-psychotic polypharmacy and absence of adjunctive anticholinergics over the course of a 10-year prospective study', *British Journal of Psychiatry, 173* (10): 325–9.

Wheeldon, T.J., Robertson, C., Eagles, J.M. and Reid, I. (1999) 'The views and outcomes of consenting and non-consenting patients receiving ECT', *Psychological Medicine, 29*: 221–3.

Psychological Interventions

DEFINITION

The use of conversations or other interpersonal methods to ameliorate mental health problems.

KEY POINTS

- Psychological interventions are outlined.
- The problematic link between psychological theory and these interventions is discussed.
- Questions about the effectiveness of psychological interventions are raised.

Psychological interventions are referred to variously in the professional mental health literature as 'psychological therapies', 'talking treatments', 'psychotherapy' or 'counselling'. They are characterised by forms of stylised conversations with patients (or 'clients'), intended to create mental health gain. There is an explicit taboo on physical contact. This provides an immediate appeal to patients, as they are seemingly less interventionist than biological treatments. However, there are some exceptions. For example, there are some 'body therapies' that involve physical contact. Also, some methods are barely conversational. An example of this would be the use of impersonally delivered positive reinforcement or aversive stimuli in the use of some behavioural techniques. By and large, though, the great bulk of what are described as 'psychological interventions' involve systematised conversations.

When psychological interventions are deployed by professionals, they negotiate therapeutic contracts with clients and deploy explicit rationales for their work. These rationales are wide and varied and reflect the lack of consensus, within both the culture of mental health professionals and of academic psychologists, about how to understand the relationship between experience and behaviour (Cheshire and Pilgrim, 2004). In very broad terms, the types of psychological approach that underpin interventions can be identified as: psychoanalysis, behaviourism, cognitivism, humanism, existentialism, general systems theory and postmodernism. Reviews of the relationship of these theoretical trends to clinical interventions can be found in Dryden (2002).

The link between psychological theory and therapeutic practice is far from straightforward. Some interventions are hybrids, which contain elements of several underpinning theories. The very commonly deployed 'cognitive-behaviour therapy' (or 'CBT' or just 'cognitive therapy') contains a particular contradiction. It is an elaboration of behaviour therapy, which can be traced to the application of behaviourism – a form of psychology which deems inner events to be difficult or impossible to study scientifically. By contrast, cognitivism (or cognitive science) privileges the study of inner events. Moreover, the link with cognitivism in contemporary academic psychology is tenuous. The original champions of cognitive therapy were not applied by cognitive psychologists but by psychiatrists who were developing pragmatic alternatives to psychoanalytical therapy (Beck, 1976; Ellis, 1994). This emphasis on the pragmatics of therapy being privileged over theory can also be found in solution-focused brief therapy, a derivative of family therapy (Hawkes et al., 1998).

Psychological interventions may be used by mental health professionals with natural groups (family therapy), stranger groups (group therapy) or with individuals. Also, therapeutic communities are whole-system treatment regimes that contain a mixture of small and large groups (with or without some individual work). The therapeutic community approach evolved in residential settings and can be traced to the 'moral treatment' of the early asylum system run by lay administrators, before medical superintendents ushered in their preferred physical approaches. The main spur for the therapeutic community movement during the 20th century was the challenge of treating a large number of 'shell-shocked' combatants, but latterly the focus has been mainly on those with a diagnosis of personality disorder or substance misuse (Kennard, 1998).

The cost-effectiveness of conversational methods of treatment has been debated at length with different reviewers offering a range of views. At the critical end of this spectrum, some argue that psychological therapies are dangerous and should be avoided by prospective clients (Masson, 1988). At the other end are those who argue that properly conducted therapy provides demonstrable benefits in response to most mental health problems (Dobson and Craig, 1998). The latter conclusion is about the evidence base supporting therapists who demonstrate 'treatment fidelity' or 'treatment integrity'. That is, they consistently conduct themselves in accordance with the rationale of a specified therapeutic approach.

The gap between the two positions of appraisal may be accounted for by the fact that *in practice* there are always some therapists who are either incompetent or abusive – they lack treatment integrity or they are exploitative. These therapists are actively harmful and provoke what the literature describes as 'deterioration effects'. This group of therapists is important to identify in services, because in psychological interventions the relationship is the main instrument of change and the benign and supportive features of the therapist predict a good outcome (Lambert and Bergin, 1983). They are also important for the overall credibility of talking treatments, because they make the difference between positive and negative aggregate outcomes. The very reputation of psychological therapies depends on competent, non-abusive practitioners.

Pilgrim (1997) noted the evidence to support the following complex picture about psychological interventions:

- The overall evidence is that benign supportive conversations are helpful to people. What is less clear is whether a particular professional *rationale* for helpful conversations is superior to any other.
- The evidence about treatment integrity suggests that professionals are more effective if they are consistently self-disciplined when applying a rationale for their work. However, lay people with no training can use conversations in an effective way to create a psychological improvement in others (they may not *want* the helping role, however).
- While there are few demonstrable differences in outcome *between* different theoretical approaches, there are wide variations in outcome achieved by therapists *within* any particular therapeutic approach. This suggests that the *quality* of a relationship is more important than the psychological theory preferred to *understand* it (reinforcing the first point above).
- There are no strong differences in the outcomes achieved by new and very experienced therapists. Again, this suggests that helpful interpersonal processes may not be linked to the sophistication of the helper but to some other factor.
- People change for the better when not in therapy. This suggests that other variables (including lay relationships) create mental health gain. What is called 'spontaneous remission' may be misleading because it implies that

psychological processes are not operating outside a professional arena – it may understate the power of informal mutual support. If this is the case, then those benefiting most from service contact are probably those whose natural networks are sparse or lacking in supportive relationships.

Despite the ambiguity surrounding the safety and mode of effectiveness of talking treatments, they are frequently a preferred alternative to biological interventions – the mainstay response offered to people with mental health problems. Underlying this grateful endorsement is the shared acculturated idea in modern Western societies that good relationships rebuild or enhance mental health. For this reason, psychological interventions, unlike biological ones, are 'anxiously sought and gratefully received'.

Some postmodern critics have noted that therapy inscribes an identity onto its clients in voluntary relationships derived from its own discourse of what it is to be properly human. For example, Rose (1996: 115) talks of the freedom offered by therapy being 'enacted only at the price of relying on experts of the soul'. Similarly, de Swaan (1991) also talks of clients being 'protoprofessionalised' by a therapy culture – learning the world view of a therapeutic ideology in advance of ever becoming a client. In other words, therapists do not simply respond neutrally to problems in living; they also seek to shape the way life should be led. Nevertheless, de Swaan concludes that: 'granted all that is wrong with the helping professions … most Europeans and Americans may still be suffering more from a lack of what these have to offer than from an overdose' (de Swaan, 1991: 67).

See also: *biological interventions; the mental health service users' movement.*

FURTHER READING

Masson, J. (1988) *Against Therapy*. London: HarperCollins.

Pilgrim, D. (2009) *A Straight Talking Introduction to Psychological Treatment*. Ross-on-Wye: PCCS Books.

REFERENCES

Beck, A.T. (1976) *Cognitive Therapy and the Emotional Disorders*. New York: Meridian.

Cheshire, K. and Pilgrim, D. (2004) *A Short Introduction to Clinical Psychology*. London: Sage.

de Swaan, A. (1991) *The Management of Normality*. London: Routledge.

Dobson, K.S. and Craig, K.D. (eds) (1998) *Empirically Supported Therapies: Best Practice in Professional Psychology*. London: Sage.

Dryden, W. (ed.) (2002) *Handbook of Individual Therapy*. London: Sage.

Ellis, A. (1994) *Reason and Emotion in Psychotherapy* (revised and updated). New York: Birch Lane Press.

Hawkes, D., Marsh, T. and Wigosh, R. (1998) *Solution-focused Therapy: A Handbook for Healthcare Professionals*. Oxford: Butterworth/Heinemann.

Kennard, D. (1998) *An Introduction to Therapeutic Communities*. London: Jessica Kingsley.

Lambert, M.J. and Bergin, A.E. (1983) 'Therapist characteristics and their contribution to psychotherapy outcome', in C.E. Walker (ed.), *The Handbook of Clinical Psychology*, Vol. 1. Homewood, IL: Dow Jones-Irwin.

Masson, J. (1988) *Against Therapy*. London: HarperCollins.
Pilgrim, D. (1997) *Psychotherapy and Society*. London: Sage.
Rose, N. (1996) *Inventing Ourselves*. Cambridge: Cambridge University Press.

Economic Aspects of Mental Health

DEFINITION

Mental health has health economic implications in two senses. First, the amount of money spent on mental health services can be calculated. Second, the economic consequences of mental health problems can be estimated.

KEY POINTS

- Using the UK at the turn of this century as a case study, the economic consequences of mental health problems are considered.
- The costs and benefits of mental health services are discussed.
- A general overview is provided of an economic case for a life course approach to prevention.

In 2013, the Chief Medical Office for public health in England and Wales published a report on evidence-based policy, which included a summary contribution from Knapp and Iemmi from the London School of Economics: 'The economic case for better mental health'. The summary from Knapp and Iemmi (2013) made the following (paraphrased) main points:

- By the turn of this century, '90% of the societal cost of depression was due to unemployment and absenteeism'.
- In relation to children with identified mental disorders in childhood, 12 times more was spent on their education than on a mental health service response.
- Dedicated programmes to support parents with children with a diagnosis of conduct disorder were cost-effective, with a return over 25 years of between 2.8 and 6.1 times the intervention cost. This was largely about crime reduction in the young.
- Early intervention services for first episodes of psychosis are cost-effective: over a ten-year period, every £1 invested avoids a further £15 in service costs.
- More than 11 per cent of the NHS budget spent on long-term conditions relates to mental health problems.

- The above direct costs need to be considered in relation to the indirect costs from unemployment, sick leave and 'presenteeism'. (The latter refer to token attendance but not working or working poorly.) These indirect costs 'totalled £30.3 billion in England in 2009/10 across all mental illnesses, compared with direct health and social care costs of £21.3 billion'. (More will be said on the costs of mental health problems for society below.)
- Regarding suicide by those of working age, the cost per annum in the UK exceeds £1.6 million.

These summary figures are gleaned from longitudinal data, and so are immediately out of date, but they give an important sense of trends and proportions. In the recent past, spending on mental health services and prevention programmes has been a constant focus of controversy, with complaints that mental health is treated poorly compared to physical health.

Although mental health is designated as a priority in healthcare policy, proportionally the growth in expenditure on it, compared to other areas in local government and the NHS, has been slower. As a result, in proportional terms, the share allocated by the local state to mental health services was falling by the turn of this century.

An indicator of that trend was the slow progress in the timetable to implement the *National Service Framework for Mental Health* (Department of Health, 1999). In 2003, the Sainsbury Centre for Mental Health report estimated that in order to meet the deadlines, resource allocation from central government would need to be doubled.

Mental health services then (as now) were subject to a range of peculiar costs or budgetary pressures. These include debt repayment, staff shortages (which lead to expensive short-term agency payments) and the increasing prescribing costs associated with the introduction of new and expensive psychotropic medications. At that time, the Sainsbury Centre for Mental Health report provided a breakdown of spending on mental health services (see Table 3.1).

Table 3.1 Expenditure by service category in 2002–03

Service category	Expenditure (%)
Community mental health teams	17.2
Access and crisis services	6.6
Clinical services, including acute inpatient care	24.6
Secure and high-dependency provision	12.3
Continuing care	12.2
Services for mentally disordered offenders	1.1
Other community and hospital professional teams/specialists	1.6

Service category	Expenditure (%)
Psychological therapy services	4.6
Home support services	2.1
Day services	5.3
Support services	1.5
Services for carers	0.3
Accommodation	10.3
Mental health promotion	0.1
Direct payments	0.1
Total direct costs	**100.0**

The salience of any item or combined items will vary from reader to reader, according to their value framework. Here one reading will be given. First, there is a sociopolitical emphasis on social control. Look at the combined items on acute facilities, secure provision and mentally disordered offenders. Between them they account for nearly 40 per cent of government spending on mental health services. This can be compared with the amount spent on mental health promotion – a mere 0.1 per cent. Second, psychological therapy services only receive 4.6 per cent of spending (suggesting a biomedical inertia in the mental health care system). Third, other non-hospital-based services, which are meant to signal a service reconfiguration towards community-based interventions, are lagging behind the political rhetoric of the chapter on mental health in *The NHS Plan* (Department of Health, 2000). Between them, the items on new assertive outreach, crisis resolution, early intervention and services for carers account for less than 7 per cent of spending.

As a result of the ongoing debate at the turn of this century about mental health having a 'Cinderella' status in health policy, the British government responded with its document *No Health without Mental Health* (Department of Health, 2011). The aspirations in the document reflected a cross-government agreement on policy priorities, although no clear and detailed investment plan, with committed money, was articulated in the document. Its aspirations included: mental health promotion; improved physical health for those with mental health problems; more patient-centred care; and a reduction in stigma and discrimination for people with identified mental health problems.

THE COST OF MENTAL HEALTH PROBLEMS

A range of studies in Europe and North America has estimated the economic cost of mental health problems. A caution when reading these is that they start from and reinforce a discourse of burden. For example, they do not include estimates of positive contributions arising from the role of creativity in society (see the entry on

Creativity) or on the role of user involvement, user-led services or the supportive or caring role some of those with mental health problems can provide to their families (Szmukler, 1996). Nevertheless, the burden discourse has legitimacy in a context in which social order and economic efficiency dominate sociopolitical priorities.

Knapp (2001) discusses the economic burden under several headings, which will be summarised here:

- *Labour market features are important* Only 20 per cent of psychotic patients are in paid employment (Foster et al., 1996). About a third of sickness absence from work is attributable to 'minor' mental health problems (Jenkins, 1985). The direction of causality is contested about labour market disadvantage (Rogers and Pilgrim, 2003) (see the entry on Social Class). For psychotic conditions, employer discrimination is clear (Campbell and Heginbotham, 1991). For anxiety states and depression, it is more likely that the primary disability of the symptoms means that patients are unable to work. Knapp (2001) summarises three main points under this heading. First, patients not working become socially excluded (like other unemployed people). Second, the welfare payments to them are a toll on the taxpayer. Third, where near full employment is the case in the economy, sickness absence due to mental health problems leads to productivity losses.
- *Some studies emphasise the economic family impact* For example, relatives may need to transport patients to and from mental health facilities or outpatient appointments (Creed et al., 1997) and may be out of pocket in their ancillary role to state provision (Schene et al., 1996). Families that have psychotic relatives are estimated to spend about 6–9 hours per day in ways which limit their social activity or which are experienced as stressful (Magliano et al., 1998). In the case of senile dementia, relatives can be involved for up to 45 hours per week in unpaid care (Cavallo and Fattore, 1997).
- *Premature death is also noteworthy* For people with a diagnosis of schizophrenia, the risk of death is 1.6 times greater (controlled for age and gender) than that for the general population. Premature death rates in all diagnostic groups are higher than in the general population (Harris and Barraclough, 1998), but especially for those who abuse substances or have an eating disorder. Much, but not all, of this mortality profile occurs because of raised rates of suicide. The premature death of those of working age removes them from both the labour market and the welfare burden, if they were unemployed. As Knapp (2001) notes, these brutal economic gains and marginal losses to productivity have to be set against the personal and social loss involved.
- Mentally disordered offenders, although small, constitute a group which creates multiple costs. There are the direct costs to victims and their insurers. Those to the criminal justice system have to be included as well. It should be emphasised, however, that both of these are also applicable to non-mentally disordered offenders. Over and above these, patient offenders have some unique costs attached to their assessment and 'disposal' into forensic mental health services. These are much more costly per capita than prison facilities.

- Welfare payments to people with mental health problems in the mid-1990s in Britain came to more than £7 billion (Patel and Knapp, 1998). People with 'mild to moderate mental health problems' are a specific burden on sickness and invalidity benefits, prompting the British government in 2007 to offer new rehabilitation services for them to work – the 'Pathways to Work' scheme. However, the National Audit Office quickly reported that the scheme was ineffective (National Audit Office, 2010). In the same year, the Department of Work and Pensions declared that the scheme had been a total failure and it was closed by the government a year later.

DRGS AND PSYCHOSOCIAL SOURCES OF COSTS

The estimate of costs to health services by economists is typically based on diagnostic-related groups, or 'DRGs', as a starting point for their calculations (such as the incidence or prevalence of 'schizophrenia' nationally or regionally). However, this has three problems in its logic. First, the conceptual validity of specific functional psychiatric DRGs is now well rehearsed (see the entries on Psychiatric Classification and Causes and Consequences of Mental Health Problems). Second, a diagnosis *per se* says little about risk or dependency. In practice, it is decision-making about both or either of these that tends to determine service activity and types of service (inpatient or community), and so explains the costs incurred. Third, rather than the cost of DRGs being calculated, we could instead trace psychosocial antecedents and their link to service utilisation, which might be more illuminating. For example, the National Society for the Prevention of Cruelty to Children (NSPCC) in the UK calculated that the outcomes of child sexual abuse cost the British government £3.2 billion in 2012. These costs accrued from demands made by survivors of the abuse on mental health and addiction services and the necessary responses of the police and social workers.

A final point to note in this section is that the political discourse about burden often focuses on 'severe and enduring mental illness' (largely a code for those diagnosed with schizophrenia). However, only 10 per cent of the global burden is accounted for by this group and over half is accounted for by anxiety and depression (Andrews and Henderson, 2000). This highlights how policy decisions about the 'burden' may sometimes be skewed by considerations other than the equity of service allocation based on diagnostic prevalence, such as the need to exercise social control over madness in general, and dangerous madness in particular. This reinforces the need to consider the topic of the economic costs of mental health problems with a political as well as a financial eye.

AN ECONOMIC CASE FOR PREVENTION

The principle of prevention is discussed in several entries in this book. Here I will note just the economic dimensions to that principle. McDaid and colleagues (2018) examined the health economic case for prevention using a life-course framework. Much of this focuses on secondary prevention (identifying life transition points that raise the probability of mental health problems emerging). It excludes more fundamental considerations of social group membership (poverty, age, race and so on), although the life-course approach helps us to focus on intra-group differences. For example, not all poor people have mental health problems, even though poverty is a strong predictor of them, so how do we account for this?

The review of McDaid et al. also covers some of the economic advantages of primary and tertiary prevention. For example, the population-level reduction of hypertension reduces the incidence of vascular dementia and thus reduces the treatment costs and carer burden. In the case of tertiary prevention, CBT and mindfulness reduce relapse in those with a diagnosis of depression, again reducing social and healthcare costs. The vulnerability of transition points in the life course largely links to the literature on life events at vulnerable transitional points (such as childbirth or becoming unemployed). In addition to this focus, I draw attention as well to the relevance of 'chronic strains' and 'daily hassles' in the entry on Secondary Prevention.

See also: *creativity; evidence-based practice; mental health promotion; public mental health; secondary prevention; social class; social exclusion; suicide; the quality of mental health care.*

FURTHER READING

Becker, T. and Kilian, R. (2006) 'Psychiatric services for people with severe mental illness across Western Europe: what can be generalized from current knowledge about differences in provision, costs and outcomes of mental health care?', *Acta Psychiatrica Scandinavica*, 429: 9–16.

Birnbaum, H.G., Kessler, R.C. et al. (2010) 'Employer burden of mild, moderate, and severe major depressive disorder: mental health services utilization and costs, and work performance', *Depression and Anxiety*, 27 (3): 78–89.

REFERENCES

Andrews, G. and Henderson, S. (eds) (2000) *Unmet Need in Psychiatry*. Cambridge: Cambridge University Press.

Campbell, T. and Heginbotham, C. (1991) *Mental Illness: Prejudice, Discrimination and the Law*. Aldershot: Dartmouth.

Cavallo, M.C. and Fattore, G. (1997) 'The economic and social burden of Alzheimer's disease on families in the Lombardy region', *Alzheimer's Disease and Associated Disorders*, 11 (4): 184–90.

Creed, F., Mbaya, P., Lancashire, S., Tomenson, B., Williams, B. and Holme, S. (1997) 'Cost effectiveness of day and inpatient psychiatric treatment: results of a randomised controlled trial', *British Medical Journal*, 314: 1381–5.

Department of Health (DH) (1999) *National Service Framework for Mental Health*. London: HMSO.

Department of Health (DH) (2000) *The NHS Plan*. London: HMSO.

Department of Health (DH) (2011) *No Health without Mental Health*. London: DH.

Foster, K., Meltzer, H., Gill, B. and Hinds, K. (1996) *Adults with Psychotic Disorder Living in the Community: OPCS Survey of Psychiatric Morbidity*. London: HMSO.

Harris, E.C. and Barraclough, B. (1998) 'Excess mortality of mental disorder', *British Journal of Psychiatry*, 173: 11–53.

key concepts in
mental health

Jenkins, R. (1985) 'Minor psychiatric disorder in employed young men and women and its contribution to sickness absence', *British Journal of Industrial Medicine*, 42: 147–53.

Knapp, M. (2001) 'The costs of mental disorder', in G. Thornicroft and G. Szmukler (eds), *Textbook of Community Psychiatry*. Oxford: Oxford University Press.

Knapp, M. and Iemmi, I. (2013) 'The economic case for better mental health', in *Annual Report of the Chief Medical Officer 2013, Public Mental Health Priorities: Investing in the Evidence*. London: Department of Health.

Magliano, L., Fadden, G., Madianos, M. et al. (1998) 'Burden on the families of patients with schizophrenia', *Social Psychiatry and Psychiatric Epidemiology*, 33: 405–12.

McDaid, D., Park, A.-L. and Wahlbeck, K. (2018) 'The economic case for the prevention of mental illness', *Annual Review of Public Health*, 40 (1): 373–89.

National Audit Office (NAO) (2010) *Support to Incapacity Benefits Claimants through Pathways to Work*. London: NAO.

Patel, A. and Knapp, M.R.J. (1998) 'Cost of mental illness in England', *Mental Illness Review Research*, 5: 4–10.

Rogers, A. and Pilgrim, D. (2003) *Mental Health and Inequality*. Basingstoke: Palgrave Macmillan.

Sainsbury Centre for Mental Health (2003) *Money for Mental Health: A Review of Public Spending on Mental Health Care*. London: Sainsbury Centre for Mental Health.

Schene, A.H., Tessler, R.C. and Gamache, G.M. (1996) 'Caregiving in severe mental illness: conceptualization and measurement', in H.C. Knudsen and G. Thornicroft (eds), *Mental Health Service Evaluation*. Cambridge: Cambridge University Press.

Szmukler, G. (1996) 'From family "burden" to caregiving', *Psychiatric Bulletin*, 20: 449–51.

The Quality of Mental Health Care

DEFINITION

The quality of mental health care is judged by the measurable achievements of its aims. The latter include mental health gain, coercive social control and the reversal of psychological impairments.

KEY POINTS

- Assessing the quality of mental health care points up its purposes.
- General criteria of quality in healthcare are applicable but particular ones have to be applied in mental health services.
- Different questions are posed about service quality depending on whether mental health gain or social control on behalf of third parties predominates.

The quality of mental health care raises many questions about its purpose. As part of a wider health service, generic criteria can be applied about such topics as hygiene, environmental safety, civility of staff, accessibility for the general public as visitors and equity of access for those referring into the service (in the case of the British NHS, this mainly means general practitioners). However, the particular functions of mental health services can be examined beyond these general features because mental health is much more controversial than physical health. The former is always open to interpretation, with many views prevailing about causes and consequences. Also, mental health services are unique in being associated with legal powers to detain and treat patients. For these reasons, at various points, mental health services might:

1. Offer to ameliorate distress or create mental health gain which is anxiously sought and gratefully received from truly voluntary patients.
2. Temporarily resolve a social crisis by removing an identified patient from a difficult interpersonal drama. All psychiatric crises are social crises.
3. Contain those posing a risk to themselves or others for varying amounts of time. These risks might be identified retrospectively by proven criminal acts (in the case of mentally abnormal offenders treated in health settings) or prospectively in detained patients who have committed no criminal act but arouse paternalistic concern in others about their welfare.
4. Enable people disabled by mental health problems, under the second and third organisational arrangements, to maximise their potential as citizens: 'psychiatric rehabilitation' is the typical description of this activity.

Only the first on this list can be judged by general health service standards about good care for those patients who enter the sick role voluntarily and act as active collaborators or acquiescent participants in treatment. At the individual level, we can simply ask whether the service is *accessible* to people who express a need for it and whether they are treated in ways that are *acceptable* to them and *appropriate* for their needs.

At the level of the health system, we can also ask whether services are *equitably available* and whether they deliver *cost-effective* treatments. These are standard criteria of success for health services and are thus measurable parameters of quality. Most patients treated for mental health problems in these circumstances are seen in a primary care setting. This suggests that the quality of primary mental health care is particularly important for the majority of us.

However, if our focus shifts to the second and third functions, which are found within the remit of specialist mental health services, then these criteria about service quality do not always fit readily. Instead, we might ask other questions about the success of the service in reducing the risk to self and others. This would be judged by measures of escape, suicide and self-harm or of patient violence (as inpatients or outpatients). These concerns about safety or *risk minimisation* take us away from the first scenario in which the mental health gain for the patient is the central purpose of the service. The main difference relates to two versions of therapeutic social control, with one responding to *expressed need* and the other responding to *defined need*.

In the case of truly voluntary patients in primary care or (less commonly) as psychiatric inpatients or outpatients, the first version entails the patient entering the sick role voluntarily. It still fulfils a role of social regulation by removing the inefficiency of sick people from society and by providing legitimate permission for this without harm or stigma to the patient.

In the second version of therapeutic social control, coercion is applied explicitly or hovers as a threat in the background for all. In these circumstances, professional action is guided by the need to avoid the risk to self and/or a nuisance or threat to others. Now the concern about economic efficiency is joined by the removal of threats to a moral order (by preventing rule infraction). It was noted above that all psychiatric crises are social crises. Coercion is used to resolve these crises and prevent their repetition. Because of this, harm and stigma are inevitable for identified patients.

Turning to the fourth on the list, since the closure of the asylum system, the main question now relates to quality of life and the surveillance of patients to check that they are not a risk to themselves or others. It is here that most ambiguity surrounds the interplay of the two types of therapeutic social control noted. Either can be in play at a moment in time for a particular patient, which creates ethical dilemmas for professionals seeking to maintain collaborative relationships with patients. The existence of community supervision orders in many countries now means that professionals face these dilemmas on a daily basis.

Thus, our understanding of service quality, when recovery is agreed to be the aim involved, would take into account those questions posed jointly about the first three scenarios. Sometimes, it will be about judging the mental health gain, especially in relation to quality of life in community settings, but at other times it may retain performance indicators about risk minimisation.

To conclude, any judgements we make about the quality of mental health care will require careful consideration about what it is we expect from them, especially in the confusion surrounding expressed and defined needs. When making these judgements, we might differ in expectations between one another. We might also change our views about what is to be expected, depending on the identified patient and different circumstances. We may differ from others in our judgements, especially if we are the patient in question. In this complex set of circumstances, it is not a simple matter of developing fixed objective criteria of service quality. 'Quality' is ultimately negotiated intersubjectively with different answers arising in different circumstances. The quality of a mental health service will be judged differently by politicians, managers, patients, significant others and clinical staff. Consequently, any discussion of the topic has to take these different perspectives into consideration.

See also: *coercion; primary care; recovery.*

FURTHER READING

Brugha, T.S. and Lindsay, F. (1996) 'Quality of mental health service care: the forgotten pathway from process to outcome', *Social Psychiatry and Psychiatric Epidemiology*, 31: 89–98.

Department of Health (DH) (2004) *Standards for Better Health*. London: DH.

Donabedian, A. (1988) 'The quality of health care: how can it be assessed?', *Journal of American Medical Association*, 12: 260.

King, S. (2010) 'Cost and impact of a quality improvement programme in mental health services', *Journal of Health Services Research & Policy*, 15 (2): 69–75.

Pilgrim, D. (2018) 'Are kindly and efficacious mental health services possible?', *Journal of Mental Health*, 27 (4): 295–7.

Evidence-based Practice

DEFINITION

Professional practice and service routines that are guided by evidence.

KEY POINTS

- Evidence-based practice is outlined.
- Assumptions about a hierarchy of evidence are outlined.
- Criticisms of evidence-based practice are rehearsed.

Evidence-based practice (EBP) has been important in healthcare generally for a number of years. Here its salience and persuasiveness will be rehearsed. Then criticisms of EBP will be noted in their particular relation to mental health services:

- *Economic rationalism* This comes at the top of the list to support EBP. With limited budgets, it is important to clarify (if we can – see later) whether a form of practice is effective (does it work?) and is cost-effective (is it the cheapest way of getting a certain result?). In the literature, these are called 'clinical effectiveness' and 'cost-effectiveness' (or 'efficiency'), respectively.
- *Risk minimisation* This is another driver of EBP. It is possible that without evidence for a positive impact of an intervention then harm may be done.
- *Service improvement* This can be achieved by the use of information gathering to check on performance. Evidence here has a double significance. EBP can be monitored to clarify whether a particular service is functioning in line with assumed best practice. Also, evidence gathering is used in systems to make such assessments. This can provide the basis for efforts at improvement and then more information can be gathered to check if the improvement has

occurred. This is called the 'audit cycle', as it is potentially an unending cycle of checking and changing.

- *Political accountability* This is another reason to support EBP. Users of services, taxpayers and politicians can demand to see evidence that their investment in services and professional interventions is worthwhile. This is partly about economic rationalism, but it is more than this because evidence can be gathered about matters other than cost-effectiveness. For example, are services equitably distributed (in socialised forms of medicine like the British NHS)? Do patients consider that interventions are appropriate for their needs? Are they acceptable to service users? Are services accessible? Evidence gathered about these sorts of questions has a democratic function.

It is common now for healthcare systems to operate a shared framework that defines evidence in hierarchical form. Systematic reviews of randomised controlled trials (RCTs) are at the top of the hierarchy (studies are pooled and overall average effects are then specified) and personal experience is at the bottom. In between are particular RCTs, cross-sectional surveys, case studies and consensus statements from groups of experts. This hierarchy is open to challenge. It is favoured by medicine but its critics argue that mental health is ultimately a social and existential matter for ordinary people, and so we require bodies of knowledge that are fitting for this picture rather than ones that are favoured by some professionals. The latter can gain power and privilege from their preferred forms of knowledge, which may arouse suspicion and criticism in disaffected service users.

EBP can be criticised, with some justification, on a number of grounds, which need to be considered not so much to discredit the concept in principle (its scientific and democratic merits were noted earlier), but to put its limits or potential into a realistic context:

- *Pragmatic considerations* If organisations or practitioners could function when evidence was available to justify their actions, then the mental health system would grind to a complete halt. Absence of evidence is not necessarily evidence of absence – although, of course, it may be. Most of the time, we do not know what works when complex systems deal with people with complex problems. EBP is derived from the logic of closed systems, whereas services and their users exist in open systems in constant flux. This implies the need for pragmatic knowledge about actual everyday services rather than evidence derived from RCTs. The latter are conducted in artificial conditions on artificial samples of patients – so, how useful are they? Maybe the assumed pecking order in the hierarchy of evidence noted earlier deserves our critical scrutiny – practical feasibility and meaningfulness are important in everyday life. Currently, most of the evidence-based practice is predicated on meta-analytic studies of treatment interventions. We know very little about the effectiveness of complex and whole systems of care delivery. We do know that overall the prevalence of mental disorders has not decreased despite their existence, implying mainly that their role is one of containment and care rather than cure. Following from this point, the methodological challenges of appraising the effectiveness of open systems (the world of politics, economic cycles and variable relationships between the intention of policies and their actual implementation) are different from the closed system world of RCTs in examining intervention compared to placebo. In practice, we know little about the precise effectiveness or efficacy of mental health systems, the precise link between service processes and service outcomes, or how to implement successful preventative rather than curative/reactive measures.

- *Political considerations* Politicians who demand EBP to warrant the financial allocation for mental health work often act in an evidence-free zone themselves. Part of this is hypocrisy (remember the 'evidence' that justified the invasion of Iraq?), but part is also warranted because policy is driven by values and not just evidence. Sometimes politicians and those they represent simply want certain things to happen as moral imperatives. Evidence has not been, and will not be, used as a justification. Take rape as an example – we do not argue that we need to check if there is any evidence that it does its victims harm before condemning it and legislating against it. Policy is about the practical allocation of values in society and evidence can be used to justify or criticise that allocation but it cannot define the values themselves.

- *Non-empirical considerations* The evidence-based medicine movement has focused overwhelmingly on clinical and cost-effectiveness. However, satisfactory patient experiences are also based on appropriate, accessible and acceptable aspects of care. How do we garner evidence about these? How do we define them? What if there are inevitable subjective and contextual differences? What works for whom and when, according to patients not staff? These imply qualitative descriptions and ethical suppositions rather than measurable variables. Thus, what is 'good care' has to take into account non-empirical, not just empirical, considerations. To extend the above point about political matters, perhaps the routines of a mental health service should be based in large part on values and not just quantifiable aggregate data about effectiveness. Perhaps we should aim to treat people with respect and dignity and maximise their rights as citizens because this is politically and morally desirable – *whether or not* we ever acquire the evidence to justify it. Not only does this values-based approach qualify any simple enthusiasm for evidence-based practice, it is supported as well by clinicians who are interested in practice-based evidence (what works for their particular patients in their particular service settings). This harks back to the pragmatic considerations noted above.

- *Pre-empirical considerations* These refer to the problem of concept definition. EBP works best when there is no dispute about the target for change. Take the question: Does a new 'anti-psychotic' medication treat schizophrenia successfully compared to a placebo? This is only meaningful if the conceptual validity of 'schizophrenia' is clear and thus its legitimacy is obvious. But, as with all functional psychiatric diagnoses, this is not the case. In these circumstances, EBP can be rendered meaningless or deemed to be illegitimate.

Evidence is a form of knowledge but not the only form. At the heart of debates about EBP in mental health is whether other forms of knowledge are as important as those derived from quantitative methods and experimental conditions in closed systems. The latter clearly are helpful but they are not sufficient to reflect on the complexities of human action and experience. The latter are also open to productive exploration by philosophers, ethnographers, artists, theologians, dramatists and novelists. The favoured methods of experimental science based on quantification and replicability do not have to define singularly our field of inquiry. If they do that, it risks setting up an assumed dichotomy between 'facts' that constitute 'evidence' on the one hand and the rest of our knowledge which is then deemed to be 'fiction', 'opinion' or just 'personal experience', and thus illegitimate, on the other. People thinking, feeling and acting in open systems cannot be properly understood if we adhere to this dichotomy.

See also: *causes and consequences of mental health problems; neuroscience; subjective and objective aspects of mental health.*

FURTHER READING

Cooper, B. (2003) 'Evidence-based mental health policy: a critical appraisal', *British Journal of Psychiatry*, 183: 105–13.

Evans, C., Margison, F. and Barkham, M. (1998) 'The contribution of reliable and clinically significant change methods to evidence based mental health', *Evidence Based Mental Health*, 1: 70–2.

Fulford, K.W.M., Peile, E. and Carroll, H. (2012) *Essential Values-based Practice: Linking Science with People.* Cambridge: Cambridge University Press.

Sackett, D.L., Richardson, W.S., Rosenberg, W. and Haynes, R.B. (1997) *Evidence-based Medicine: How to Practice and Teach EBM.* New York: Churchill Livingstone.

Williams, D.D.R. and Garner, J. (2002) 'The case against the "evidence": a different perspective on evidence-based medicine', *British Journal of Psychiatry*, 180: 8–12.

Recovery

DEFINITION

Recovery refers to the extent to which a person with mental health problems regains or attains a meaningful life, with or without their symptoms.

KEY POINTS

- Recovery is a contested concept.
- For professionals, it is about successful treatment or rehabilitation but for critical service users, it is about survival and emancipation.

Despite the succinct offer of a definition above, in recent years, 'recovery' became contested as quickly as it became popular. Its current popularity among all stakeholders taking an interest in mental health problems risks a misleading picture of agreement. As Davidson and Roe note: 'There is an increasing global commitment to recovery as *the* expectation for people with mental illness. There remains, however, little consensus on what recovery means in relation to mental illness' (2007: 459, emphasis in the original).

In the 1990s, Anthony (1993) described recovery as the 'guiding vision' for mental health services. The term started to gain popularity in the late 1980s, reflecting the great push to replace large-scale institutional care with community care. Any analysis of recovery needs to take into account the various factors relevant to that shift. These include: the cost to the state of long-term large hospital care; criticisms from radical professionals about the anti-therapeutic impact of this care; the new social movement of disaffected service users with their demands for citizenship; the widespread impact of consumerism in health and welfare policies; and professional claims about therapeutic optimism. The latter include professional preferences for chemical or conversational correctives to mental health problems and an emphasis on the 'pharmacological revolution' or 'increasing access to psychological therapies'.

This recent therapeutic optimism is not new (Pilgrim and McCrainie, 2013). Before the pessimism associated with the eugenic consensus of the late 19th century, those running the asylums and madhouses would make ambitious claims about cures. What constrains such optimism about recovery from mental health problems today is the modern emphasis upon risk minimisation. Thus, therapeutic optimism and an emphasis on citizenship for those previously put away, out of sight and out of mind, are limited by the presence of 'mental health law'. This is specifically designed to control risk and nuisance. As a consequence, when applied effectively and legitimately, it does not produce social inclusion (one defining expectation of successful recovery) but social exclusion.

Therefore, hopes for a simple consensus about recovery are confounded by two challenges at present. The first is that open-ended expectations about full citizenship for those with mental health problems are constrained by this risk emphasis enshrined in 'mental health law' and compounded by public prejudice and discrimination against those who are psychologically different in society.

The second challenge is that 'recovery' is relatively new and, for now, conceptually elastic. In the latter regard, one distinction made by Davidson and Roe (2007) to correct their own caution against the concept being over-inclusive is between 'recovery from' and 'recovery in' mental illness. The former is akin to a cure (the removal of symptoms and a return to full psychosocial functioning), while the latter is akin to recovery in the sense used by Alcoholics Anonymous. Mental health problems are viewed as long-term conditions that people live with daily, and try to make progress about, despite their vulnerability to relapse to various degrees or even despite the ongoing presence of symptoms. If a problem cannot be 'cured', it might be endured and coped with. It might even provide a special source of meaning.

Elsewhere (Pilgrim, 2009), I make a further distinction between three versions of recovery:

1. Recovery from illness, i.e. an outcome of successful *treatment*.
2. Recovery from impairment, i.e. an outcome of successful *rehabilitation*.
3. Recovery from invalidation, i.e. an outcome of successful *survival*.

In the first, an 'old wine in new bottles' approach can be adopted from biomedical psychiatry. Recovery is about patients complying with medical treatment and getting better. Those not complying are lacking in insight about the need to take their medication, or if they do comply, but remain symptomatic, they are deemed to be 'treatment resistant'.

In the second, social psychiatry encourages contracts with patients to tailor treatment packages, emphasising social skills training, which enables them to stay out of hospital for as long as possible.

In the third, service contact may be seen as part of the problem rather than part of the solution. Here, critical service users see recovery as the struggle to cope with and overcome a form of triple invalidation – an emancipatory emphasis. Psychiatric patients have survived the insults in childhood that gave rise to their psychological problems. They have survived the coercion and clinical iatrogenesis of service contact (hence the term 'psychiatric survivors'). And they have survived stigma and social exclusion in an intolerant society.

Hopper (2007) suggests that recovery entails: renewing a sense of possibility (the politics of hope from psychiatric survivors); regaining competencies (the rehabilitation emphasis of social psychiatrists); reconnection and finding a place in society (endorsed by all three conceptions of recovery noted earlier); and 'reconciliation work' (the rebuilding of self-confidence and individual agency, lost or fragile, emphasised by psychiatric survivors). However, Hopper also goes on to note that what is missing from this overly personal discourse about recovery is social structure: 'race, gender and class tend to fade away into unexamined background realities, underscoring (intentionally? inadvertently?) the defining centrality of psychiatric disability in these lives' (Hopper, 2007: 868).

Hopper encourages a refocusing of recovery on to a 'capabilities approach' (World Health Organization, 2001). This makes a link between decrements in health and increments in disability for all of us and so it does not split off disabled people from the rest of humanity (sometimes called 'othering'). It also emphasises the impact of the social structural factors on recovery noted by Hopper. These can be ignored if the only focus is one of human agency and human rights. The latter tend to be at the centre of the libertarian user criticisms of psychiatric theory and practice, described earlier.

Recovery from mental disability is not simply or mainly about professional interventions or degrees of individual compliance with, or resistance to, them. It is instead about the availability of meaningful daily activity (including employment), access to independent living and the availability of social support. This is the virtuous circle of increased social capital leading to improvements in health and the latter then improving confidence and competence in social engagement. Thus, the availability of community resources to facilitate this virtuous circle is independent of the actions of professionals or patients as individuals. A risk of focusing on recovery as a personal journey is that, paradoxically, it over-personalises the responsibility of the patient for stasis and change. The wider context of mental health problems shapes the latter in ways which are not about individual-level action but social causation and evaluation.

See also: *causes and consequences of mental health problems; evidence-based practice; social models of mental health.*

FURTHER READING

Davidson, L. and Roe, D. (2007) '"Recovery from" and "recovery" in serious mental illness: one strategy for lessening confusion plaguing recovery', *Journal of Mental Health*, 16 (4): 459–70.
Pilgrim, D. and McCrainie, A. (2013) *Recovery and Mental Health: A Critical Sociological Account*. Basingstoke: Palgrave Macmillan.

REFERENCES

Anthony, W.A. (1993) 'Recovery from mental illness: the guiding vision of the mental health system in the 1990s', *Psychosocial Rehabilitation Journal*, 16: 11.
Davidson, L. and Roe, D. (2007) '"Recovery from" and "recovery" in serious mental illness: one strategy for lessening confusion plaguing recovery', *Journal of Mental Health*, 16 (4): 459–70.
Hopper, K. (2007) 'Rethinking social recovery in schizophrenia: what a capabilities approach might offer', *Social Science & Medicine*, 65 (5): 868–79.
Pilgrim, D. (2009) 'The role of recovery in modern "mental health" policy', *Chronic Illness*, 4 (4): 295–304.
Pilgrim, D. and McCrainie, A. (2013) *Recovery and Mental Health: A Critical Sociological Account*. Basingstoke: Palgrave Macmillan.
World Health Organization (WHO) (2001) *International Classification of Functioning Disability and Health*. Geneva: WHO.

Coercion

DEFINITION

The use or threat of force in order to ensure a human being complies with the wishes of others. In the context of mental health services, coercion ensures compulsory detention, compulsory treatment or compulsory isolation.

- The circumstances under which psychiatric coercion occurs are described.
- A continuum of engagement between voluntarism and coercion is discussed.
- Ethical challenges to psychiatric coercion are highlighted.

One of the most controversial aspects of mental health services is their association with coercion. At the centre of this controversy is the ethical norm that adult human beings do not coerce others. The typical lawful exception to this is when people break the criminal law. Under these circumstances, the police are given delegated lawful powers of coercive detention. What makes mental health services unique is that equivalent powers are lawfully delegated to health workers to control mental disorder and that liberty may be deprived without trial, even when no crime has been committed.

Broadly, there are three circumstances when this happens. First, mentally disordered offenders may be compulsorily detained in forensic mental health services. Second (and more frequently), people with mental health problems, who have not committed a criminal offence, are detained or treated against their wishes. At the time of writing, in Britain, the conditions under which these groups are coerced are described under the 1983 Mental Health Act, with sections of the Act, which refer to 'mentally disordered offenders', being separated from those about 'civil' patients. Third, in some countries, there are legal powers to provide involuntary treatment in community settings.

The probability of coercion is predicted, to some extent, by diagnosis. Those with diagnoses of functional psychosis or antisocial personality disorder are treated more coercively – the former in acute mental health services and the latter in forensic mental health services. The other group of patients who are subject to raised levels of coercion are those who are profoundly depressed and actively suicidal.

Szmukler and Appelbaum (2001) point out that coercion is the most extreme point on a continuum of engagement between mental health professionals and patients. At the other end of the continuum is completely voluntary contact, initiated and maintained by the client. Some commentators, such as de Swaan (1991), have noted that even this point involves patients being acculturated to expect and demand treatment from professionals ('protoprofessionalisation'), raising a question about the nature of voluntarism.

Further towards coercion, from pure voluntarism, are four gradations of influence, on what Szmukler and Appelbaum describe as a 'spectrum of pressures':

- *Persuasion* A patient may be reasoned with and reminded of the consequences of not cooperating with treatment in the past.
- *Leverage* Here a professional might express disappointment in the client's non-cooperative stance. This might lead to cooperation if the client is dependent on the professional.

coercion

183

- *Inducements* The patient may be offered advantages related to community living in exchange for treatment compliance.
- *Threat* Here the patient is told that, regretfully, if they do not agree to treatment or hospitalisation, then formal powers of compulsion will be invoked; they are made an offer they cannot refuse.

This spectrum or continuum between voluntary and involuntary personal engagement exists in a formal legal context in developed countries. Libertarian critics of mental health law point out that as long as the threat of involuntary detention and treatment exists, then the point of genuine voluntary contact on the continuum becomes meaningless (Szasz, 1970). Certainly, patient accounts of officially entering hospital informally or voluntarily suggest that the common use of threat of coercion leads to many being recorded as being voluntary, but they are really 'pseudo-voluntary' patients (Rogers, 1993). This also raises a more general point about conceptualising the spectrum noted above: it has subjective as well as objective indicators. For example, a voluntary patient may *feel* coerced even when there is no formal record of coercion being evident and coercion is denied by the treating professionals (Hiday, 1992).

Coercion is thought to be warranted, by professionals and others, on two broad grounds. First, there is the paternalistic justification that psychiatric patients often do not recognise the need for treatment, and therefore others have to act in their interests to protect their health and wellbeing. Second, sometimes there is a need to protect third parties. (Together, these two points are also captured in the phrase 'risk to self or others'.)

Ethical questions arise on both fronts about discrimination against people with mental health problems. In relation to the preventative paternalistic motive, there are many examples of those without mental health problems who act in a self-injurious way and where enforced medical paternalism could play an effective preventative role. Common examples are cigarette smoking and excessive eating. However, smokers and obese people are not detained without trial or treated compulsorily. With regard to a danger to others, speeding driving and drunken violence can lead to detention (though even here not inevitably). However, when this occurs, it is after due legal process has been applied and only in relation to past proven action, not *potential* action, on the part of the perpetrator. Thus, although ethical grounds can be invoked to justify psychiatric coercion, these grounds can be substantially challenged. It is also clear that the ways in which rules of coercion are differentially applied to people with mental health problems mean that they suffer discrimination.

Coercion has played a role in discussions of both the secondary and tertiary prevention of mental illness. Secondary prevention involves nipping an illness in the bud, when early symptoms appear. Tertiary prevention is about staving off a relapse in those already ill. An example of the latter point is the professional eagerness to ensure a compliance with medication in psychotic patients, in order to prevent a relapse and the need for hospitalisation. With regard to secondary prevention, there has been a recent controversy about early intervention in psychosis. Those in favour of this would like to have powers to ensure treatment compliance in those seen to be at risk. Those against this aspiration point out that prediction of actual psychosis in individuals is difficult and it places those who would not go on to become psychotic at risk of the adverse effects of medication (Bentall and Morrison, 2002; cf. Miller and McGlashan, 2003).

For the foreseeable future, it is likely that in developed societies legal powers will be maintained and occasionally reformed in order to ensure that people with mental health problems are removed from society and are obliged to accept treatment. It is also likely that substantial ethical controversy and some political opposition will continue to surround both of these trends. Aside from the question of human rights violations, when coercion is applied by one human being on another, mental health professionals also struggle with the knowledge that the more they are seen to coerce the less likely it is that patients will contact them for help voluntarily. The known presence of recurrent coercion in mental health services encourages people with mental health problems to evade contact.

See also: *mental health policy; risks to and from people with mental health problems; segregation.*

FURTHER READING

Atkinson, J. (2007) *Advance Directives in Mental Health: Theory, Practice and Ethics.* London: Jessica Kingsley.

Szmukler, G. and Appelbaum, P. (2001) 'Treatment pressures, coercion and compulsion', in G. Thornicroft and G. Szmukler (eds), *Textbook of Community Psychiatry.* Oxford: Oxford University Press.

REFERENCES

Bentall, R.P. and Morrison, A.P. (2002) 'More harm than good: the case against using antipsychotic drugs to prevent severe mental illness', *Journal of Mental Health, 2*: 351–6.

de Swaan, A. (1991) *The Management of Normality.* London: Routledge.

Hiday, V. (1992) 'Coercion in civil commitment: process, preferences and outcome', *International Journal of Law and Psychiatry, 15*: 359–77.

Miller, T.J. and McGlashan, T.H. (2003) 'The risks of not intervening in pre-onset psychotic illness', *Journal of Mental Health, 12* (4): 345–9.

Rogers, A. (1993) 'Coercion and voluntary admission: an examination of psychiatric patients' views', *Behavioral Sciences and the Law, 11*: 259–67.

Szasz, T.S. (1970) *Ideology and Insanity.* New York: Doubleday.

Szmukler, G. and Appelbaum, P. (2001) 'Treatment pressures, coercion and compulsion', in G. Thornicroft and G. Szmukler (eds), *Textbook of Community Psychiatry.* Oxford: Oxford University Press.

Corruption of Care

DEFINITION

'By this is meant the fact that primary aims of care – the cure or alleviation of suffering – have become subordinate to what are essentially secondary aims, such as the creation and preservation of order, quiet and cleanliness' (Martin, 1984: 102).

KEY POINTS

- The main features of 'scandal hospitals' are described.
- The potential role of corruption of care in prompting hospital run-down is discussed.

The entry on Malpractice discusses this phenomenon at the level of the individual practitioner. In this entry, a higher-level description is given about the ways that care *systems* can fail. The term 'corruption of care' was coined by John Martin (1984) in his book *Hospitals in Trouble*. Martin was interested in reviewing the conclusions of reports on recurrent neglect and abuse in mental illness and mental handicap hospitals (the terminology of the time). He looked at a period between 1965 and 1980 and drew some overall conclusions or lessons:

- *Chronicity of client group* A characteristic of these hospitals was that they dealt with long-term patient populations. The chronicity of the groups of people with learning disabilities or with a range of long-term mental health problems meant that they were socially devalued and voiceless. It also meant that they were unrewarding to the staff responsible for them. The fact that the patient groups were diverse (in terms of diagnosis) suggests that problems of neglect and abuse could be largely accounted for by the failure of policy-makers, managers and practitioners to respond efficiently and humanely to chronic deviance.
- *Geographical isolation* The policy in the Victorian period was to build large institutions in rural places or on the outskirts of urban areas. These places were typically marked off by perimeter walls. Their distance from others in society meant that lay visiting was infrequent and in controlled periods. Ordinary external scrutiny was therefore limited. Another aspect of geographical isolation was that it was common for staff to be drawn from a relatively closed local population. Staff could work all of their lives in one place and their children could repeat this process.
- *Ward isolation* The hospitals were so large that they were divided into many separate units or wards. A feature of 'scandal hospitals' was that they manifested a 'fiefdom mentality': that is, those running the individual wards

enjoyed a sense of separateness and autonomy, with senior staff having the discretion to use their personal power as they wished. A neglectful norm could then readily develop. Staff could ignore patients and their needs and relate predominantly to one another instead. They could ensure that daily ward routines were attended to without reference to the needs of patients.

- *Personal staff isolation* An extension of ward isolation was that the wards had long periods with low staffing levels. A few staff members might be left alone to look after large numbers of difficult-to-manage or unrewarding patients for long periods of time.

- *Medical isolation* A feature of hospitals with problems was that medical staff would be distant from ward activity. Consultants would visit wards infrequently. The more unrewarding and chronic the group, the more this tendency occurred. As with infrequent lay scrutiny from visitors, this meant that the beginnings of bad practice were not spotted by outsiders to the daily ward environment.

- *Intellectual isolation* Because staff might work on wards for many years on end with little or no updated training, they had a tendency to become isolated from professional knowledge. This meant that they lost touch with changes in both technical knowledge and professional ethics.

- *Privacy* While neglect was typically an insidious process, whereby standards of care might deteriorate over time, quite openly, within a ward fiefdom, abuse was a different matter. The latter (which was typically about physical mistreatment) required conditions of privacy, where one or two staff members were alone with a victim or victims. Ward and personal isolation, noted above, created the conditions for this possibility of privacy.

Martin's account of organisational failure can itself be placed in a political and historical context. The history of the Victorian hospitals involved mental health nurses coming from a legacy of manhandling: that is, the psychiatric branch of nursing, which became professionalised in the 20th century, was not connected to the medical or physical branch of the profession. The latter, championed by Florence Nightingale, was middle class, genteel and female. By contrast, the asylum attendants of the 19th century were male and working class, with many of them moving in and out of other forms of unskilled manual work (Carpenter, 1980). Nightingale and her successors actively resisted this group entering the profession of nursing for many years. Thus, the roots of hospital-based mental health nursing were characterised by a norm of physical (and of necessity) rough handling.

Another contributory feature of the historical context was the use of physical restraint and treatment. This is a medical not a nursing feature. Alienists, mad-doctors and the early psychiatrists established a norm of bodily interference. Mechanical restraints, such as straitjackets, were common in the asylum system. Cold compresses and dunking in cold baths were often medically prescribed in response to agitated or disruptive patient behaviour well into the 20th century.

The biomedical preference for medicinal responses meant that it became common for patients to be restrained and forcibly injected with tranquillisers. This increasing practice, during the late 20th century, at times led to the death of patients. These professional norms about physical interference were only a short distance away from physical abuse, with 'use' and 'abuse' being difficult to distinguish. Once physical interference became a norm, then treatment, the pragmatic management of disruption or threat and punishment were easily jumbled in the minds and actions of staff.

By and large, these scandals appear to be a thing of the past (at least in those countries with a programme of large hospital closure). However, many of the features of systemic isolation still apply in two senses. First, with re-institutionalisation (the tendency for chronic cases now to reside in long-term small nursing homes or private hospitals) the corruption of care remains possible. Second, in Britain and other countries, which closed most of their large mental hospitals, forensic facilities are retained. For example, in Britain, we still have four large high-security hospitals (Ashworth, Broadmoor, Carstairs and Rampton). The final report discussed by Martin (1984) was about abuse at Rampton Hospital. During the 1980s and 1990s, further official inquiries into neglect and abuse emerged in the high-security hospitals (previously called the Special Hospital system) (Kaye and Franey, 1998; Pilgrim, 2007). Some of these were prompted by the death in seclusion of patients who had been manhandled and forcibly tranquillised. Black patients were disproportionately represented in these deaths.

Given the public shock and professional shame created by scandals involving the neglect or abuse of psychiatric patients, it is tempting to ascribe particular causal powers to the inquiries summarised by Martin (1984). They could be seen as an important political determinant of hospital closure policy ('desegregation'). However, this would be misleading for three reasons. First, competing accounts of desegregation do not place a large emphasis on official inquiries into maltreatment but suggest other factors, such as technical changes in care and cost (Rogers and Pilgrim, 2005). Second, some of the recent inquiry reports explicitly recommended hospital closure but no action then ensued. This was the case not once but twice, during the 1990s, in relation to Ashworth Hospital, which remains open (although its patient numbers have been reduced). Third, the wider critique of institutional psychiatry (hospital-based, dehumanising and biomedically orientated), known as 'anti-psychiatry', acquired little government credibility in most Western countries (except Italy). As a consequence, it had scant influence on mainstream government decision-making about mental health policy. Basically, states abandoned large hospitals only when they were politically and economically ready to do so, not because conditions in them were scandalous. After all, they had been highly oppressive places for over 100 years. With good cause, they were feared by those on the outside and certainly suffered by those on the inside – hence the concept of being a 'psychiatric survivor'. Although injected tranquillisation created a new source of patient death in the last quarter of the 20th century (Kellam, 1987), from the outset, the asylums were a threat to life. In the mid-19th century, when the asylum system was burgeoning, around 40 per cent of admissions to hospital were soon dead (Russell, 1985).

Together, these three points reinforce a fundamental and persistent aspect of mental health policy: it has been driven, by and large, by the need for social order. This means that the social control of deviance, if necessary with the use of staff force and without care for the human rights of patients, has been central to government concerns. This conclusion suggests that inquiries investigating *organisational failures* might also be recording the dark side of a *political success* in controlling incorrigible deviance. If this conclusion is correct, then it is unlikely that the 'corruption of care' will disappear in the foreseeable future.

See also: *anti-psychiatry; forensic mental health services; malpractice; segregation.*

FURTHER READING

Martin, J.P. (1984) *Hospitals in Trouble*. Oxford: Blackwell.
Szasz, T.S. (2007) *Coercion as Cure*. New Brunswick, NJ: Transaction.

REFERENCES

Carpenter, M. (1980) 'Asylum nursing before 1914: a chapter in the history of nursing', in C. Davies (ed.), *Re-writing Nursing History*. London: Croom Helm.
Kaye, C. and Franey, A. (eds) (1998) *Managing High Security Psychiatric Care*. London: Jessica Kingsley.
Kellam, A.M.P. (1987) 'The neuroleptic syndrome, so-called: a survey of the world literature', *British Journal of Psychiatry*, 150: 752–9.
Martin, J.P. (1984) *Hospitals in Trouble*. Oxford: Blackwell.
Pilgrim, D. (ed.) (2007) *Inside Ashworth: Professional Accounts*. London: Radcliffe.
Rogers, A. and Pilgrim, D. (2005) *A Sociology of Mental Health and Illness* (3rd edn). Maidenhead: Open University Press.
Russell, R. (1985) 'The lunacy profession and its staff in the second half of the 19th century, with special reference to the West Riding Lunatic Asylum', in W.E. Bynum, R. Porter and M. Shepherd (eds), *The Anatomy of Madness*, Vol. 3. London: Tavistock.

Malpractice

malpractice

DEFINITION

Malpractice refers to improper professional behaviour. It includes wilful neglect and any form of exploitation of the client to gratify the practitioner.

KEY POINTS

- Malpractice in healthcare is discussed.
- The particular significance of malpractice for people with mental health problems is highlighted.
- Responses to the phenomenon of malpractice from different interest groups are summarised.

Malpractice is one part of a series of ways in which mental health professionals might fail their clients. Both physical and psychological mental health interventions are researched under ideal conditions of randomised controlled trials in which optimal practice is being observed. In routine service provision or in private practice, the chances of sub-optimal professional practice are multiple.

First, practitioners may make mistakes. Errors of judgement and memory are ordinary human failings and so all health and social care professionals are thus susceptible, some of the time, to this risk. Second, practitioners may be careless and demonstrate poor practice. For example, they may keep poor records or prove lax in breaking the rule of strict confidentiality. As with errors, carelessness may be unintentional but sometimes this is not the case. Also, carelessness may be a product of organisational failures and not just individual shortcomings (or the latter may flow from the former). For example, practitioners may be poorly trained or their employers may not provide the time and resources for them to keep their practice up to date and well supervised. Thus, when negligence does occur, there may be uncertainty about whether it is a moral or organisational failure (or both). Third, the practitioner may deliberately exploit clients. In formal terms, this third area is definitely about malpractice but its ethical and legal status is not neatly separable from wilful negligence.

In mental health services, errors and poor practice are dealt with mainly by a process of audit. That is, 'critical incidents' or 'near misses' are routinely logged and discussed by service managers and corrective action considered and at times implemented. For example, error rates in the administration of drugs by nurses can be monitored and new safeguards introduced. Mistakes, carelessness and poor practice are mainly dealt with as organisational failures, although occasionally they may lead to disciplinary action against individual practitioners.

The shift from a framework that mainly emphasises *organisational determinism* to one which places *moral culpability* centre stage is important. A problem about the whole area of bad practice is that lay people and professionals do not always agree about the balance to be struck between these two. This has led to the anomalous position of healthcare organisations emphasising the need for a 'no blame' culture, while at the same time using internal and external disciplinary mechanisms to make poor practitioners individually accountable for their actions. (This contradiction reflects a deeper ambivalence in modern society about determinism and human agency. The common uncertainty about how to understand and respond to professional neglect and abuse is symptomatic of this wider ambivalence.)

The peculiar ways in which people with mental health problems are open to abuse are discussed in the entry on Corruption of Care, but here it should be noted that they are particularly vulnerable to exploitation for a number of reasons:

- Some people with mental health problems may lack the capacity to appreciate that they are being exploited.
- Their primary mental health problems may lead to a highly dependent stance in relation to professionals. For example, patients who are highly anxious may become childlike in their dependency on fellow adults, including mental health professionals. In another example, some patients are highly suggestible. Histrionic patients are particularly vulnerable in this regard.
- Even if a person with a mental health problem properly reflects on abusive professional action and proceeds to complain legitimately, their mental state may undermine their credibility in the eyes of third-party adjudicators. A variant of this is that even if the latter are credulous about a patient's account, the patient may lack the confidence that they will be believed.
- The tradition of individual casework, in counselling and psychotherapy, sets up the physical conditions in which abuse may be more likely. This has resonances with other healthcare scenarios, where unchaperoned intimate meetings occur. For example, most publicised cases of sexual malpractice will involve GPs, psychological therapists or gynaecologists. This is not to say that privacy causes exploitation – it is a necessary but not a sufficient condition. Most healthcare workers do not use this condition of privacy to exploit their clients, but the exploitative minority are not insignificant. Estimates of psychological therapists who admit, in anonymous surveys, to sexual relationships with one or more clients varies from 4 to 8 per cent. This may be an underestimation, as even in anonymous surveys, professionals are likely to underreport malpractice. In the USA, over half of the malpractice actions against mental health workers are about sexual contact with clients.

Ideas about correcting or minimising malpractice vary. Some would be of the opinion, for example, that psychotherapy has such a poor track record in relation to financial, emotional, physical and sexual abuse that it should be avoided at all costs. The argument for this radical suggestion is developed in *Against Therapy* by Jeffrey Masson (1992). Users who have survived malpractice argue for more stringent and quicker judgements about exploitative professionals once a complaint has been lodged. The professional response has tended to emphasise more effective supervision and training (continued professional development). Governmental responses have focused more on legal regulation. There are international differences in the latter regard. For example, in many states in the USA, sexual malpractice is criminalised, but in the UK, it is not dealt with under criminal law but only as a professional disciplinary matter.

A major challenge faced by mental health professional bodies is that an emphasis on extensive training, supervision and legal registration (the traditional web of safeguards offered to the public) has not always been persuasive to disaffected service users. Abusive therapists who are exposed are often found to be well qualified and appropriately registered to practise. Moreover, the disciplinary proceedings used when complaints are made are often protracted and distressing. Even when a practitioner is expelled for malpractice ('struck off'), this is rarely a lifelong ban. These processes can give the impression that professional interests, rightly or wrongly, are privileged when legitimate complaints are made by abused clients.

The question of physical abuse is complicated. For example, mental health workers are lawfully permitted to impose physical treatments on dissenting bodies. In any other circumstance, this would be common assault. By contrast, physical contact is considered to be unethical in codes of practice governing psychological therapies (and even here there are exceptions, as in the case of 'body therapies').

Emotional abuse is also not always easy to define and demonstrate in the quasi-judicial setting of disciplinary proceedings triggered by client complaints. In a very broad sense, any psychological therapist must be gaining some emotional gratification from their work. They listen privately to one after another problematic personal account of others, week in, week out, for years on end. This unusual professional lifestyle must be sustained by some personal gain for the therapist, begging the question: At what point are a therapist's emotional needs being privileged over their client's needs?

The notion of financial exploitation is even more open to interpretation because of the norms of private practice in mental health work. Some forms of psychotherapy are long term and so cumulatively take large quantities of money from paying clients. Also, value for money is a consumer judgement. But the latter in some forms of psychotherapy is simply seen as one of many symbolic communications to discuss in the therapy. The client who pays late or complains about paying is not simply seen as a rational customer with consumer rights. Instead, these communications about the fee are simply material to interpret, along with others, about the person and their life. In this context, financial exploitation is difficult to define in clear terms. Given these complexities in relation to the physical, emotional and financial norms of therapist action, it is not surprising that sexual malpractice tends to be investigated more (both in disciplinary proceedings and in research).

See also: *biological interventions; capacity and culpability; coercion; corruption of care; psychological interventions; risks to and from people with mental health problems.*

FURTHER READING

Barker, P. (ed.) (2011) *Mental Health Ethics*. London: Routledge.
Bersoff, D.N. (1995) *Ethical Conflicts in Psychology*. Washington, DC: American Psychological Association.
Masson, J. (1992) *Against Therapy*. London: Fontana.

REFERENCE

Masson, J. (1992) *Against Therapy*. London: Fontana.

key concepts in
mental health

Challenges for Practitioners

DEFINITION

Mental health work poses both general challenges common to all healthcare practitioners and particular ones related to dealing with distress and unintelligibility in society and the risks these might pose to self or others. Moreover, these challenges are immediate and personal, as well as collective and longstanding for service providers.

KEY POINTS

- All human services settings pose challenges for practitioners about maintaining and improving mental health and these are discussed.
- In specialist mental health services, this broad intention is jeopardised often by the contradictions created by the competing expectation of risk management.
- Given this wider contradiction, challenges for individual practitioners need to be understood and resolved within the collective expectations about public order created by those who are sane by common consent.

In developed societies today, a range of human service organisations contain professionals who deal with or reflect upon the mental health of their clients or employees. For example, managers in any work setting and teachers in any school tend to be mindful of the psychological welfare of those they are paid to be responsible for. The bridge to specialist mental health work can then be found in other systems, such as primary care (where up to a third of patients have some degree of explicit or underlying mental health problem), and in the voluntary sector of civil society, which deals with a range of challenges for those coming to them. From the Samaritans to Rape Crisis Centres, some parts of that sector will be dealing disproportionately with distressed people.

The personal and other resources needed to deal with the challenges posed will vary from setting to setting. We can think in terms of the following:

1. *Will the practitioner be confident and competent in their role?* In general health and social care settings, professionals will generally be mindful about the limits of competence and, when in doubt, will refer on to those they judge to be more suited to the task. This of course assumes the ready availability of those more specialist workers, raising the question of resources in systems.
2. *Will the practitioner be sensitive to matters of risk to self and others?* The driver of risk assessment and management may be foremost in their minds.

challenges for practitioners

Risk-averse decision-making may communicate distrust to the client, thereby undermining successful contract formation to engender personal change. Given that most service relationships are based upon voluntarism and mutual respect, mental health services are marked by different norms that can, and do at times, undermine trust. The latter are formally recognised when they are governed by legal arrangements. Mental health services are thus clouded, more than others, by the matter of risk-averse social control. This is highlighted by three simple points. First, employees of the state are offered immunity in mental health services from accusations of false imprisonment and assault by the provision of mental health law, so-called. Second, healthcare professionals at times impose bodily constraint ('restraint') and social isolation ('seclusion') on their client group. In penal contexts, solitary confinement is considered injurious or a risk to mental health, or even a punishment. Third, mental health services cannot demonstrate, unequivocally and case by case, that in exchange for deprivation of liberty, personal constraint and iatrogenic risk, mental health gain in the identified patient can be demonstrated. Merely to detain and treat is no guarantee of client improvement; indeed, the reverse may accrue. This expected moral exchange is called the 'principle of reciprocity' and to date mental health services regularly fail its expectations.

3. *Following from this point, can practitioners distinguish their success at minimising risk in their work with clients from their effectiveness at improving mental health?* Matters of effectiveness and acceptability to the client may or may not be readily reconcilable with efforts at risk management. For example, making medication compliance a condition of community living may be driven by risk minimisation for staff rather than improved client satisfaction. This is why community treatment orders have been controversial.

4. *Can practitioners maintain their personal boundaries at all times when dealing with vulnerable people?* A particular dilemma when communicating to clients in the above ambiguous context, in which benevolence and risk minimisation interweave contingently from moment to moment, relates to boundary maintenance. Should professionals ever touch their clients? What happens if sexual feelings arise between the professional and the client? While such ethical considerations are relevant in all service contexts where there are discrepancies of power and status and where one party is a professional and the other is a client, in mental health contexts these matters are thrown more clearly into relief.

5. *What stance should practitioners take towards past adversity in their client group?* People with mental health problems often report adverse histories of neglect and abuse, some of it severe and beyond the immediate experience of the practitioner. Professionals may ward off the personal impact of this by ignoring it (and, say, focusing on 'diagnose and treat' biomedical routines instead). However, if these personal accounts from clients are listened to credulously and compassionately, what impact might this have, especially cumulatively, on the professional? We vary in our capacity to absorb and contain the feelings expressed by others who are distressed and who report stories of past adversity.

Strategies for coping with this are implicated in service organisation (such as mentoring, supervision and personal therapy). Some cope by leaving client contact and moving into managerial, training or research roles.

6. *Can absolute confidentiality be guaranteed in mental health services?* Normal considerations of client confidentiality can become complicated in mental health services by the matter of criminality. In forensic mental health services, the latter may be a common consideration about risk management, for example when considering discharge (see point 2 above), but across all services there is also the matter of clients being victims of historical crimes (see point 5 above). Survivors of physical and sexual abuse in childhood are over-represented in mental health services. What do professionals do with client reports of that criminality, especially if the perpetrator is still alive and may be a risk to new victims? One answer is to evade the task because of the overwhelming emotional and ethical implications of acknowledging the historical legacy involved.

7. *How honest are practitioners about their points of agreement and disagreement in relation to how they conceptualise mental health problems?* The above questions imply a strong pragmatic need for collaboration in multidisciplinary teams to balance care and control when managing patients under their professional and legal jurisdiction. This pragmatic group-think may obscure fundamental epistemological differences and their implied preferences about assessment and intervention. In turn, those unresolved matters may interfere with efficiency and mutual trust in the staff culture.

The above seven questions are offered as a checklist for discussion, without any clear answers being provided in response. Sometimes there are simply no clear general answers, as the contingencies of the dilemma are particular and require situated reasoning and reflection. Following from this, trainers and managers of services should provide time and space for the implications of the challenges listed, because of their gravity and complexity. Squaring the circle of care and control is often beyond the capability of individual practitioners but throws into relief the wider expectation in modern societies of the role and purpose of 'mental health services'. Practitioners in the latter swim in unusual ethical waters, related to risk management and (dis)trust between practitioners and their clients. Sometimes distrust between practitioners also colours the workings of a mental health service.

Of course, challenges about clients exist in a range of human service settings, but mental health services bring with them unusual dilemmas for practitioners. In those circumstances, there may be a tendency to rely mechanistically upon the '3P' routines – 'policies, protocols and procedures' – in the abstract or on paper, without working through their complexity in practice. Mental health service quality in part is a function of how successfully this process of working through is seen to be done genuinely, rather than rhetorically, by staff and clients alike. Given the complexity of these challenges and the particular contradictions surrounding care and control in mental health services, collective responsibility for their regular discussion is important.

Leaving them as mere ethical challenges for individual practitioners ignores their wider contradictory systemic context. That context has been generated for a range of reasons, including public safety and public order, endorsed by politicians and a wider electorate who are sane by common consent. Mental health practitioners are beholden to these third parties and so cannot put themselves unambiguously at the service of the identified patients they encounter in their work. This unusual scenario, in a service supposedly deemed to be about the health of identified patients, implies the need for a depth and extent of professional reflection not typically necessitated in other healthcare settings.

See also: *coercion; corruption of care; malpractice; philosophical aspects of mental health; the quality of mental health care.*

FURTHER READING

Araci, D. and Clarke, I. (2017) 'Investigating the efficacy of a whole team, psychologically informed, acute mental health service approach', *Journal of Mental Health*, 2: 307–11.

Barker, P. (2011) *Mental Health Ethics: The Human Context*. London: Routledge.

Bean, P. (1980) *Compulsory Admissions to Mental Hospitals*. London: Wiley.

Bowles, A. (2000) 'Therapeutic nursing care in acute psychiatric wards: engagement over control', *Journal of Psychiatric and Mental Health Nursing*, 7: 179–84.

Eastman, N. (1994) 'Mental health law: civil liberties and the principle of reciprocity', *British Medical Journal*, 308: 43.

Fabris, E. (2011) *Tranquil Prisons: Chemical Incarceration Under Community Treatment Orders*. Toronto: University of Toronto Press.

Hepworth, I. and McGowan, L. (2013) 'Do mental health professionals enquire about childhood sexual abuse during routine mental health assessment in mental health settings?', *Journal of Psychiatric and Mental Health Nursing*, 20 (6): 473–83.

More, W.K. (2010) 'Restraints and the code of ethics: an uneasy fit', *Archives of Psychiatric Nursing*, 24 (1): 3–14.

Pilgrim, D. (2012) 'Final lessons from the Mental Health Act Commission for England and Wales: the limits of legalism-plus-safeguards', *Journal of Social Policy*, 41 (1): 61–81.

Pilgrim, D. and Vassilev, I. (2007) 'Risk, trust and mental health services', *Journal of Mental Health*, 16 (3): 347–57.

Ramsany, S. (2001) *Caring for Madness: The Role of Personal Experience in the Training of Mental Health Nurses*. London: Whurr.

Riley, H., Fagerjord, G.L. and Høyer, G. (2018) 'Community treatment orders – what are the views of decision makers?', *Journal of Mental Health*, 27 (2): 97–102.

Schilling, E.A., Aseltine, R.H. and Gore, S. (2008) 'The impact of cumulative childhood adversity on young adult mental health: measures, models, and interpretations', *Social Science & Medicine*, 6 (5): 1140–51.

Shaw, I., Middleton, H. and Cohen, J. (2007) *Understanding Treatment without Consent*. Aldershot: Ashgate.

Szasz, T.S. (2007) *Coercion as Cure: A Critical History of Psychiatry*. New Brunswick, NJ: Transaction.

Szmukler, G. and Appelbaum, P. (2001) 'Treatment pressures, coercion and compulsion', in G. Thornicroft and G. Szmukler (eds), *Textbook of Community Psychiatry*. Oxford: Oxford University Press.

Part IV

Mental Health and Society

Mental Health Policy

DEFINITION

This refers to any society's attempts to promote mental health and to ameliorate mental health problems. It includes legislative arrangements and politically pre-scribed forms of professional duty and service response.

KEY POINTS

- Mental health policy changes over time in the developed countries of the world are summarised.
- Some differences between these policy trends and policy events in the less developed countries are discussed.

The notion of mental health policy is relatively recent. Until the 20th century, there was a lunacy policy, which gave way gradually to a mental illness policy. It was noted in the first section (Mental Health) that the use of the term 'mental health', as a prefix to 'policy', 'problems' or 'services', is a recent euphemism. However, it is our current discourse and so this entry will use the term as if it is not problematic.

What this initial disclaimer does do, however, is help us unpick layers of rele-vant policies which have accumulated over time. Also, this story is not fixed and universal. Most of the research on mental health policy has been about mapping changes in Western Europe, North America and Australasia. In the developing countries, much of this historical pattern is inapplicable. For this reason, the dominant picture in the developed countries will be summarised and then some counter-examples will be given from other parts of the world. An international summary of mental health policy development at the time of writing is presented in Figure 4.1 from the World Health Organization.

SUMMARY OF SHIFTS IN MENTAL HEALTH POLICY IN THE DEVELOPED COUNTRIES

Western Europe contains the old colonial powers and so has the longest history to summarise. The export of European cultures to the Americas and Australasia, after the Middle Ages, means that not all of the following applies to them. In the 16th and 17th centuries in Europe, the insane either wandered free or were constrained or cared for in religious dwellings. Madness at this point was not seen as a medical problem but as a social and supernatural one.

The next change was the loose development of many small private madhouses in the 18th century. A few famous large madhouses, like Bedlam in London (1408),

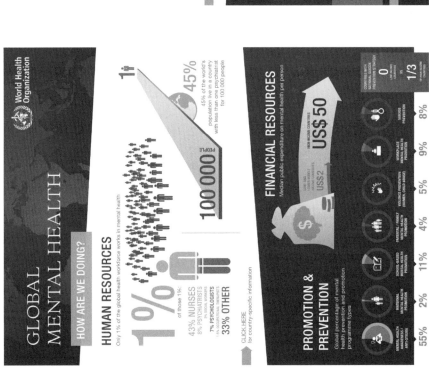

Figure 4.1 International summary of mental health policy

the Casa de Orates in Valencia (1408) and the Hospital General in Paris (1656), predated this period. Although Michel Foucault (1965) in his *Madness and Civilization* dates the 'Great Confinement' of madness in Europe to the Paris institution, in England a full state system of lunatic asylums did not emerge until the 19th century (Goodwin, 1997; Rogers and Pilgrim, 2002).

The First World War brought neurosis within the ambit of psychiatry and enlarged its activities to community-based interventions. However, between the First and Second World War (and after the latter), it was still hospital-based psychiatry, with its preference for biological interventions, which predominated. What the 20th century then saw was two cultures of patients being treated – one in the community (with access sometimes to psychological interventions) and another which was still warehoused for long periods in large, old asylums and treated wholly with physical interventions. The latter represented the persistent biomedical position of hospital-based psychiatry, dating from the mid-19th century and still existing today.

During the 20th century, the psychiatric jurisdiction over psychotic and neurotic patients was enlarged further, as those with personality problems and addictions were added. This is why we now see this admixture of diagnoses in mental health services. Running alongside these changes in professional jurisdiction were formal adjustments to mental health legislation, which defined professional powers of detention and intervention and stipulated safeguards both for patients and against the unfair detention of the sane. In Britain, these legislative changes occurred in 1930, 1959, 1983 and 2007. In the past 50 years, another and more nebulous layer of mental health policy has been in relation to mental health promotion (see the entry with this title).

Hospital run-down in Western Europe occurred rapidly in the 1980s (see the entry on Segregation), with community care being both the great hope of radical reformers and a focus for anger and derision from paternalistic interest groups seeking a return to greater institutional control of mental disorder. The phase of post-hospital closure we currently inhabit is characterised by three key policy processes:

- First, there is *the tendency towards re-institutionalisation*. This refers to the tendency to return to the days of smaller private madhouses (albeit now including, and built outwards from, the state-funded acute units).
- Second, there is now *evidence of trans-institutionalisation*. This refers to the evidence that some patients who previously would have been contained in the Victorian asylums now spend long periods of time in jail. Another area of policy debate is in relation to the adequacy of housing, employment and other aspects of social inclusion, for community-based patients (see the entry on Social Exclusion).
- A third policy challenge for those still committed to social inclusion is in relation to *public education about the range and nature of mental health problems*. Negative stereotypes are currently being maintained by the hostile and deriding coverage of mental health problems in the mass media (see the entry on The Mass Media).

MENTAL HEALTH POLICY IN DEVELOPING COUNTRIES

The colonial impact of European states was reflected in mental health policy in a particular way. On the one hand, Western (especially Germanic) views about insanity were exported. On the other hand, the mass segregation of the pauper insane by the state was absent. For example, in India, there was an immediate but weak mirroring of the English asylum concept. However, the provision was overwhelmingly for *white* patients. There were regional differences in the administration of these lunatic asylums and they were financially driven. Also, the class composition of imperial power meant that the Indian asylum system had to make unusual provision to respond to the social status of British rulers who became insane (Ernst, 1985). While European asylums overwhelmingly dealt with pauper lunatics, on colonised soil abroad, the mad were more likely to be from a much higher social class. By the end of the 19th century, the scale of 'European asylums abroad' had declined radically, as the colonial power steadily withdrew its presence.

Most developing countries have had much less hospital-based psychiatry. In some, it was simply absent during the 20th century (for example, Laos; see Westermeyer and Kroll, 1978). In others, it arrived very late (for example, not until 1961 in Nepal; see Nepal, 2001). By the time that asylum beds were peaking in Europe in the mid-20th century, the Indian sub-continent had few hospitals or mental health workers. For example, by 1947, England had 15 times more psychiatric beds than India with only 10 per cent of its population (Murthy, 2001).

A paradoxical advantage of this lack of resources for mental health care development in the developing world is that there was less of an institutional infrastructure to remove or displace when community models of care came into favour (German, 1975; Wig, 1999). A community-based or primary care-driven mental health policy was a socio-economic necessity, created by a scarcity of resources. Because madness was segregated with less frequency, recovery rates for those with a diagnosis of schizophrenia have been higher in developing countries than in Western Europe and the USA (Warner, 1985).

In light of the discrepancies in resources for mental health policies between the developed and developing countries, the World Health Organization (2000) has suggested a three-pronged global policy. First, there should be more resources allocated to mental health care in all countries, but especially in the developing ones. Second, resource redistribution is needed *within* healthcare systems to benefit mental health services (the latter is typically relatively under-funded). Third, programmes of collaborative shared care should be developed between state-funded mental health services and voluntary bodies, religious bodies, families, community organisations and patients.

See also: *coercion; mental health; mental health promotion; segregation.*

FURTHER READING

Glasby, J. and Tew, J. (2015) *Mental Health Policy and Practice*. Basingstoke: Palgrave Macmillan.
Rogers, A. and Pilgrim, D. (2002) *Mental Health Policy in Britain*. Basingstoke: Palgrave Macmillan.

REFERENCES

Ernst, W. (1985) 'Asylums in alien places: the treatment of the European insane in British India', in W.F. Bynum, R. Porter and M. Shepherd (eds), *The Anatomy of Madness*, Vol. 3. London: Tavistock.

Foucault, M. (1965) *Madness and Civilization*. New York: Random House.

German, A. (1975) 'Trends in psychiatry in Black Africa', in S. Arieti and G. Chrzanowshi (eds), *New Dimensions in Psychiatry: A World View*. New York: Wiley.

Goodwin, S. (1997) *Comparative Mental Health Policy*. London: Sage.

Murthy, R.S. (ed.) (2001) *Mental Health in India 1950–2000*. Bangalore: People's Action for Mental Health.

Nepal, M.K. (2001) 'Mental health in Nepal', in R.S. Murthy (ed.), *Mental Health in India 1950–2000*. Bangalore: People's Action for Mental Health.

Rogers, A. and Pilgrim, D. (2002) *Mental Health Policy in Britain*. Basingstoke: Palgrave Macmillan.

Warner, R. (1985) *Recovery from Schizophrenia: Psychiatry and Political Economy*. London: Routledge.

Westermeyer, J. and Kroll, J. (1978) 'Violence and mental illness in a peasant society: characteristics of violent behaviours and folk use of restraints', *British Journal of Psychiatry*, 133: 529–41.

Wig, N.N. (1999) 'Development of regional and national mental health programmes', in G. de Girolamo (ed.), *Promoting Mental Health Internationally*. London: Royal College of Psychiatrists.

World Health Organization (WHO) (2000) *World Health Report, Health Systems: Improving Performance*. Geneva: WHO.

Segregation

DEFINITION

The imposed separation of one social group from another or from the general population. The term sometimes refers to the isolation of one person.

KEY POINTS

- The history of the segregation of madness is outlined.
- Competing ideas about segregation and desegregation policies are discussed.
- The trans-historical trend of the public rejection of madness is noted.

The mass segregation of pauper lunatics took place over the final three centuries of the second millennium in Europe and North America. Psychiatric historians do not agree on the precise timing of this societal shift or on the exact explanation for its occurrence (Foucault, 1965; Rothman, 1971; Grob, 1973; Scull, 1979). Some would argue that the segregation of lunacy reflected a moral shift in an industrial age of increasing rationality and efficiency (which, of its nature, madness defies). Others would hold that class interests in capitalist societies dictated the need to split off and control an economically burdensome underclass (the 'lumpenproletariat'). The destitute, old, sick and infirm were taken into workhouses. The mad and foolish were eventually accommodated in the asylum system during the 19th century. Prior to that, they could be found in workhouses and in private or charitable madhouses.

The volume of segregated madness peaked during the 1950s in most countries. It then steadily declined, with a sharp drop-off after 1980. The latter marked the eventual implementation of 'desegregation', which has also been called 'decarceration', 'de-institutionalisation' and 'community care'. In Britain, the term 'community care' was first mentioned in the 1930 Mental Treatment Act, but only developed common currency in the 1980s. The explanations for desegregation have also been varied (Scull, 1983; Busfield, 1986; Goodwin, 1997; Rogers and Pilgrim, 2005). These competing (or sometimes additive) explanations have included: the introduction of new psychiatric drugs; the fiscal crisis created for the welfare state of costly large institutions; and a shift in professional concerns about appropriate treatment and its setting.

A tension that has been inherent to both the segregation and desegregation policy trends relates to the possibility of social reintegration. That is, therapeutic pessimists have argued for the need to manage chronicity. The therapeutic optimists have argued for the cure or rehabilitation of madness. The pessimists were content to permanently warehouse madness from society, with lunatics permanently living and then dying in the asylum. The optimists hoped to reverse madness and permit liberty. Examples of the latter in the 19th century included the moral treatment used by religious, non-medical administrators of asylums (such as the Quaker Retreat at York) and the early efforts at physical treatment offered by the medical superintendents, who formed the early profession of psychiatry after the mid-19th century (Digby, 1985).

Despite the hopes of lunacy policy reformers, the moral treatment of the older charitable asylums, like the Retreat, failed to transfer to the state-run asylum system and custodialism prevailed (Donnelly, 1983). Moreover, although moral treatment was ostensibly more humane, it was still a form of social control and even used physical restraint at times (Castel, 1985; Tomes, 1985). Similarly, during the 20th century, there were therapeutic optimists championing both biological and psychological interventions. At the same time, others have argued that the quality of life of chronic patients and the need for genuine asylum, and not cure, should be policy priorities.

Moreover, the shift from custodialism to professional therapeutic optimism in the second half of the 20th century was not always appreciated by patients, especially electroconvulsive therapy (ECT), insulin coma therapy and psychosurgery. Other innovations, such as industrial therapy, were less offensive but were often menial and arguably exploitative. The old segregated asylums had advantages, however (compared to the poor urban environments occupied by many chronic patients today). They were typically in large, semi-rural spacious grounds with an estate often including a farm, which occupied some patients and provided produce for the hospital. Also, the internal living areas were more spacious than the cramped, low-ceilinged environment of many acute mental health units today.

An indication that madness, once segregated, was deemed to reflect a form of lesser humanity was the concern expressed in society, at the turn of the 20th century, about unfair detention. This showed the willingness of society to split off one group, which could be incarcerated and assaulted with impunity (the insane), from another, whose personal sensitivities and right to autonomy, privacy and physical safety should be fully respected (the sane). Most of the concerns about segregation, thereafter, have not been about the *existence* of segregation but about its proper application. Since the 1920s, reforms of mental health legislation have resonated with this point, as they spell out the circumstances and safeguards required for the imposition of legitimate rather than unfair psychiatric detention.

Another manifestation of this 'two groups of humanity' mentality was the concern expressed after the 1970s about the 'political abuse of psychiatry' (Bloch and Reddaway, 1977). Reports of psychiatrists using enforced psychiatric diagnosis and life-diminishing treatments (major tranquillisers) on political dissidents created an international scandal. However, an implication of the outrage it produced was that enforced psychiatric treatments, which were life-diminishing, were legitimate impositions on those who were truly mentally ill. The lack of outrage about the latter indicates that the general public are still prone to accept that the insane do not warrant the rights of full humanity.

Another example about the mass mentality of the sane, faced with madness in their midst, is given by Jodelet (1991). In a social experiment since 1900, at Ainay-le-Château in France, patients have been fostered by families in the community. However, they are still separated psychologically by their hosts, who fear contagion and violence and who do not permit sexual relationships between patients and non-patients. On the rare occasion that a sexual relationship has developed, the couple has been banished from the community.

A final historical continuity to mention under this entry is individual segregation. In the 18th century, chains were used to restrain mad individuals. By the end of the 19th century, padded cells and straitjackets were used. By the end of the 20th century, unpadded strip cells or seclusion rooms had come into fashion in secure hospitals and acute mental health settings. This remains the case today, although 'seclusion' (in prison, the same process is called 'solitary confinement') is seen as a problematic practice and so its minimal use is preferred by mental health professionals. Even today, there are parts of the former Communist Eastern bloc (the Czech Republic, Slovenia and Slovakia) where cages are found in large psychiatric institutions. Seclusion rooms and cages indicate that physical segregation is still very much part of the current institutional landscape of psychiatry.

Current mental health services, in developed societies, still fulfil a function of segregation. However, their bed capacity is much more restricted. Acute mental health services only have a fraction of the beds of the old large institutions and they are charged with moving people on as soon as possible. By contrast, the old large hospitals were places of permanent residence, and by the end of their days they were often called 'long-stay' institutions. The forensic system, of high and medium secure mental health services, offers this residual long-stay function of the Victorian asylum system but is not on the same scale as the old network of asylums.

The reduction in the number of beds in the state sector of mental health services has been compensated for, to some extent, by the development of private facilities to segregate those with mental health problems whose disruptiveness or economic burden cannot be dealt with in community settings. This can be thought of as 're-segregation' or 're-institutionalisation' and may mark a return to a form of residential policy similar to that of the 18th century (Pilgrim and Rogers, 1996). Also, rates of mental disorder in prison populations have increased, suggesting that a deviant group who were once in the asylum system may now be detained elsewhere. A second readjustment made about the function of segregation, the closure of the majority of the large hospitals, has been legal. Mental health legislation has been adapted to include forms of surveillance and options for the rapid rehospitalisation of patients now living in the community. Services now are a mixture of small acute units, assertive outreach, outpatient clinics, home treatment services and day centres. The new Mental Health Act (2007) for England and Wales reflects this readjustment, as it focuses on the control of patients in a range of settings other than in hospital (the emphasis of prior mental health legislation in 1890, 1930, 1959 and 1983).

See also: *biological interventions; forensic mental health services; madness; mental health; mental health policy; risks to and from people with mental health problems.*

FURTHER READING

Busfield, J. (1986) *Managing Madness.* London: Hutchinson.

Fabris, E. (2011) *Tranquil Prisons: Chemical Incarceration under Community Treatment Orders.* Toronto: University of Toronto Press.

Scull, A. (1979) *Museums of Madness: The Social Organization of Insanity in 19th Century England.* London: Allen Lane.

REFERENCES

Bloch, S. and Reddaway, M. (1977) *Psychiatric Terror: How Soviet Psychiatry is Used to Suppress Dissent.* New York: Basic Books.

Busfield, J. (1986) *Managing Madness.* London: Hutchinson.

Castel, R. (1985) 'Moral treatment: mental therapy and social control in the nineteenth century', in S. Cohen and A. Scull (eds), *Social Control and the State.* Oxford: Basil Blackwell.

Digby, A. (1985) 'Moral treatment at the retreat 1796–1846', in W.F. Bynum, R. Porter and M. Shepherd (eds), *The Anatomy of Madness,* Vol. 2. London: Tavistock.

Donnelly, M. (1983) *Managing the Mind.* London: Tavistock.

Foucault, M. (1965) *Madness and Civilization.* New York: Random House.

Goodwin, S. (1997) *Comparative Mental Health Policy: From Institutional to Community Care.* London: Sage.

Grob, G. (1973) *Mental Institutions in America: Social Policy to 1875.* New York: Free Press.

Jodelet, D. (1991) *Madness and Social Representations.* London: Harvester Wheatsheaf.

Pilgrim, D. and Rogers, A. (1996) 'Something old, something new ... sociology and the organization of psychiatry', *Sociology, 28* (2): 521–38.

Rogers, A. and Pilgrim, D. (2005) *A Sociology of Mental Health and Illness* (3rd edn). Maidenhead: Open University Press.

Rothman, D. (1971) *The Discovery of the Asylum: Social Order and Disorder in the New Republic*. Boston, MA: Little Brown.

Scull, A. (1979) *Museums of Madness: The Social Organization of Insanity in 19th Century England*. London: Allen Lane.

Scull, A. (1983) *Decarceration*. Oxford: Polity Press.

Tomes, N. (1985) 'The great restraint controversy: a comparative perspective on Anglo-American psychiatry in the nineteenth century', in W.F. Bynum, R. Porter and M. Shepherd (eds), *The Anatomy of Madness*, Vol. 3. London: Tavistock.

Eugenics

DEFINITION

Eugenics proposes that human society can be improved by limiting or eliminating the transmission of proved or assumed defective genes.

KEY POINTS

- The history of eugenics is summarised in relation to people with mental health problems.
- The implications for psychiatry and psychology are discussed.

The profession of psychiatry emerged in the 19th century, when the eugenic movement was becoming respectable in both Europe and North America. This was also a time when the founders of differential psychology (the academic basis for testing intelligence and personality in clinical psychology today) began to incorporate eugenic ideas into psychological theories. As MacKenzie (1971) notes, eugenics was a mainstream ideology of the professional middle classes of Europe and North America at the turn of the 20th century. At first, it was promoted strongly by the political left in Britain. Key early eugenicists included social democrats, such as the writers George Bernard Shaw and H.G. Wells, Sidney and Beatrice Webb (two co-founders of the London School of Economics and Political Science) and the esteemed mathematician Karl Pearson. Although a self-professed socialist, Pearson frequently propounded racist, and especially anti-Semitic, views. Many of today's methods in behavioural statistics are derived from Pearson, who drew upon and promoted the work of Francis Galton. The latter was the British father of eugenics and his philosophy was soon central to a global movement across the full political spectrum (Galton, 1881). Before eugenics fell from respectability in the wake of the Nazi era, to be discussed, its mid-20th-century advocates included the economist John Maynard Keynes, Neville Chamberlain, the British prime minister at the outbreak of the Second World War, and William Beveridge, who is usually credited with being the 'architect' of the British welfare state in general, and the National Health Service in particular.

A core assumption of eugenics was that human society could be improved by regulating the genetic make-up of the population. A corollary of this was that some groups were assumed to be particular threats to this programme of social improvement, especially those deemed to be physically or psychologically imperfect. At the turn of the 20th century, a common assumption in the educated classes of Europe and North America was that a 'tainted gene pool' existed, which could manifest itself in a range of deviant conduct – madness, epilepsy, idiocy, prostitution, alcoholism and criminality (Marshall, 1990). Thus, the social problems associated with poverty were not seen as ones of political and economic inequality. Instead, they were viewed as outcomes of biological degeneracy.

The Anglo-German version of this ideological formation was then reflected in the Kraepelinian legacy, which was explicitly eugenic (Kraepelin, 1883). However, the eugenic trend was not limited to that German diagnostic tradition alone (Mott, 1912). One notable eugenist was Aubrey Lewis, an Australian and the first Medical Director of the Institute of Psychiatry in London after the Second World War, even though he was largely committed to a Meyerian and not a Kraepelian viewpoint (Lewis, 1934). He and others at the Institute, like H.J. Eysenck who founded the first British clinical psychology there in 1952, continued to support the British Eugenics Society, which began life as the Eugenics Education Society in 1907; its name was changed to the 'Galton Institute' in 1989 (Mazumdar, 1992).

The core Kraepelinian trajectory of genetic bio-reductionism was shaped by, and part of, the eugenic assumptions that culminated in the Nazi Holocaust. This was reflected in both the psychiatric research of Rudin (1916) and Luxenburger (1928) and German health policy more generally in the early 20th century (Binding and Hoche, 1920; Weindling, 1989). Rudin and Luxenburger were students of Kraepelin, and together they led the 'Munich School' of psychiatric genetics. The German work was promoted in the UK and the USA in the mid-20th century by Eliot Slater and Franz Kallmann, respectively, who were temporary members of the Munich group. After the Second World War, Rudin was found guilty at the de-Nazification tribunal at Nuremberg. In the 1930s, Kallmann ironically had to migrate to the USA (he was part Jewish) and Slater returned to his native London. For the rest of his career, he advocated the Munich position about the genetic determination of mental disorders (Slater, 1936; Mayer-Gross et al., 1954; Slater and Cowie, 1971; Gottesman and McGuffin, 1996). Kallmann's twin study samples continued to be used as evidence for the genetic determination of 'schizophrenia' in post-war Anglo-American psychiatry (Kallmann, 1953). Slater's work gained formal post-war native respectability, when he was the Director of the MRC Psychiatric Genetics Unit at the Institute of Psychiatry London, from 1959 to 1969. This Anglo-American resonance and legacy of the

Munich School is still cited and endorsed today in psychiatric textbooks (Roelcke, 2007; Pilgrim, 2008).

The 'mercy killing' by medical practitioners of psychiatric patients and others who were deemed to be 'life devoid of meaning' in German clinical settings prefigured the 'Final Solution' of the death camps in Poland (Weindling, 1989). The so-called 'involuntary euthanasia' of psychiatric patients, and other disabled people, was the last element in a collusive relationship between the Nazis and the German Doctors' Association. This had started with a wider enthusiasm for the involuntary sterilisation of mentally and physically disabled people. That policy was commonplace in European society generally at the time (e.g. Dowbiggin, 1985), and the reach of the coercive eugenic message could also be found in the USA, where psychiatrists seriously debated 'involuntary euthanasia' in 1942 (Joseph, 2005).

An indication of the mainstream policy influence of eugenic thinking, continuing well into the 20th century in Britain, was the report to the government of the Wood Committee (HMSO, 1929). It signalled that the racial focus of Nazism was by no means unique, although Mazumdar (1992) argues that the British wing of eugenics was focused on class not race. The Wood Committee talked of the need to prevent the 'racial disaster of mental deficiency' and, as Stone (2001) notes, the notion of 'race' in Britain probably reflected a form of post-colonial ethnocentricity, which assumed a social hierarchy based on a blend of both race and class.

Mental deficiency was considered by eugenicists to mark the final stage of the inheritance of degeneracy. Around this time, a whole range of social reform activities in Europe and North America, including the birth control and mental hygiene movements, as well as programmes to sterilise psychiatric patients and those with learning disabilities, reflected eugenic ideas. The association today of birth control and abortion ('family planning') with feminist ideology can divert our attention from these older political concerns, which were primarily eugenic, although in the social democratic circles of Fabianism noted earlier, the two ideologies were entwined.

A remaining question relates to the current resonance of eugenic ideas within the culture of mental health professionals. The strong biological determinism, which makes a link between madness and the defective genetic make-up of patients, still dominates modern psychiatry, although epigenetic reasoning has tended to displace it in the academy. Biodeterminism was central to the bids for scientific legitimacy by the psychiatric profession in the 19th century, and it continued to resonate in the next. Thus, there is a traceable link between the original eugenic-genetic model of madness and taken-for-granted aspects of current psychiatric thinking.

To conclude, although eugenic ideas may now seem to be outmoded and discredited, they have three forms of recent relevance. First, the current orthodoxy within psychiatry that madness is genetically preprogrammed can be traced, in large part, to eugenically orientated research during the Nazi era and before. Second, much of the current personality and intelligence testing in clinical psychology is traceable to a form of late Victorian psychology (the 'psychology of individual differences' or 'differential psychology') that was promoted by British eugenicists. Third, many of the recent ethical and political debates about euthanasia, genetic counselling, abortion, cloning and *in vitro* fertilisation resonate with those for and against a eugenic position. For example, abortion in the wake of detected foetal abnormality is not only opposed by some religious groups, but it also offends many in the disability movement.

See also: *causes and consequences of mental health problems; intellectual disability.*

FURTHER READING

Mazumdar, P. (1992) *Eugenics, Human Genetics and Human Failings: The Eugenics Society, Its Sources and Critics in Britain*. London: Routledge.
Meyer, J.E. (1988) 'The fate of the mentally ill during the Third Reich', *Psychological Medicine*, 18: 575–81.

REFERENCES

Binding, K. and Hoche, A.E. (1920) *Die Freigabe der Vernichtung Lebenunwerten Lebens*. Leipzig: Verlag von Felix Merner.
Dowbiggin, I. (1985) 'Degeneration and hereditarianism in French mental medicine 1840–90: psychiatric theory as ideological adaptation', in W.F. Bynum, R. Porter and M. Shepherd (eds), *The Anatomy of Madness*, Vol. 1. London: Tavistock.
Galton, F. (1881) *Natural Inheritance*. London: Macmillan.
Gottesman, I.I. and McGuffin, P. (1996) 'Eliot Slater and the birth of psychiatric genetics in Great Britain', in H. Freeman and G. Berrios (eds), *150 Years of British Psychiatry*, Vol. 2: *The Aftermath*. London: Athlone.
HMSO (1929) *Report of the Wood Committee on Mental Deficiency*. London: HMSO.
Joseph, J. (2005) 'The 1942 "euthanasia" debate in the *American Journal of Psychiatry*', *History of Psychiatry*, 16 (2): 171–9.
Kallmann, F.J. (1953) *Heredity in Health and Mental Disorder*. London: Chapman and Hall.
Kraepelin, E. (1883) *Compendium der Psychiatrie*. Leipzig: Abel.
Lewis, A. (1934) 'German eugenic legislation: an examination of fact and theory', *Eugenics Review*, 26: 183–91.
Luxenburger, H. (1928) 'Vorlaufiger Bericht uber psychiatrische Seriennuntersuchungen an Zwilligen', *Zeitschrift fur die Gesamte Neurologie und Psychiatrie*, 116: 297–326.
MacKenzie, D. (1971) 'Eugenics in Britain', *Social Studies of Science*, 6: 499–532.
Marshall, R. (1990) 'The genetics of schizophrenia', in R.P. Bentall (ed.), *Reconstructing Schizophrenia*. London: Routledge.
Mayer-Gross, W., Slater, E. and Roth, M. (1954) *Clinical Psychiatry*. London: Cassell.
Mazumdar, P. (1992) *Eugenics, Human Genetics and Human Failings: The Eugenics Society, Its Sources and Critics in Britain*. London: Routledge.
Mott, F. (1912) *Heredity and Eugenics in Relation to Insanity*. London: Eugenics Society.
Pilgrim, D. (2008) 'The eugenic legacy in psychology and psychiatry', *International Journal of Social Psychiatry*, 54 (3): 272–84.
Roelcke, V. (2007) 'The establishment of psychiatric genetics in Germany, Great Britain and the USA, c. 1910–1960, to the inseparable history of eugenics and human genetics', *Acta Historica Leopoldina*, 48: 173–90.
Rudin, E. (1916) *Zur Vererbung und Neuenstehung der Dementia Praecox*. Berlin: Springer.
Slater, E. (1936) 'German eugenics in practice', *Eugenics Review*, 27 (4): 285–95.

key concepts in
mental health

Slater, E. and Cowie, V. (1971) *The Genetics of Mental Disorders*. London: Oxford University Press.
Stone, D. (2001) 'Race in British eugenics', *European History Quarterly, 31* (3): 397–425.
Weindling, P. (1989) *Health, Race and German Politics between National Unification and Nazism, 1870–1945*. Cambridge: Cambridge University Press.

Capacity and Culpability

DEFINITION

'Capacity' is a legal term referring to the ability of a person to make sound rational judgements. A closely related notion is that of 'culpability' – the extent to which a wrong-doer is deemed to be responsible for their actions. Both involve notions of personal responsibility and imply autonomous human action.

KEY POINTS

- Considerations about mental disorder and personal capacity are discussed.
- Legal considerations about the culpability of mentally disordered offenders are outlined.

A vexed question for all concerned in mental health policy and practice relates to human agency – the quality most of us have, as we mature, to reflect on our actions and anticipate in advance their consequences. As the above definition indicates, it is common for judgements to be made by third parties that some patients are incapable of understanding the nature and consequences of their own actions, or the impact of the actions of others on them. Also, personal agency may be queried when wrongdoing occurs at the hands of people who are deemed to be mentally abnormal. This complexity will be discussed now under a number of points:

- *Capacity as a relative concept* Generally, capacity is attributed to adults but not to children. However, the attribution of personal capacity to a 13-year-old is greater than that to a 3-year-old, even though, legally, both are children. Similarly, a person in the early stages of dementia will be deemed to have more capacity than another individual in its later stages.
- *Neurological and psychiatric cases* The example of dementia points up a common reason for a person being deemed to lack capacity. Some of the dispute around mental disorder and capacity hinges on the legitimacy of medical diagnoses. In the case of organic mental illnesses – which are true neurological diseases – arguments against paternalism are less strong and less common.

Disputes tend to arise in relation to functional psychiatric diagnoses, including personality disorder. Moreover, whether a condition is judged to be organic or functional, a medical judgement still has to be made about the *extent* to which a person's disorder might impair their capacity.

- *Judgements about incapacity have consequences* Once the judgement is made about a lack of capacity, consequences will flow. For example, if a person is deemed to lack capacity, third parties are expected to make decisions on their behalf. An example here might be of a parent deciding that a young adult with learning disabilities, who is sexually active, should be sterilised. The operation then proceeds with that parent's consent. Less dramatic examples are of third parties receiving pension payments on behalf of a dementing patient. In the case of patients with functional diagnoses, such as schizophrenia, third parties (relatives, social workers and psychiatrists) may frequently negotiate desirable outcomes on their behalf. In all of these cases, medical ethicists tend to use the notion of 'impaired autonomy' rather than the legal notion of 'capacity'. This takes us on to the next point.

- *Impaired autonomy is a social judgement* Medical ethics relies for its guidance on principles developed by the philosopher and economist John Stuart Mill. He argued that, in a civilised society, the autonomy of law-abiding citizens should be respected and protected at all times *except* in the cases of children, the insane and idiots – 'those who are still in a state to require being taken care of by others must be protected against their own actions, as well as against external injury' (1980: 137). This gives the green light for mental health professionals to act in a warranted paternalistic way towards their patients. Indeed, according to Mill, they are *obliged* to act in that way.

Problems arise, however, when disputes are introduced about the *extent* to which a person is deemed to lack capacity and about the *consequences* of restraint. In the first case, anti-paternalists would argue that mentally disordered people can and should make judgements on their own behalf. Paternalists would point out that they cannot and that doctors are obliged to intervene, as a duty of care. In the second case (about restraint), there is a different dispute. Paternalists would say that a failure to restrain in order to treat risks a deterioration of the mental disorder. Anti-paternalists would argue that (metaphorically) the cure may be worse than the disease. An example here would be of a deluded patient who is coping on their own but, by the agreement of all, is mad or 'suffering from a severe mental illness'. They are detained in hospital involuntarily under the Mental Health Act and forcibly medicated. They lose their accommodation. They lose their liberty. They are put at risk of the adverse effects of anti-psychotic medication. Which is ethically preferable – intervening or letting them be?

Another example is the problem in making decisions about the anorexic patient whose body weight drops to a life-threatening level. These patients are not typically psychotic. In all normal respects, they are sane and can reason logically. The risk to the self is very high, though – should medical intervention be imposed? If so, should it be limited to life-saving, nutritional first aid or should it extend to a longer compulsory period of psychiatric detention? If it is the latter, for how long should this continue?

- *Inconsistency in decision-making about culpability* When it comes to dangerousness to others, rather than to the self, there are examples of inconsistency. For example, some sex offenders are sent to prison while others are sent to a secure hospital. Inside mental health facilities, psychotic patients who act in an antisocial way are tolerated by staff but those with a diagnosis of personality disorder acting in a similar fashion are not. Both are being treated within a paternalistic medical regime, but one group are still deemed to be responsible for their actions and so are treated moralistically and critically whereas the other are not.
- *Variants of impaired legal culpability* While arguments about capacity are often about the risk of impaired judgement jeopardising the health or even the life of the patient, those concerning culpability refer to criminal acts against others. In criminal law, for a person to be judged guilty, the court must be satisfied that there was malicious intent on the part of the perpetrator. In the case of the accused not being mentally disordered, an act may be judged to be unintentional or accidental. This may lead to the perpetrator not being tried or being acquitted. Unintended but reckless or negligent acts (such as manslaughter) are lesser crimes than those where 'malice aforethought', 'intention' or *mens rea* is evident. For this reason, they tend to lead to less severe sentencing. In the case of British mentally disordered offenders, these decision-making processes may be overridden in a variety of ways:

  - First, the perpetrator may not be deemed fit to stand trial – they lack a 'fitness to plead'. In these circumstances, they may be sent to a secure hospital without trial, provided that their role in the offence is clear to the court. If their mental disorder is treatable or recovery emerges naturally with time, then they may be recalled at a later date to face trial.
  - Second, whether or not the patient is deemed fit to plead, they may be judged to be 'not guilty by reason of insanity'. When this is the case, then the court, having taken psychiatric advice, decides that the person was sufficiently mentally disordered *at the time of the offence* that they were unaware that their actions were wrong. The insanity defence is more common in some countries than others. It is rare in Britain, where the third contingency is more likely to operate, when a case of homicide is being considered by the court.
  - Third, the defence of 'diminished responsibility' can be invoked, when mentally disordered offenders commit murder, but not in the case of other crimes in current English law. The legal term used in this context is suffering from 'abnormality of mind', which does not map neatly onto diagnostic categories preferred by psychiatrists.
  - Fourth, the most contentious decision is in relation to a temporary loss of reason and intention. This might apply to automatism (crimes committed while sleepwalking) and more commonly, but also more controversially,

crimes committed while under the influence of drugs or alcohol. Substance abuse is particularly contentious. On the one hand, it is deemed to be a mental disorder. On the other hand, in some crimes, such as dangerous driving, the intoxicated driver is typically treated much more harshly, by the courts, than the sober one. When this happens, the presence of a mental disorder, where the offender can demonstrate their long-term substance dependence, does not mitigate the action but the reverse occurs. This is against the trend of general decision-making in relation to mentally disordered offenders. However, it does not imply that a hospital 'disposal' by the courts necessarily leads to a lesser period of detention than imprisonment for the perpetrator, merely that the conditions of detention are likely to be more humane.

See also: *forensic mental health services; intellectual disability; substance misuse.*

FURTHER READING

Gillon, R. (1997) *Philosophical Medical Ethics*. London: Wiley.

Greaney, N., Morris, F. and Taylor, B. (2009) *Mental Capacity: A Guide to the New Law*. London: The Law Society.

Gunn, J. and Taylor, P. (eds) (1993) *Forensic Psychiatry: Clinical, Legal and Ethical Issues*. London: Butterworth/Heinemann.

Markham, D. (2003) 'Attitudes towards patients with a diagnosis of "borderline personality disorder": social rejection and dangerousness', *Journal of Mental Health*, 12 (6): 595–612.

Mill, J.S. (1980) *On Liberty*. London: Clarendon Press.

REFERENCE

Mill, J.S. (1980) *On Liberty*. London: Clarendon Press.

Anti-psychiatry

DEFINITION

'Anti-psychiatry' describes the work of a range of professional critics of orthodox psychiatric theory and practice.

KEY POINTS

- The character of anti-psychiatry is described.

- The main themes that connect anti-psychiatry with more recent views from post-psychiatry and the mental health service users' movement are described.

'Anti-psychiatry' can be heard as a term of hostile contempt from some who defend traditional theory and practice in psychiatry. It may be used resentfully or dismissively about, or against, any idea or person critical of the profession and its norms. Less emotively, it is also used to describe the output of a range of thinkers from a variety of countries in the 1960s, who offered a set of critiques about psychiatry. These included the published work of the psychiatrists Thomas Szasz (USA), Franco Basaglia (Italy), David Cooper (England), Ronald Laing (Scotland), Frantz Fanon (Algeria) and Jacques Lacan (France). Also, some North American sociologists, particularly those promoting labelling theory, contributed to this constellation of ideas, such as Erving Goffman and Thomas Scheff. The work of the French philosopher Michel Foucault also added to the mix, although some of his later ideas fitted less readily. Most of these thinkers are now dead but their criticisms remain influential.

With the exception of David Cooper, none of these luminaries embraced the label of 'anti-psychiatry'. Thomas Szasz actively rejected the term. To him, it implied being opposed to *everything* that psychiatry does and so it was logically absurd. As most of those associated with the intellectual leadership of 'anti-psychiatry' were *psychiatrists*, Szasz had a point. By and large, though, the label was *about* the critics rather than from them. Despite this ambivalence from the critical group, the label stuck – an irony given that the hazards of labelling were central to its critique. The notion of a 'constellation of ideas' is used here neutrally because when the term 'anti-psychiatry' was utilised by defenders of the profession, there was more than a strong hint of an organised global attack.

In support of this conspiracy theory, it is true that contributors came from all over the world and they often referenced and supported one another's work. However, this trend was inconsistent and the political ideology of the group was mixed. It included liberals like Goffman, Marxists like Cooper, left-leaning humanists like Laing, and strident anti-communists like Szasz. Indeed, the latter can be considered a right-wing libertarian because of his consistent hostility to the role of the state, as an enemy of individual freedom, and his support for the free market. By contrast, Foucault was a left-wing libertarian and some of his work was out of sync with the strong humanist current apparent in many of the other thinkers. The evidence of attack from different parts of the world probably says more about the vulnerability of psychiatric theory and practice than the conspiratorial motives of its critics. Psychiatry was, and remains, an easy target for criticism and so its practitioners are understandably wary and weary of being attacked.

The anti-establishment and libertarian culture of the 1960s was also reflected in the fiction of the period, which included themes resonant with the 'anti-psychiatric' position. Examples included Hannah Green's *I Never Promised You a Rose Garden*, Doris Lessing's *Golden Notebooks* and Ken Kesey's *One Flew*

Over the Cuckoo's Nest. The latter, starring Jack Nicholson, became an international box office success at the cinema.

The 'anti-psychiatric' clinicians in diverse ways promoted a radicalised version of psychoanalysis (Lacan, Szasz and Laing were psychoanalysts). Marxist and Weberian social science (Marcuse and Goffman, respectively) was influential. Also, the influences of existentialism (Sartre) and phenomenology (Merleau-Ponty) were evident. Laing's work also drew upon Eastern ways, especially Buddhism. In the 1970s, a range of feminist writers began to address 'anti-psychiatric' themes, particularly critiques of the modern family (for example, Kate Millet and Shulamith Firestone), as well as exploring the confluence of psychoanalysis and feminism (for example, Juliet Mitchell).

The summary above does not imply that the 1960s was the first period when psychiatry's knowledge base and role in society had attracted criticism. 'Anti-psychiatry' came in the immediate wake of the publication in 1958 of Barbara Wootton's influential book *Social Science and Social Pathology*. This attacked value judgements masquerading as science in diagnosis and the interfering role of psychiatric professionals. Also, there had been a long tradition, since the early 1920s, of critical theory derived from the work of the Frankfurt School – a range of writers discussing the implications of the confluence of Marxian and Freudian thinking.

There is evidence of the continuing influence of 'anti-psychiatry'. Many disaffected users, who during the 1970s and 1980s began to organise themselves into a new social movement to oppose orthodox psychiatric theory and practice, drew heavily on 'anti-psychiatric' work. Also, a new generation of 'critical psychiatrists' emerged during the 1990s, which now focuses on very similar concerns to those of its predecessors. Sometimes, this intellectual position, which has been mainly influenced by the work of Michel Foucault and other founders of postmodern social science, is called 'post-psychiatry'.

Here are a series of critical concerns that connect 'anti-psychiatry', the mental health service users' movement and 'post-psychiatry':

- *The meaning of madness* While the traditional medical view of madness is that it is an illness, probably resulting from a genetically programmed deterioration of the brain, critics query this or offer alternative views. For example, Laing and Cooper were keen to explore the ways in which unintelligible conduct might make sense within a person's social situation (particularly in the family). Similarly, critical service users have more recently organised Hearing Voices groups. These do not pre-judge the meaning of auditory hallucinations, as the pathological by-product of a schizophrenic illness. Instead, people are helped to examine the role of the voices in their particular biographical context. This is a central theme of 'anti-psychiatry': the shift from patients as examples of an assumed general pathology (say, 'schizophrenia') to people with problems requiring individualised forms of understanding.
- *The problem of coercion* Critics of psychiatry have questioned its coercive role. Coercion is rarely used to enforce medical treatment. By contrast, psychiatry

uses coercion on a daily basis. Because coercive powers are delegated lawfully to psychiatry, the profession accepts their legitimacy and is often unreflective about their implications. More than that, coercion takes medical paternalism to its furthest point by emphasising the doctor's right to treat rather than the patient's right to liberty.

- *The problem of stigmatisation* Critics of psychiatry complain that it makes an active contribution to the stigmatisation of psychological difference by the use of devaluing diagnoses, such as 'schizophrenia'.
- *The problem of social exclusion* A consequence of coercive removal from society and stigmatising diagnoses is that psychiatric patients have their citizenship undermined. This focus has been less evident since the run-down of the old asylum system, but newer services are criticised for their biomedical character and their lack of concern for the advocacy of social inclusion for patients.
- *The psychiatric preoccupation with physical treatments* A final theme in the views of critics is the unimaginative over-use of drug treatments and electro-convulsive therapy (ECT) by psychiatry. The less common psychosurgery is a particular focus of opposition but ECT also comes in for recurrent criticism. Campaigns can still be found to outlaw both ECT and psychosurgery. Alternatives suggested by critics range from non-intervention to various forms of psychotherapy.

These themes remain live in current debates about mental health services and the professional priorities of those who work in them. They are also still evident in the demands made for service improvements by local user groups.

See also: *coercion; stigma; the myth of mental illness*.

FURTHER READING

Clare, A. (1976) *Psychiatry in Dissent*. London: Tavistock.
Cooper, D. (1968) *Psychiatry and Anti-psychiatry*. London: Tavistock.
Fanon, F. (1963) *The Wretched of the Earth*. London: Granada.
Foucault, M. (1967) *Madness and Civilization*. London: Tavistock.
Goffman, E. (1961) *Asylums*. Harmondsworth: Penguin.
Laing, R.D. (1967) *The Politics of Experience and the Bird of Paradise*. Harmondsworth: Penguin.
Millet, K. (1970) *Sexual Politics*. New York: Doubleday.
Roth, M. (1973) 'Psychiatry and its critics', *British Journal of Psychiatry*, 122: 174–6.
Scheff, T. (1966) *Being Mentally Ill: A Sociological Theory*. New York: Aldine.
Sedgwick, P. (1980) *PsychoPolitics*. London: Pluto Press.
Wing, J. (1978) *Reasoning about Madness*. Oxford: Oxford University Press.
Wootton, B. (1958) *Social Science and Social Pathology*. London: Routledge and Kegan Paul.

REFERENCE

Wootton, B. (1958) *Social Science and Social Pathology*. London: Routledge and Kegan Paul.

Labelling Theory

DEFINITION

Labelling theory is a sociological approach to the study of deviance, which empha-sises the ways in which rule breaking and role failure are maintained by the reactions of others. For this reason, labelling theory is also known as 'societal reaction theory'.

KEY POINTS

- The strengths and weaknesses of labelling theory are described.
- The more recent development of 'modified labelling theory' is outlined.

Labelling theory developed from one wing of the Chicago School of Sociology, 'symbolic interactionism', which understands society by studying the ways in which humans exchange meanings in their interactions. Within this general approach, labelling theory focuses on the reaction of others to deviance. It accepts that the origin of *primary deviance* (say, being mentally disordered) may include a variety of biological, psychological and social causes. The focus for labelling theo-rists, though, is mainly on the maintenance and amplification of *secondary devi-ance*. The reactions of others shape the latter. Others may ignore or focus on devi-ant conduct, depending on a range of social contingencies.

Yarrow et al. (1955) found that the wives of men eventually labelled as schizo-phrenic ignored and rationalised symptoms for varying periods of time before seeking help. Rosenhan (1973) showed that 'pseudo-patients' were admitted to psychiatric facilities for simply reporting hearing the words 'empty', 'hollow' and 'thud'. In all other respects, they behaved rationally. The psychiatric staff recorded all of their behaviour, as if it was indicative of mental illness.

In these studies, there was confusion about the significant labellers. For Scheff (1966), it was psychiatrists. For Goffman (1961), it was the family, psychiatrists and staff in the mental hospital. However, there was an agreement that labelling irrevocably alters the person's identity and social status. Once a person is seen to have lost their reason, their credibility is permanently undermined (Garfinkel, 1956). Their old identity is cast off and a new one takes its place (a 'status degrada-tion ceremony'). Part of such a process then leads to the labelled person internalising the new identity ascribed to them. This is then maintained by self-labelling and the expectations of others.

After the 1960s, labelling theory fell out of favour because of a number of criticisms:

- Gove (1975) argued that it understates the underlying power of the causes of primary deviance. Moreover, Gove claimed that labelling has the positive consequence of giving patients access to help to reduce their deviance.

- If lay people play such an important role in deviance amplification, then we would expect everyday stereotypes of mental illness to match psychiatric diagnoses. However, Jones and Cochrane (1981) found that stereotypes conform very poorly to what psychiatrists diagnose in their work. The typical stereotype of a wild and deranged patient is wholly inaccurate. The most common diagnosis of 'depression' tends not to be mentioned in lay stereotypes of mental illness. Also, Rosenhan's pseudo-patients did not go on to actually take on the role of psychiatric patients after their discharge from hospital.
- Labelling theory does not really provide us with a clear picture of what the salient contingencies are that make the difference between deviance being ignored or being ascribed.

On this last point, some circumstances do seem to predict the ascription of mental illness. Women are more likely to be labelled than men in lay networks. Also, the greater the personal gap between labellers and the potentially labelled (in relation to race, culture, gender and class), the greater the chances of mental illness being ascribed and the more negative the label (Horwitz, 1982).

Despite the demise in popularity of labelling theory in the 1970s, more recent favourable appraisals have emphasised the substantial evidence for labelling theory, albeit in a modified form. Link and Phelan (1999) have drawn attention to a number of studies, which clearly demonstrate the negative effects of labelling:

- Some studies indicate that disvalued social statuses, such as prostitution, epilepsy, alcoholism and drug abuse, form a hierarchy of stigma, with mental illness being near to the bottom (e.g. Skinner et al., 1995).
- Some experimental studies also show that knowledge of a person's psychiatric history predicts social rejection and that these tendencies start in childhood (e.g. Harris et al., 1990).
- Surveys of the general public show that fear of violence and the need to keep a social distance diminish with increasing contact with people with a psychiatric diagnosis (Alexander and Link, 2003).
- Some studies, even at the time that labelling theory was losing its popularity, demonstrated that a psychiatric history reduced a person's access to housing and employment (e.g. Farina and Felner, 1973).

These types of findings have led to 'modified labelling theory'. Link and Phelan (1999) confirmed two main findings in a series of studies. First, provided that best practice is offered in mental health services, people with mental health problems can derive positive benefits (supporting Gove's claim about the positive opportunity created by labelling). Second, whether or not specialist mental health services have positive or negative effects (a function of their range of quality), independent effects of stigma and social rejection persist in the community.

The theory Link and colleagues have developed to account for this second finding relates not to direct prejudicial action by others (the 'classical' position of labelling theory) but to a shared cultural expectation. The latter entails mental illness leading to suspicion, a loss of credibility and social rejection. All parties, including and *especially* the person who *develops* a mental health problem, share this assumption from childhood. Consequently, the patient enters, or considers entering, interactions with others with this shared negative assumption. Non-patients also expect patients to be expecting social distance. This shared view then leads to both parties lacking confidence in their interaction, creating a self-fulfilling prophecy. The patient keeps their distance and the non-patient expects this and lets it occur. Subsequently, this creates social disability and isolation in the patient.

Modified labelling theory is also supported by the work of Thoits (1985), who noted that classical labelling theory was preoccupied with involuntary relation-ships, whereas most consultations for mental health problems occur voluntarily, mainly in primary care services. Thoits demonstrated how we learn from a young age to self-monitor emotional deviance.

For example, we begin to learn when it is appropriate to be happy, sad or fear-ful. Consequently, we can also identify in ourselves when our emotional conduct might be considered inappropriate by others. Thoits describes this as a shared awareness of the compliance with, or transgression of, 'feeling rules'. For example, the phobic patient knows that their fear is irrational but they also feel as though their conduct is not within their control. The depressed adult knows that their low mood and lack of confidence disable them from carrying out the normal fam-ily and work obligations expected of them, and this knowledge may fuel their depression further.

See also: *causes and consequences of mental health problems; social exclusion; stigma; the mass media.*

FURTHER READING

Link, B.G. and Phelan, J.C. (1999) 'The labeling theory of mental disorder (II): the consequences of labeling', in A.V. Horwitz and T.L. Scheid (eds), *A Handbook for the Study of Mental Health*. Cambridge: Cambridge University Press.
Scheff, T. (1966) *Being Mentally Ill: A Sociological Theory*. Chicago, IL: Aldine.

REFERENCES

Alexander, L.A. and Link, B.G. (2003) 'The impact of contact on stigmatizing attitudes toward people with mental illness', *Journal of Mental Health*, 12 (3): 271–90.
Farina, A. and Felner, R.D. (1973) 'Employment interview reactions to former mental patients', *Journal of Abnormal Psychology*, 82: 268–72.
Garfinkel, H. (1956) 'Conditions of successful degradation ceremonies', *American Journal of Sociology*, 61: 420–4.
Goffman, E. (1961) *Asylums*. Harmondsworth: Penguin.
Gove, W. (1975) 'The labeling theory of mental illness: a reply to Scheff', *American Sociological Review*, 40: 242–8.
Harris, M.J.R., Millich, E.M. and Johnson, D.W. (1990) 'Effects of expectancies on children's social interactions', *Journal of Experimental Social Psychology*, 26: 1–12.
Horwitz, A.V. (1982) *The Social Control of Mental Illness*. New York: Academic Press.
Jones, L. and Cochrane, R. (1981) 'Stereotypes of mental illness: a test of the labelling hypothesis', *International Journal of Social Psychiatry*, 27: 99–107.

Link, B.G. and Phelan, J.C. (1999) 'The labeling theory of mental disorder (II): the consequences of labeling', in A.V. Horwitz and T.L. Scheid (eds), *A Handbook for the Study of Mental Health*. Cambridge: Cambridge University Press.

Rosenhan, D.L. (1973) 'On being sane in insane places', *Science, 179*: 250–8.

Scheff, T. (1966) *Being Mentally Ill: A Sociological Theory*. Chicago, IL: Aldine.

Skinner, L.J., Berry, K.K., Griffiths, S.E. and Byers, B. (1995) 'Generalizability and specificity of the stigma associated with the mental illness label: a reconsideration twenty-five years later', *Journal of Community Psychology, 23*: 3–17.

Thoits, P. (1985) 'Self-labeling processes in mental illness: the role of emotional deviance', *American Journal of Sociology, 91*: 221–49.

Yarrow, M.J., Schwartz, C., Murphy, H. and Deasy, L. (1955) 'The psychological meaning of mental illness', *Journal of Social Issues, 11*: 12–24.

Stigma

DEFINITION

Stigma refers to the social consequences of negative attributions about a person based upon a stereotype. In the case of people with mental health problems, it is presumed that they lack intelligibility and social competence and that they are dangerous.

KEY POINTS

- The features of stereotyping and stigma are outlined.
- The particular ways in which people with mental health problems are stereotyped and stigmatised are discussed.

Stigmatisation has two main aspects. First, the person stigmatised is perceived stereotypically as an example of a social group (rather than tentatively and respectfully as an individual). Second, this stereotyping or 'social typing' has negative connotations. (It happens occasionally that there is *positive* stereotyping. This does not lead to stigma but it is still illogical.) These two features are associated with emotional reactions in others, such as fear, contempt and disgust, although pity and concern may also be evoked. In the case of the stereotyping of people with mental health problems, all of these reactions may be present in different proportions from one situation to another. Thus, stereotyping has both cognitive and emotional aspects.

What then arises from these inner processes of stereotyping is a social reaction, whereby one party rejects the other or reacts towards them in a way that is significantly different. As a result, the stigmatised person is set apart and they suffer the consequences of the social distance created. The person feels depersonalised, rejected and disempowered. As a consequence, they may develop what Goffman (1963) called a 'spoiled identity'. Rogers and Pilgrim (2015) note that people with mental health problems are stigmatised in a particular way, which refers to three presumed qualities in the target: a lack of intelligibility, a lack of social competence and the presence of violence. The strongest cultural stereotype is the spectre of a homicidal madman – a deranged being who explodes violently, erratically and inexplicably (Foucault, 1978). This scenario remains a focus of fascination for news-reporting even today, when it is singled out sporadically, against a wider backdrop of completely unreported homicides. In the USA, this aspect of reporting is important in relation to gun crime (as it makes mental state, not gun ownership, the focus of the reporting).

In order to establish that stereotyping is irrational, it is necessary to examine the evidence that may or may not support it. In our case here, do mentally ill people always lack intelligibility? Are they always socially incompetent? Are they always violent?

- *The question of intelligibility* In most social situations, participants have an obligation, if called upon, to render their speech and conduct intelligible about any rule transgression or role failure (Goffman, 1971). If we break a rule, then we should be able, if called upon, to give an account. If asked, we must be able and willing to provide a persuasive reason or an explanation (Scott and Lyman, 1968). If we do not, then that itself represents a form of rule breaking. With specific regard to madness, then, this rule breaking does indeed occur. Lay judgements about the emergence of madness refer primarily to a person's lack of intelligibility and inability to explain their oddity in an acceptable or persuasive manner (Coulter, 1973). Of critical importance here is that judgements about the social obligation to explain oneself occur in context. Take the example of talking to oneself. Generally, this might be the main piece of behavioural evidence that a person is mad. However, if it happens in church or when the person is holding a mobile telephone to their ear, then madness is much less likely to be attributed. Also, the presence of auditory hallucinations may be considered intelligible in one context but not another.

Thus, there *is* some empirical evidence to suggest that the stereotype of people with mental health problems lacking intelligibility is valid. Generally, it is fair to say that mad people act in a way that others do not understand and that they are unable or unwilling to give credible accounts to others of their thoughts and actions. However, there is also evidence that this generalisation (the key to stereotyping) is flawed. First, mad people may be unintelligible sometimes and not at other times. For example, it is common for psychosis to occur episodically, with periods of recovery and sanity. Another example is in relation to persistent paranoid delusions. In this case, the person may act completely intelligibly all of the time *except* when the delusional material emerges in conversation. Second, many people with mental health problems (those with a diagnosis of neurosis rather than psychosis) are highly aware of their problems – indeed, they may be preoccupied with giving accounts to others about their feelings and actions. The attribution of unintelligibility only applies to madness, not all mental disorder, and even then, not all of the time.

- *The question of social competence* Lay judgements about mental health problems and their formal medical codification in psychiatric diagnoses include an attribution of failed social competence. The mad person loses their credibility because they have lost their reason. Because they are not taken seriously, they are socially disabled – they are not permitted to be competent. The depressed or anxious person is unable to carry out their normal role obligations. As with the previous point about intelligibility, there is evidence to undermine these generalisations about the loss of competence (and its associated credibility). First, some people with mental health problems are disproportionately creative. Second, some symptoms create greater competence at some tasks. For example, those with a diagnosis of obsessive-compulsive disorder or obsessive-compulsive personality disorder are more likely to perform above average on tasks requiring a close attention to detail. Third, religious leaders may enjoy heightened credibility even though they may manifest symptoms of mental illness.

There is therefore some evidence that some people with mental health problems act in an unintelligible way some of the time. There is no evidence that all people with mental health problems are unintelligible all of the time. Likewise, there is some evidence that some people with mental health problems have diminished social competence, some of the time, to warrant diminished social credibility. However, this is not true all of the time for all people with mental health problems. Indeed, some of the time their competence and credibility are actually raised and not diminished. In addition, some patients are at increased risk of being violent to others. However, these are in the minority. The vast majority of people with a psychiatric diagnosis are not more violent than those without a diagnosis. In some cases, for example in anxious people or in psychotic patients with 'negative symptoms', the probability of violence is actually lower than would be the case in the general population.

The persistence of these three elements of stigmatisation of those with mental health problems is historically rooted in the generalisations made about madness. Not only were these historically based stereotypes always questionable on empirical grounds, but they are also now applied inappropriately and unfairly to many patients who are not mad. This is because the jurisdiction of contemporary mental health services extends beyond the management of madness. Solutions offered to reverse stigmatisation include patients demanding citizenship rights and professionals pleading for mental illness to be treated with the same respect as physical illness. (These points are explored further in the entry on Social Exclusion.)

See also: *creativity; labelling theory; madness; mental health; social exclusion; the mass media.*

FURTHER READING

Rogers, A. and Pilgrim, D. (2015) *A Sociology of Mental Health and Illness* (5th edn). Maidenhead: Open University Press.

stigma

Sartorius, N. (ed.) (2008) *Understanding the Stigma of Mental Illness: Theory and Interventions.* London: John Wiley & Sons.

REFERENCES

Coulter, J. (1973) *Approaches to Insanity.* New York: Wiley.

Foucault, M. (1978) 'About the concept of the "dangerous individual" in 19th-century legal psychiatry', *International Journal of Law and Psychiatry,* 1: 1–18.

Goffman, E. (1963) *Stigma: Some Notes on the Management of Spoiled Identity.* Harmondsworth: Penguin.

Goffman, E. (1971) *Relations in Public.* Harmondsworth: Penguin.

Rogers, A. and Pilgrim, D. (2015) *A Sociology of Mental Health and Illness* (5th edn). Maidenhead: Open University Press.

Scott, M.B. and Lyman, S.M. (1968) 'Accounts', *American Journal of Sociology,* 33: 12–18.

Social and Cultural Capital

DEFINITION

Social and cultural capital refer to the objective features of social and cultural networks and the subjective experiences and advantages accruing from them.

KEY POINTS

- The origins of the concept are summarised.
- The relationship between economic, cultural and social capital is noted.
- Social and cultural capital have a proven impact on mental health.

In social science, the concept of social capital has been mainly linked to the work of Coleman (1988), Putnam (2000) and Bourdieu (1984), with the latter offering the concept within his wider discussion of forms of capital. Reviewing this work, Crossley (2005) notes that capital can have economic, social and cultural forms and that it entails:

> different sorts of resources that social agents can mobilize in pursuit of their projects and which, on account of their value, agents will tend to seek to pursue and accumulate. (Crossley, 2005: 53)

Most of us are familiar with money as a resource for people (regular income, savings, inheritance and so on), but the use of 'capital' in other senses may be less obvious. Cultural capital is discussed by Bourdieu in terms of accumulated artefacts in a person's life (such as books, recorded music or works of art), as well as their particular socialisation in school and the family (their 'upbringing'). An expression of cultural capital is the social competence bestowed by the latter, which is then reflected in variable degrees of self-confidence, depending on the person's particular background. Put simply, richer, privately educated people will tend on average to be more self-confident than poorer and less well-educated people.

This embodied form of cultural capital overlaps with another concept used by Bourdieu, that of 'habitus' – the learned habits, attitudes and skills of a person. Habitus provides the basis for cultural capital: the latter is one of its possible outcomes but it is not inevitable. It is only when the outcome involves a *relationship*, to the advantage of the person, that habitus bestows cultural capital. Cultural capital, mediated by habitus, and economic capital, typically reflecting a person's class position, can also affect the accumulation and expression of social capital.

Social capital can refer to objective descriptions of social networks (say, in a locality) and subjectively to a person's experience of social contacts or meaningful relationships. Thus, social capital is a *current* description of a social connectivity, affected by external contingencies, whereas cultural capital refers to the *legacy* of confidence, competence and status that accrue from upbringing and are then expressed in particular current life circumstances. All three forms of capital are mutually supportive but they do not totally determine one another. For example, people from a rich background with a good job and higher educational credentials may find themselves in life circumstances of social isolation and so will still have poor social capital. The ramifications of social capital are indicated in Figure 4.2.

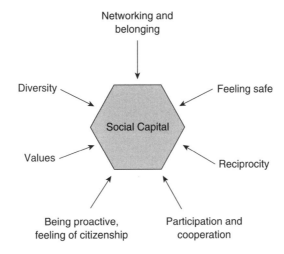

Networking and belonging

Diversity

Feeling safe

Social Capital

Values

Reciprocity

Being proactive, feeling of citizenship

Participation and cooperation

Figure 4.2 The ramifications of social capital

Social networks are a fairly good predictor of health status and not just of mental health status (Milne et al., 2004). This is also true of socio-economic status or class, stable employment and educational level. It is another illustration of the interweaving of economic, cultural and social forms of capital. However, if people, whatever their upbringing or economic worth, find themselves to be socially isolated and so depleted of social capital, then their poor mental health is a likely outcome. In other words, social networks, *independent* of the wealth and upbringing of individuals, can affect wellbeing (Cassel, 1976; Cobb, 1976; Henderson, 1992). Perceived social support is positively correlated with mental health (e.g. Sarason et al., 1990; Veil and Baumann, 1992; Thoits, 1995). Henderson (1992) reported 35 separate studies of the relationship between social support and depression, which demonstrated the consistent link between the two.

Marital status is another product of economic, social and cultural capital which predicts mental health status. Mental health problems are commoner in people living alone. (However, in the case of divorced single people, men show decrements in mental health but women do not.) Overall, the rich get richer in two senses: those with an intimate partner tend to enjoy more personal support than single people, and those with more disposable income tend to have richer social networks. Also, work brings with it direct opportunities for social connections (Turner and Marino, 1994; Ross and Mirowsky, 1995).

This does not rule out the direct (i.e. unmediated) impact of poverty on mental health (Rogers and Pilgrim, 2003). However, it strongly suggests that lower levels of income provide fewer *opportunity structures* for people to develop social contact and thereby experience personal support (House et al., 1988). These opportunity structures entail access to social events, as well as the increased confidence to interact with others with increasing social status. A criticism that has been levelled against politicians now emphasising social capital is that they use it as a way of avoiding the distal but direct relationship with structural inequality just noted. The process of social capital building can be offered as a low-cost policy substitute for dealing with structural inequalities about power and wealth.

To conclude, social capital, like cultural and economic capital, is a good predictor of mental health. These three forms of capital often interact and affect mental health in individual circumstances but sometimes these effects can operate separately from each other. The competence, confidence and financial resources to obtain and sustain meaningful relationships underpin good mental health. Consequently, these mutually influencing forms of capital are important to understand by those studying or treating people with mental health problems.

See also: *social class; social exclusion; wellbeing*.

FURTHER READING

Crossley, N. (2005) *Key Concepts in Critical Social Theory*. London: Sage.

Phongsavan, P., Chey, A., Bauman, R., Brooks, R. and Silove, D. (2006) 'Social capital, socio-economic status and psychological distress among Australian adults', *Social Science & Medicine*, 63: 2546–61.

REFERENCES

Bourdieu, P. (1984) *Distinction*. London: Routledge and Kegan Paul.

Cassel, J. (1976) 'The contribution of host environment to host resistance', *American Journal of Epidemiology, 14*: 107–23.

Cobb, S. (1976) 'Social support as a moderator of life stress', *Psychosomatic Medicine, 38*: 300–14.

Coleman, J. (1988) *Foundations of Social Theory*. Cambridge, MA: Harvard University Press.

Crossley, N. (2005) *Key Concepts in Critical Social Theory*. London: Sage.

Henderson, A.S. (1992) 'Social support and depression', in H.O.F. Veil and U. Baumann (eds), *The Meaning and Measurement of Social Support*. New York: Hemisphere.

House, J.S., Umberson, D. and Landis, K.R. (1988) 'Structures and processes of social support', *Annual Review of Sociology, 14*: 293–318.

Milne, D., McAnaney, A., Pollinger, B., Bateman, K. and Fewster, E. (2004) 'Analysis of the forms, functions and facilitation of social support in one English county: a way for professionals to improve the quality of health care', *International Journal of Health Care Quality Assurance, 17* (6): 294–301.

Putnam, R. (2000) *Bowling Alone*. New York: Touchstone.

Rogers, A. and Pilgrim, D. (2003) *Mental Health and Inequality*. Basingstoke: Palgrave Macmillan.

Ross, C.E. and Mirowsky, J. (1995) 'Does employment affect health?', *Journal of Health and Social Behavior, 36*: 230–43.

Sarason, B.R., Pierce, G.R. and Sarason, I.G. (1990) 'Social support: the sense of acceptance and the role of relationships', in B.R. Sarason, I.G. Sarason and G.R. Pierce (eds), *Social Support: An Interactional View*. New York: Wiley.

Thoits, P. (1995) 'Stress, coping and social support processes: where are we? What next?', *Journal of Health and Social Behavior, 2* (Suppl.): 53–79.

Turner, J.R. and Marino, F. (1994) 'Social support and social structure: a descriptive epidemiology', *Journal of Health and Social Behavior, 35*: 193–212.

Veil, H.O.F. and Baumann, U. (1992) 'The many meanings of social support', in H.O.F. Veil and U. Baumann (eds), *The Meaning and Measurement of Social Support*. New York: Hemisphere.

Social Exclusion

DEFINITION

Social exclusion refers to the various ways in which an individual or group of individuals are denied access to levels of citizenship, social association and wealth available to others.

KEY POINTS

- Examples are given of the social exclusion of people with mental health problems.
- A focus on social exclusion is contrasted with the traditional emphasis on stigma.

A number of entries in this book emphasise the negative social consequences of receiving a psychiatric diagnosis and having service contact. While the causes of mental health problems may remain contested, their consequences (whether viewed as direct impairment or constructed disability) are very clear (Secker, 2011). Those with mental health problems experience social exclusion on a number of fronts:

- *Labour market disadvantage* Psychiatric patients are often unemployed and their history may jeopardise any future employment. Only a minority of psychotic patients will find work (Jenkins and Singh, 2001). Neurotic patients are four times more likely to be unemployed than non-patients and five times more likely to be receiving invalidity benefits than the general population (Rogers and Pilgrim, 2003). People with mental health problems are nearly three times as likely as physically disabled people to be unemployed (Department for Education and Employment, 1998). Chronic unemployment feeds demoralisation and, in the case of psychotic patients, increases their chances of relapse (Warner, 1985).
- *Derision and hostility from the mass media* The mass media both reflect and encourage public hostility and distrust towards people with mental health problems. In particular, newspapers are disproportionately prone to publish stories that link mental health problems to violence (Philo et al., 1994). By contrast, little is said about patients as victims of violence or as productive or creative members of society. The norms about discriminatory reporting are evident in headlines such as 'Schizophrenic kills …' (newspapers would not print 'Black kills …'). Also, the mass media will use ordinary language descriptions of madness in a silly, humorous way in stories ('Looney council …'). This tendency to make mental health a source of either anxiety or trivial humour creates the conditions under which media audiences are more likely to reject and distrust people with mental health problems.
- *Poverty* This is wider than labour market disadvantage but in part flows from it. People with mental health problems are more likely to live in socially disorganised and poor localities. In the latter are high levels of noise, pollution, litter and traffic congestion. In addition to these environmental stressors, social networks are weak and crime rates high. Those with mental health problems who remain chronically unemployed have to suffer the shared consequences with others in this situation. Daily life is unstructured and meaningful activity may be unavailable. The comforts of substance misuse may fill the void that this desolate culture creates. Substance misuse amplifies mental health problems and undermines physical health. Poverty means that stress-reduction activities (such as holidays) are restricted. Thus, a whole range of cultural and economic processes impinge on poor people. Those with pre-existing mental health problems are particularly vulnerable to these negative social forces.
- *Lawful discrimination* People who have inpatient stays in acute mental health services are detained in unusual circumstances. Typically, they will have committed no crime. No one will have acted as an advocate to argue against their

admission – all of the professional procedures are aimed at formalising a consensus for the decision. Although they may be recorded, officially, as being a 'voluntary' or 'informal' patient, they may have been given no genuine choice. It is common for patients to enter hospital in a pseudo-voluntary state. They are told that if they do not 'come quietly', then powers of involuntary detention will be invoked (Rogers, 1993). If they resist detention or seek to leave the hospital, then staff members are provided with legal powers to physically restrain them. If they refuse medication, it may be imposed upon them. They may be isolated in a room ('secluded'). While there are safeguards against excesses and misuse in these regards, there is clear daily empirical evidence that a psychiatric diagnosis brings with it a range of risks to any patient's privacy and autonomy. Together, these legal powers also create particular ways in which people with mental health problems are excluded from society. Once limited to hospitals, they are now being extended increasingly to community settings (Dennis and Monahan, 1996).

It is therefore clear that, on a number of fronts, people with mental health problems are socially excluded. Evidence about this broader set of social forces constraining the welfare and citizenship of patients has led some commentators to criticise the stigma framework. For example, Sayce (2000) argues that the latter reduces the field of inquiry to that of the characteristics and plight of stigmatised *individuals*. Sayce holds that we should instead examine the *collective* discriminatory response of others. The four areas of discrimination noted above together provide this collective response.

Sayce points out that although the frame of individual stereotyping needs to be widened to look at collective responses, the cognitive features of the latter are still an important starting point from which to understand a range of stances in society about the social inclusion or exclusion of people with mental health problems. She notes that different interest groups manifest different assumptions about three interrelated aspects of discrimination towards people with mental health problems: the nature of mental health problems; the causes of mental health problems; and what should be done about discrimination.

If a psychiatrist or the relative of a patient considers that the latter is suffering from a genetically caused disturbance of brain biochemistry, they will argue that discrimination will be reduced by campaigning for us all to accept mental illness to be like any other illness. Moreover, they would also demand more research into the (putative) genetic causes of mental illness, now framed as a brain disease, in order to reduce the prevalence of future 'sufferers'. The latter term is common within this approach because patients are seen as the diseased victims of biological misfortune (namely, being born with the wrong genes). By contrast, a service user who argues that psychological difference is caused by a variety of oppressive factors will argue for social change and the right to full citizenship, and thereby the reduction or abolition of compulsory psychiatric treatment.

Take another example. A biological view of depression might lead to an educational campaign to encourage patients to seek antidepressant treatment. For this reason, the drug companies in their marketing strategies depict depression in a matter-of-fact way as a biological illness. Social inclusion in this context would be limited to an equal right to medical treatment. By contrast, an environmental etiological view would give rise to calls for reductions in social stressors (like poverty, work stress and so on) (Goldstein and Rosselli, 2003). Social inclusion in this context would be about people with mental health problems having access to benign and supportive living environments and to satisfying work roles.

The representations of different diagnostic groups by others can also affect degrees of treatment equity within mental health services. For example, mental health workers tend to be paternalistic towards psychotic patients but distrusting and rejecting towards those with a diagnosis of personality disorder (Markham, 2003). Both are stigmatised groups but different attributions about personal 'fault' from professionals lead to differential levels of personal acceptance and support.

See also: *labelling theory; social class; stigma; the mental health service users' movement.*

FURTHER READING

Huxley, P. and Thornicroft, G. (2003) 'Social inclusion, social quality and mental illness', *British Journal of Psychiatry*, 182: 289–90.

Secker, J. (2011) 'Mental health problems, social exclusion and social inclusion', in D. Pilgrim, A. Rogers and B. Pescosolido (eds), *The SAGE Handbook of Mental Health and Illness*. London: Sage.

REFERENCES

Dennis, D.L. and Monahan, J. (eds) (1996) *Coercion and Aggressive Community Treatment*. New York: Plenum Press.

Department for Education and Employment (DfEE) (1998) *Labour Force Survey: Unemployment and Activity Rates for People of Working Age*. London: DfEE.

Goldstein, B. and Rosselli, F. (2003) 'Etiological paradigms of depression: the relationship between perceived causes, empowerment, treatment preferences and stigma', *Journal of Mental Health*, 12 (4): 551–64.

Jenkins, R. and Singh, B. (2001) 'Mental disorder and disability in the population', in G. Thornicroft and G. Szmukler (eds), *Textbook of Community Psychiatry*. Oxford: Oxford University Press.

Markham, D. (2003) 'Attitudes towards patients with a diagnosis of "borderline personality disorder": social rejection and dangerousness', *Journal of Mental Health*, 12 (6): 595–612.

Philo, G., Secker, J., Platt, S., Henderson, L., McLaughlin, G. and Burnside, J. (1994) 'The impact of the mass media on public images of mental illness', *Health Education Journal*, 53: 271–81.

Rogers, A. (1993) 'Coercion and voluntary admissions: an examination of psychiatric patients' views', *Behavioural Sciences and the Law*, 11: 259–68.

Rogers, A. and Pilgrim, D. (2003) *Inequality and Mental Health*. Basingstoke: Palgrave.

Sayce, L. (2000) *From Psychiatric Patient to Citizen: Overcoming Discrimination and Social Exclusion*. Basingstoke: Macmillan.

Secker, J. (2011) 'Mental health problems, social exclusion and social inclusion', in D. Pilgrim, A. Rogers and B. Pescosolido (eds), *The SAGE Handbook of Mental Health and Illness*. London: Sage.

Warner, R. (1985) *Recovery from Schizophrenia: Psychiatry and Political Economy*. London: Routledge.

The Mental Health
Impact of Social Media

DEFINITION

The emergence and expansion of the use of social media since the turn of the 21st century have altered our relationship with ourselves, one another and technology. This has affected our psychological functioning in a range of ways.

KEY POINTS

- The growth of social media use, which has altered our relationships to ourselves, one another and technology, is discussed.
- These changes, which have brought costs and benefits to our mental health, are examined.

The emergence of the internet and the mass availability of devices for its daily use have altered those societies using it in recent years. This has afforded a range of changes to our experience and conduct. Information that once took hours, days or weeks to transfer can now occur instantly. This has affected norms about the speed of life (making it more exciting but also more challenging or anxiety-provoking). The technology itself has now become an expected accompaniment, especially among young people, with the mobile phone now being used as a palm-top computer, not merely a device to make calls to others. The displacement of telephone calls by text messaging has altered the expectation of direct one-to-one conversations and with it the skills and confidence associated with the older form of communication.

These changes have brought with them an emerging literature about the risks to our mental health of social media, although the benefits of it have also been noted.

RISKS OF SOCIAL MEDIA USE

Because of the relatively recent mass usage of social media, a range of risks to mental health have been identified, although we can distinguish expressed *concerns* about such risks from *empirical evidence* of harm. Here I list those concerns and make reference where applicable to studies recording harm. The daily reliance on social media use can alter sleep patterns, cause moodiness and raise general anxiety levels in users (Young and Lo, 2012; Kross et al., 2013; Hormes et al., 2014).

It is an ongoing professional debate as to whether social media engagement is a form of addiction; differentiating it from a norm is problematic, given the prevalence and range of positive and negative experiences of it being reported (Andreassen et al., 2012; Cash et al., 2012; Brailovskaia, 2017). Demoralising exchanges online can lower mood and cyber-bullying creates distress in its victims (in individual cases, an outcome of suicide might be reported in the mass media) (Williford et al., 2013; Steers et al., 2014; Spears et al., 2015; Primack et al., 2018; Twenge et al., 2019). The last of these studies is from the USA and points to an upward trend in young suicide. However, a caution in attributing this to social media use is that recently there has also been an increase in opioid use in the USA.

When experiences are reported as negative by users, this in turn leads to them reporting increased social isolation; a paradox given that social media is allegedly about social connectivity (Primack et al., 2019). Social comparisons about appearance and opinion can alter self-worth and generate envy (Vogel et al., 2015). The immediate relationship with the technology itself might encourage a new form of narcissism. For example, 'selfies' have only become possible because of a camera that is turned on the self, which can then be admired by both the user and the people who might receive the image immediately or eventually. The admiration of self images also now extends to the presentation of self to others. Photo-shopping can alter our features aesthetically. (This moment-to-moment narcissism might extend to photographs of food about to be consumed.) This image manipulation and the confusion of electronic social contact with authentic sociability have prompted wider philosophical questions about the nature of relationality in modern society and the prospect of a shift towards self-objectification in young women, reversing the gains of second-wave feminism (Turkle, 2012; De Vies and Peter, 2013). The emerging evidence on the negative impact of social media on their users is currently being reviewed by politicians in the UK (House of Commons Science and Technology Committee, 2019). The latter have already suggested that legislation should be introduced to regulate social media use and that its impact on children should be a priority for discussions in British schools.

In informal groups, the intermittent and sometimes predominant use of 'screen time' in the presence of others has altered. Today, we are in the midst of testing out new norms about the acceptability of this disruption to traditional expectations about courteous respect for those in our immediate presence. In some formal contexts, social media use is considered transgressive, with authority figures in the group instructing others to 'turn off your phones'.

The changes of presentation of self in everyday life noted above mean that we can manipulate others in a range of ways apart from deceiving them about our physical appearance. We can also create artificial identities that can be passed off as being authentic. Apart from people on 'hook up' sites discovering in practice that the person present is different from the photo previously seen, criminals can exploit others. For example, given the unambiguous evidence about the long-term impact of child sexual abuse on mental health, the impact of the internet is now salient, with the police being overwhelmed in their efforts to identify offenders. The latter groom their victims online and may negotiate eventual sexual contact.

This also extends to *in vivo* offending online: a man in one country can direct the rape of a child on camera by a third party in another country thousands of miles away. A by-product of this law enforcement challenge created by internet use has been the counter-manipulative activity of vigilantes pursuing child sex offenders, who use social media to lure them into public spaces for their arrest (Martellozzo, 2012; Pilgrim, 2018).

Finally, in this section we can note specific concerns expressed about the use of social media by distressed people. These include the potential harm created by pro-anorexia websites, but also the link between volume of use of social media in young people and their risk of eating problems (Sidani et al., 2016). Apart from dedicated pro-anorexia sites, there are similar ones related to self-harm and suicide (Wilson et al., 2007; Mörch et al., 2018). An ambiguity here is about the moral worth of these sites. Their critics point to the increased risks to mental health, whereas their enthusiastic users would argue that they are forms of social support and personal validation. This ambiguity prompts the next section.

BENEFITS OF SOCIAL MEDIA

Read alone, the section above produces a fairly negative picture about the impact of social media on our relationship to self and others. Social media now mandate our attention and this might lead to our psychological distress or it could prompt action that has a detrimental impact on our mental health. To use it brings risks, but not using it also creates the risk of 'fear of missing out' or 'FOMO' on knowledge or entertainment being enjoyed by peers. This creates a bind on all of us today because approach-avoidance conflicts are inherently stressful.

Despite this bind, the Pandora's Box effect of social media means that their very availability broadly is considered a beneficial necessity in modern life. (The philosophical term for a taken-for-granted norm is 'doxa'.) Our current doxa is to endorse, maybe unreflectively, the overall benefit of social media in principle. Those promoting internet use have a commercial interest in only emphasising its benefits, but its mass usage suggests that they are kicking at an open door, within post-industrial consumer societies. The latter would apply even to those claiming a Marxist-Leninist ideology not just in liberal democracies. For example, in China the internet is restricted but it is still used widely in practice.

Commercial transactions have been rendered faster and more effective by the internet and so its advantages to consumers is self-evident. Its advantages to commercial providers complement this consumer demand, affording them opportunities to market their wares and keep transactional costs down. Online research (in all its senses) has now been rendered fast and efficient by the presence of the internet and professional researchers enjoy immediate updates in their area of interest by using platforms like Twitter. The distress online noted above is more about the impacts on relationality in personal interactions, with many being with people whom the users have never met personally, and where their hostile comments can be anonymous. If users were only to use social media for information transfer and neutral or positive communications, then social media use would be benign and beneficial. However, this would require a normative shift towards courteous restraint, analogous to the rules that we traditionally associate with face-to-face meetings with others. How that restraint is to be encouraged or ensured remains unclear at the time of writing.

Combining these points, web-based interactions arguably reflect mass democratisation (because they rely on user-generated content) and they create opportunities for increased social networking (a form of social capital). As we become aware of the debates about the costs and benefits of social media, the balance sheet about mental health can be thought of as an aggregate question (does it make whole or sub-populations mentally healthier or not?) and an individual question (does it benefit or psychologically injure this particular individual?).

Social media use is only one facet of the utility of the internet. At present, people are making their own judgements about its risks to them. Discussions of 'detox' are common and pride emerges for some who manage to leave common platforms or reduce their 'face time'. Social media use may be emerging as a risk that is analogous to smoking: enjoyable to its users but potentially injurious.

See also: *economic aspects of mental health; secondary prevention; social and cultural capital.*

REFERENCES

Andreassen, C.S., Torstein, T., Bromberg, G.S. and Palliser, S. (2012) 'Development of a Facebook Addiction Scale', *Psychological Reports, 110* (2): 501–17.

Brailovskaia, J. (2017) 'Facebook Addiction Disorder (FAD) among German students – a longitudinal approach', *PLoS One, 12* (12): 2423–78.

Cash, H., Rae, C.D., Steel, A.H. and Winkley, A. (2012) 'Internet addiction: a brief summary of research and practice', *Current Psychiatry Review, 8* (4): 292–8.

De Vies, D. and Peter, J. (2013) 'Women on display: the effect of portraying the self online on women's self-objectification', *Computers in Human Behavior, 29* (4): 1483–9.

Hormes, J.M., Kearns, B. and Timko, C.A. (2014) 'Craving Facebook? Behavioral addiction to online social networking and its association with emotion regulation deficits', *Addiction, 109* (12): 2079–88.

House of Commons Science and Technology Committee (2019) *Impact of Social Media and Screen-Use on Young People's Health.* Fourteenth Report of Session 2017–19. London: House of Commons.

Kross, E., Verduyn, P., Demiralp, E., Park, J., Lee, D.S., Lin, N. et al. (2013) 'Facebook use predicts declines in subjective well-being in young adults', *PLoS ONE, 8* (8): e69841.

Martellozzo, E. (2012) *Online Child Sexual Abuse: Grooming, Policing and Child Protection in a Multi-Media World.* London: Routledge.

Mörch, C.-M., Côté, C.-L., Laurent, C.-L. et al. (2018) 'The Darknet and suicide', *Journal of Affective Disorders, 1* (241): 127–32.

Pilgrim, D. (2018) *Child Sexual Abuse: Moral Panic or State of Denial?* London: Routledge.

Primack, B.A., Bisbey, M., Shensa, A., Bowman, N., Karim, S.A., Knight, J. and Sidani, J.E. (2018) 'The association between valence of social media experiences and depression', *Depression and Anxiety, 35* (8): 784–94.

Primack, B.A., Karim, S.A., Shensa, A., Bowman, N., Knight, J. and Sidani, J.E. (2019) 'Positive and negative social media experiences and social isolation', *American Journal of Health Promotion* (online), 21 January, https://doi.org/10.1177/0890117118824196

Sidani, J.E., Shensa, A., Hoffman, B. and Primack, B.A. (2016) 'The association between social media use and eating concerns among US young adults', *Journal of American Academy of Nutrition and Dietics*, *116* (9): 1465–72.

Spears, B.A., Taddeo, C.M., Daly, A.L., Stretton, A. and Karklins, L.T. (2015) 'Cyberbullying, help-seeking and mental health in young Australians: implications for public health', *International Journal of Public Health*, *60* (2): 219–26.

Steers, M.L-N., Wickham, R.E. and Acitella, L.K. (2014) 'Seeing everyone else's highlight reels: how Facebook usage is linked to depressive symptoms', *Journal of Social and Clinical Psychology*, *33* (8): 701–31.

Turkle, S. (2012) *Alone Together: Why We Expect More from Technology and Less from Each Other*. New York: Basic Books.

Twenge, J.M., Cooper, A.B., Joiner, T.E., Duffy, M.E. and Binau, S.G. (2019) 'Age, period, and cohort trends in mood disorder indicators and suicide-related outcomes in a nationally representative dataset, 2005–2017', *Journal of Abnormal Psychology*, *128* (3): 185–99.

Vogel, E.A., Rose, J.P., Okdie, B.M., Eckles, K. and Franz, B. (2015) 'Who compares and despairs? The effect of social comparison orientation on social media use and its outcomes', *Personality and Individual Differences*, *86*: 49–56.

Williford, A., Elledge, L.C., Boulton, A.J., DePaolis, K.J., Little, T.D. and Salmivalli, C. (2013) 'Effects of the KiVa antibullying program on cyberbullying and cybervictimization frequency among Finnish youth', *Journal of Clinical Child and Adolescent Psychology*, *42*: 820–33.

Wilson, J., Peebles, R., Hardy, K.K. and Litt, I. (2007) 'Surfing for thinness: a pilot study of pro-eating disorder web site usage in adolescents with eating disorders', *Pediatrics*, *118* (6): 1635–43.

Young, C.M.Y. and Lo, B.C.Y. (2012) 'Cognitive appraisal mediating relationship between social anxiety and internet communication and adolescents', *Personality and Individual Differences*, *52* (2): 78–83.

Risks to and from People with Mental Health Problems

DEFINITION

People with mental health problems may be a source of risk to themselves and others. They are also subject to particular risks from others and their environment.

KEY POINTS

- The evidence for and against the stereotype that psychiatric patients are dangerous is reviewed.

- The evidence about psychiatric patients being at risk from others is reviewed.

The dominant cultural image of mental disorder (dating back to antiquity) is one of violence. The problem with this dominant image is that it is stereotypical. It is empirically inaccurate and, for the majority of people with mental health problems, also a source of unfair treatment (in its widest sense).

In order to bring both accuracy and justice into the debates about mental health problems and dangerousness, a number of points can be made:

- *Because the concept of mental disorder is now very wide, it includes some highly dangerous people* The continued association between violence and psychiatric diagnosis does now have some empirical basis. The reason for this is that two broad diagnostic groups (those who abuse substances and those with a diagnosis of antisocial personality disorder) have significantly high rates of violence. Indeed, in the case of antisocial personality disorder, violence (sexual or otherwise) is central to its circular definition. As psychiatry developed in the 20th century, its jurisdiction extended from lunacy to include personality disorder and substance misuse. This now means that people with these diagnoses are psychiatric patients and so encourage and maintain the stereotype that *all* psychiatric patients are dangerous (Pilgrim and Rogers, 2003).
- *Substance abuse and personality disorder, not psychosis, are the best predictors of violence* The above point begs a question: are people with a diagnosis other than substance misuse or antisocial personality disorder prone to violence? The answer is 'no'. Indeed, most psychotic and the overwhelming majority of neurotic patients are no more violent than the general population (Steadman et al., 1998). This point is also true of many forms of personality disorder. There is an important exception to this trend, however: those with 'co-morbidity' or 'dual diagnosis'. Psychotic patients who abuse substances are significantly more violent than either the general population or psychotic patients who do not abuse substances. Similarly, some mentally disordered offenders are given a dual diagnosis of mental illness and personality disorder. Substance misuse and antisocial personality disorder are highly predictive of violence to others. Psychotic patients with positive symptoms (hallucinations and delusions) who abuse substances are significantly more dangerous (Soyka, 2000). Thus, the key issue here is that psychosis alone is not an indicator of risk to others, despite the longstanding stereotype implying such a relationship. It is the co-presence of substance abuse and/or personality problems that raises the probability of violence in psychiatric populations. This co-presence is important for another reason: psychiatric patients live in circumstances in which the comforts of substance abuse are common. They are three to four times more likely to abuse substances than the general population (Regier et al., 1990). Between 20 and 30 per cent of psychotic patients living in the community are likely to abuse substances (Hambracht and Hafner, 1996).

- *Iatrogenic damage and loss of liberty* The largest risk to patients is from service contact. Most admissions to acute units are now involuntary so patients are at a high risk of losing their liberty without trial. Also, all forms of treatment, both biological and psychological, carry risks (see the entries on Biological Interventions and Psychological Interventions). Apart from the risk created by professional action, patients are also at risk of stigma from service contact. Hospitalisation also disrupts community living and may even jeopardise tenancy arrangements.
- *Crime* Because psychiatric patients are often poor, they tend to live in poor community contexts with higher crime rates. For this reason, patients run a high risk of being the victims of both acquisitive and violent crime. They are also at risk of becoming criminals because of local cultural norms. Patients typically live in what Silver and colleagues (1999) call 'concentrated poverty'. These living conditions contain more 'violence-inducing social forces' which impact upon patients as potential victims and perpetrators (Hiday, 1995). For this reason, discussions about patients in either role need to take into account ecological factors, not just the clinical and personality characteristics of individuals (Rogers and Pilgrim, 2003).
- *Risks associated with poverty* In addition to the risk of being the victims of crime, poor living circumstances also bring with them peculiar stressors: congested traffic, litter, air pollution, poorer access to healthcare and education, and fewer leisure facilities. They also mean that stress-reducing options (such as holidays) are reduced.
- *Suicide* This is discussed in a separate entry. Here it will simply be noted that people with mental health problems live shorter lives than others. Most of this loss of years alive is as a result of suicide.
- *'The manner in which one is dangerous'* This phrase was used by Szasz (1963) to make the point that psychiatric patients suffer discrimination. Some dangerous roles are highly rewarded and bring with them raised social status (for example, boxers, mountaineers, racing drivers and astronauts). Also, some forms of injurious and self-injurious behaviour do not lead to the actors being readily detained without trial (for example, smoking, fast driving). Moreover, the rules of detention about dangerousness are applied differently to patients. They may lose their liberty without trial for *predicted future action*. By contrast, other violent citizens only risk the loss of liberty as a consequence of *proven past action*. The due process of a court trial allows the accused to argue for their innocence and freedom, and they are provided with an advocate to support these arguments. By contrast, the civil detention of psychiatric patients occurs without court proceedings and the patient is not provided with the opportunity to argue for their continued liberty with the support of a legal advocate.

To conclude, any comprehensive discussion of the issue of risk and mental health problems has to consider a two-way process. While media reports and public prejudice may focus disproportionately on one aspect (violent risk to others), the reality is that it is risks to patients that are more prevalent – those concerning iatrogenic damage, poverty and premature death. Moreover, patients enjoy less legal protection than others when their risk to others is being investigated and dealt with.

See also: *biological interventions; psychological interventions; stigma; suicide; the mass media.*

FURTHER READING

Pilgrim, D. and Rogers, A. (2003) 'Mental disorder and violence: an empirical picture in context', *Journal of Mental Health*, 12 (1): 7–18.

Szasz, T.S. (1963) *Law, Liberty and Psychiatry*. New York: Macmillan.

REFERENCES

Hambracht, M. and Hafner, H. (1996) 'Substance abuse and the onset of schizophrenia', *Biological Psychiatry*, 40: 1155–63.

Hiday, V. (1995) 'The social context of mental illness and violence', *Journal of Health and Social Behavior*, 36: 122–37.

Pilgrim, D. and Rogers, A. (2003) 'Mental disorder and violence: an empirical picture in context', *Journal of Mental Health*, 12 (1): 7–18.

Regier, D.A., Farmer, M.E., Rae, D.S., Locke, B.J., Keith, S.J., Judd, L.L. and Godwin, F.K. (1990) 'Comorbidity of mental disorders with alcohol and other drug use: results from the epidemiologic catchment area (ECA) study', *Journal of the American Medical Association*, 264: 2511–18.

Rogers, A. and Pilgrim, D. (2003) *Mental Health and Inequality*. Basingstoke: Palgrave.

Silver, E., Mulvey, E.P. and Monahan, J. (1999) 'Assessing violence risk among discharged psychiatric patients: towards an ecological approach', *Law and Human Behavior*, 23: 237–55.

Soyka, M. (2000) 'Substance misuse, psychiatric disorder and violent and disturbed behaviour', *British Journal of Psychiatry*, 176: 345–50.

Steadman, H.J., Mulvey, E.P., Monahan, J., Robbins, P.C., Applebaum, P.S., Grisso, T., Roth, L.H. and Silver, E. (1998) 'Violence by people discharged from acute psychiatric facilities and by others in the same neighbourhood', *Archives of General Psychiatry*, 55: 109.

Szasz, T.S. (1963) *Law, Liberty and Psychiatry*. New York: Macmillan.

The Mass Media

DEFINITION

The mass media refer to outlets of information and entertainment, such as radio, television, cinema and newspapers. The role of the mass media in maintaining negative images of people with mental health problems has been the focus of substantial criticism.

KEY POINTS

- The role of the mass media in reinforcing and maintaining prejudice against people with mental health problems is examined.
- Some recent counter-examples from radio programmes and the cinema are described.

The definition above refers to 'outlets of information and entertainment'. The blurring of the boundaries between the two is reflected in the notion of 'infotainment' – the tendency of the mass media to maximise audience levels by mixing information with strategies of shock and titillation. The more serious the intention of the journalist and the ethos of particular outlets within the media, the more likely it is that empirical findings and even-handed analysis are privileged over entertainment. The longstanding stereotypes of mental health problems being linked to violence and derision mean that they are ready-made topics for journalistic interest. People with mental health problems are also vulnerable when distressed and lack credibility because of their defined loss of reason. This makes them easy targets for negative news stories and storylines.

Historically, negative images about madness preceded the emergence of the mass media (Rosen, 1968). For this reason, it is not logical to argue that the latter simply create negative images of mental health problems in modern society. It is relevant, though, to examine the role played by the mass media in maintaining and amplifying such images and to provide an empirical and ethical critique of this role. The educational role of the mass media about mental health problems is significant. For example, surveys of public opinion about mental illness reveal that the mass media are the main source of information for lay people (Wahl, 1995). Moreover, negative media reports are a source of stress and distress for people who have mental health problems (Mind, 2000).

Within media depictions, there is an overwhelming emphasis on violence. This is true of newspaper news stories (e.g. Angermeyer and Schulze, 2001) as well as TV fictional portrayals (e.g. Signorielli, 1989). This trend seems to be consistent and global for the various countries studied: the USA (Diefenbach, 1997), Canada (Day and Page, 1986), Germany (Angermeyer and Schulze, 2001), New Zealand (Nairn et al., 2001) and Britain (Philo et al., 1994; Rose, 1998). The trend of violent portrayal may be amplifying, with people with mental health problems being depicted as being even more dangerous than was the case 50 years ago (Phelan et al., 2000). Sieff (2003) points out that while there has been a recent increase in the occurrence of positive images, these tend to be limited to people with anxiety or depressive symptoms. The link between psychosis and violence and unpredictability remains very strong.

Cinematic presentations of mental health problems have tended to reflect and reinforce this stereotype of violence but, recently, more positive or sympathetic images can be found in mainstream film-making (for example, *A Beautiful Mind*). They can also be found in some films where a minor character has a mental health problem (for example, *Just a Boy*). These are a recent corrective to a long tradition of film-making in which mental health problems are associated only with either violence or ridicule.

The mass media have also provided an occasional opportunity for mental health issues to be discussed seriously. For example, two of the public inquiries into the mistreatment of patients in the two English Special Hospitals of Rampton (1980) and Ashworth (1991) were triggered by investigative TV programmes.

An earlier example was the interest taken by the *That's Life* programme in the 1970s about tranquilliser use. It is noteworthy that this began as a collaborative campaign with Mind (the National Association of Mental Health) about the problems of anti-psychotic medication (*major* tranquillisers). However, the programme was deluged with interest from the watching public about addiction to benzodiazepines (*minor* tranquillisers). This indicates that the role of the mass media has to be understood as an interaction with its recipient audiences rather than as a one-way source of influence. It also reflects the power differential between the two medicated groups, with psychotic patients being displaced by neurotic patients.

Other examples of serious consideration about mental health matters in the mass media in recent years have been programmes such as *All in the Mind* and *In the Psychiatrist's Chair* on the BBC's Radio 4. These allow professionals and patients to offer the general public a voice and to discuss research about mental health issues. They are not sensationalist and nor do they contribute to scaremongering and public prejudice. Indeed, it is the newspapers (especially, but not uniquely, the tabloids) that are most prone to these negative interventions.

See also: *labelling theory; social exclusion; stigma.*

FURTHER READING

Carpiniello, B., Girau, R. and Orrù, M.G. (2007) 'Mass-media, violence and mental illness: evidence from some Italian newspapers', *Epidemiology and Psychiatric Sciences*, 16 (3): 251–5.

Cutcliffe, J.R. and Hannigan, B. (2001) 'Mass media, "monsters" and mental health clients: the need for increased lobbying', *Journal of Psychiatric and Mental Health Nursing*, 8 (4): 315–41.

REFERENCES

Angermeyer, M.C. and Schulze, B. (2001) 'Reinforcing stereotypes: how the focus on forensic cases in news reporting may influence public attitudes towards the mentally ill', *International Journal of Law and Psychiatry*, 24: 469–86.

Day, D.M. and Page, S. (1986) 'Portrayal of mental illness in Canadian newspapers', *Canadian Journal of Psychiatry*, 31: 813–17.

Diefenbach, D. (1997) 'The portrayal of mental illness on prime-time television', *Journal of Community Psychology*, 43 (4): 51–8.

Mind (2000) *Counting the Cost*. London: Mind Publications.

Nairn, R., Coverdale, J. and Claasen, D. (2001) 'From source material to news story in New Zealand print media: a prospective study of the stigmatizing processes in depicting mental illness', *Australian and New Zealand Journal of Psychiatry*, 35 (5): 654–9.

Phelan, J.C., Link, B.G., Stueve, A. and Pescosolido, B.A. (2000) 'Public conceptions of mental illness in 1950 and 1996: what is mental illness and is it to be feared?', *Journal of Health and Social Behavior*, 41: 188–207.

Philo, G., Secker, J., Platt, S., Henderson, L., McLaughlin, G. and Burnside, J. (1994) 'The impact of the mass media on public images of mental illness: media content and audience belief', *Health Education Journal*, 53: 271–81.

Rose, D. (1998) 'Television, madness and community care', *Journal of Applied Community Social Psychology*, 8: 213–28.

Rosen, G. (1968) *Madness in Society*. New York: Harper.

Sieff, E.M. (2003) 'Media frames of mental illnesses: the potential impact of negative frames', *Journal of Mental Health*, 12 (3): 259–69.

Signorielli, N. (1989) 'The stigma of mental illness on television', *Journal of Broadcasting and Electronic Media*, 33 (3): 325–31.

Wahl, O.F. (1995) *Media Madness: Public Images of Mental Illness*. New Brunswick, NJ: Rutgers University Press.

Social Models of Mental Health

DEFINITION

These refer to an emphasis on the social as the primary source of causes and meanings in relation to mental health and mental disorder.

KEY POINTS

- A number of sociological accounts can be found in relation to mental health and mental disorder.
- They include: social causationism; critical theory; social constructivism; social realism; and social reaction (or labelling) theory.

'The social' has been invoked in a number of ways in relation to mental health and mental disorder. This invocation has led to competition between sociological accounts as well as variants on the particular salience of the social. Thus, we find a range of views from the social being singularly important, to it being considered in interaction with others, especially biological, psychological and spiritual factors. Given this mixed picture, although it is common to hear of 'the social model', as we also hear of 'the medical model', we need to take account of pluralism and complexity. For this reason, it is more appropriate to describe and explore social factors and arguments in the field, rather than assume a single 'social model'. The latter often signals complex and cross-cutting arguments about social causation, socially-derived identities and culturally-specific norms and meanings (for example, see Rosenfield, 2012).

An emphasis on 'the social' can lead to forms of sociological reductionism, just as much as biology and psychology have manifested their version of this risk. In relation to meanings, a singular emphasis on the social can lead to arguments that 'everything is socially constructed' or that mental health or mental disorder are merely contingent by-products of professional activity of the 'psy complex' or 'the mental health industry'. Arguing against this position, Craib (1997) (a sociologist) describes radical social constructionism as a form of 'social psychosis' because it is out of touch with the psychological and biological reality. In relation to causes, a social emphasis can lead to the conclusion that mental health problems can be understood and rectified simply by paying attention to the stressors associated with poverty, race, age and gender.

While there is, indeed, a strong case to be made about the social sources of meanings and causes, both risk sociological reductionism. For example, all societies have some notions of madness and misery, suggesting that they are not merely socially constructed and contingent. In the case of misery, there are fairly predictable circumstances that invoke this (especially loss and entrapment) in all mammalian species. Thus, we can garner evidence to demonstrate that misery is not socially constructed, even if the lay and professional words used for it across time and space are variable. Instead, there is evidence that misery is real and that it has predictable psychological and physiological antecedents and consequences.

In the case of causes, if social factors are all-important, why then are there individual differences *within* social groups – for example, why are only some poor people depressed? Explanations for within-group differences draw our attention to the importance of variable social stressors, but they also point up the peculiar psychological circumstances enjoyed by some of us but not others. The importance of the variable quality of relationships in families of origin and differences in individual attributions about similar events suggests that psychological, not social, arguments might at times be privileged. And although biological factors may have been over-valued in the history of psychiatry, they might also explain individual differences in psychological functioning some of the time.

Social group membership is therefore important. However, in understanding the emergence of wellbeing or mental disorder, it cannot account for individual differences. The latter imply the legitimate need to examine personal and biological factors. With all of these cautions in mind, a number of trends about the social in our field can be described (Rogers and Pilgrim, 2014):

- *Social causationism* Refers to models that emphasise social stressors alone or in combination, leading to a mental health outcome. A good, sophisticated version of this can be found in the work of Brown and Harris (1978) on depression in working-class women.
- *Critical theory* Refers to the integration of Freudian and Marxian explanations of psychopathology (the 'Frankfurt School'). It emphasises the interplay between inner, especially unconscious, events and historically contingent outer social contexts (Slater, 1977). This enabled its early theorists to understand the authoritarian personality, the mass psychology of fascism and everyday

culture and psychopathology. Its later theorists focused on family socialisation and ego development, the mass media and culture, the cessation of political protest in capitalist societies and critiques of science and positivism (Marcuse, 1964; Offe, 1984; Habermas, 1989).

- *Social constructivism (or constructionism)* According to Brown (1995), this has taken three forms in social science. The first focuses on social problems and the ways in which social forces define their salience and existence (Spector and Kituse, 1977). This is clearly relevant to mental health problems. The second is associated with French post-structuralism and, in the field of mental health in particular, the work of Foucault (1965, 1981). The third has been associated with the sociology of scientific knowledge (Latour, 1987) and applied infrequently to our field of interest here.

- *Social realism* Refers to the approach which argues that madness and misery are real and multiply determined but that the knowledge used to describe them is socially constructed. This is associated with the philosophical position of critical realism (Bhaskar, 1989) and emphasises that it is not madness and misery which are socially constructed but the ways that we describe them (Greenwood, 1994; Pilgrim and Rogers, 1994).

- *Social reaction (or labelling) theory* Has been particularly influential in the field of mental health (Scheff, 1966; Fabrega and Manning, 1972; Link and Phelan, 1999). It argues that primary deviance arises from many sources (biological, psychological and social) but that the ultimate fate of individual rule breakers is determined by contingent social-psychological factors. The latter then shape secondary deviance – namely, the extent to which rule breaking is tolerated or labelled and controlled. The latter processes occur in both the lay and professional arenas and consolidate and amplify the role and identity of deviant individuals, such as those with a psychiatric diagnosis.

See also: *causes and consequences of mental health problems; gender/sex; labelling theory; race; social class; stigma.*

FURTHER READING

Brown, G. and Harris, T. (1978) *Social Origins of Depression*. London: Tavistock.
Rogers, A. and Pilgrim, D. (2014) *A Sociology of Mental Health and Illness* (5th edn). Maidenhead: Open University Press.

REFERENCES

Bhaskar, R. (1989) *Reclaiming Reality*. London: Verso.
Brown, G. and Harris, T. (1978) *Social Origins of Depression*. London: Tavistock.
Brown, P. (1995) 'Naming and framing: the social construction of diagnosis and illness', *Journal of Health and Social Behavior*, 1 (Suppl.): 34–52.
Craib, I. (1997) 'Social constructionism as a social psychosis', *Sociology*, 31 (1): 1–15.
Fabrega, H. and Manning, P.K. (1972) 'Disease, illness and deviant careers', in R.A. Scott and J.D. Douglas (eds), *Theoretical Perspectives on Deviance*. New York: Basic Books.
Foucault, M. (1965) *Madness and Civilisation*. New York: Random House.

Foucault, M. (1981) *The History of Sexuality*. Harmondsworth: Penguin.

Greenwood, J.D. (1994) *Realism, Identity and Emotion: Reclaiming Social Psychology*. London: Sage.

Habermas, J. (1989) 'The tasks of a critical theory of society', in S.E. Bronner and D.M. Kellner (eds), *Critical Theory and Society: A Reader*. London: Routledge.

Latour, B. (1987) *Science in Action: How to Follow Scientists and Engineers*. Cambridge, MA: Harvard University Press.

Link, B. and Phelan, J. (1999) 'The labeling theory of mental disorder: the consequences of labeling', in A.V. Horwitz and T.L. Scheid (eds), *A Handbook for the Study of Mental Health*. Cambridge: Cambridge University Press.

Marcuse, H. (1964) *One Dimensional Man*. London: Routledge and Kegan Paul.

Offe, C. (1984) *Contradictions of the Welfare State*. London: Hutchinson.

Pilgrim, D. and Rogers, A. (1994) 'Something old, something new … sociology and the organisation of psychiatry', *Sociology, 21* (2): 521–38.

Rogers, A. and Pilgrim, D. (2014) *A Sociology of Mental Health and Illness* (5th edn). Maidenhead: Open University Press.

Rosenfield, S. (2012) 'Triple jeopardy? Mental health at the intersection of gender, race, and class', *Social Science & Medicine, 74* (1): 1791–6.

Scheff, T. (1966) *Being Mentally Ill: A Sociological Theory*. Chicago, IL: Aldine.

Slater, P. (1977) *Origin and Significance of the Frankfurt School*. London: Routledge.

Spector, M. and Kituse, J. (1977) *Constructing Social Problems*. Menlo Park, CA: Cummings.

Suicide

DEFINITION

Deliberate, self-imposed death.

KEY POINTS

- The error of conflating suicide with mental disorder is noted.
- A range of points is summarised about the complexity of the topic.

The paradox of this entry is that it contributes further to a criticism about to be made – that suicide is seen, all too readily and singularly, as a mental health problem. The entry makes a small further contribution to this fundamental error of reasoning but, in its defence, it will also try to correct the error. Suicide is a complex topic and will be discussed here under a number of points:

- *Suicide is a crude and at times misleading proxy for mental health* There are a number of problems with any policy measure which conflates suicide and mental disorder. Suicide is not necessarily irrational. There are many circumstances in which a resolution of personal suffering is for the individual to make a logical decision to end his or her life. Also, in some cultures or circumstances, suicide has been seen as an honourable, not a dysfunctional, act. For example, the traditional Japanese phenomena of *hara-kiri* and *kamikaze* indicate that death at one's own hands can be both appropriate and honourable (and certainly not a symptom of psychopathology). Another example of this question of rationality and honour is in relation to *jauhar*. This was a ritual of collective female suicide in Hindus in medieval India, when faced with invading Muslim hordes. Death was a preferred option to degradation and slavery.

More ambiguously, some religious cults have attracted attention when their leaders have demanded obedience about mass suicide (for example, the Waco suicides in Texas and the Heaven's Gate suicides in California). The ambiguity surrounds value judgements about cults. Are they an example of mass mental disorder? Are their leaders grandiose and sadistic and their followers dependent and masochistic? Did all of the current accepted major world religions start as small cults?

The main point here is that there is a danger of irrationality being imputed retrospectively in all cases. That is, when and if a person commits suicide, it is easy to argue that the 'balance of their mind' was faulty at the fatal moment or that they had a prior mental disorder which made them particularly prone to self-sacrifice. Such a conclusion is by no means always logically warranted. Moreover, in older people with multiple physical illness, there may be an understandable wish to die. This can lead to the *post hoc* psychiatric attribution of mental illness (depression) in this group, which is deemed to warrant treatment. This is not to say that suicide some of the time may well reflect irrational reasoning. What cannot be legitimately claimed, however, is that suicide *always and necessarily* reflects irrationality.

- *There are international and intra-national differences in suicide profiles* Differences occur in the preferred type of suicide and the rate of suicide (see Figure 4.3, which depicts the global map of suicide rates from the World Health Organization). In the USA, guns are the preferred option (reflecting their availability). By contrast, in relatively gun-free cultures like Britain, carbon monoxide poisoning from car exhaust fumes is the main option used by men (women are more likely to use pills to self-poison). Suicide rates are at their highest in Northern, Central and Eastern Europe (including Russia) and North America. They are at their lowest in the Mediterranean and Islamic countries. These patterns may change over time. For example, Durkheim in his classic sociological study of suicide noted that during wartime the suicide rate drops. It increases during peaks in both prosperity and relative poverty. More recent evidence suggests that areas with high rates of poverty, poor employment, unemployment and poor local social cohesion witness higher suicide rates. There are also occupational differences, with medical practitioners and farmers being at a higher risk than the general population.

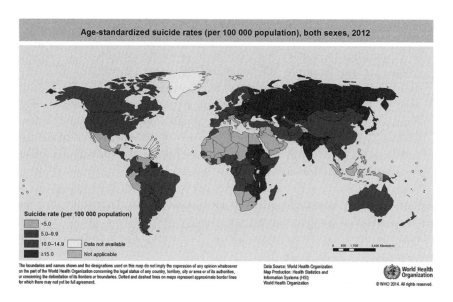

Figure 4.3 Global map of suicide rates, 2012

- *There are age and gender differences in suicidal behaviour* Across the life span, there is a global pattern of men completing suicide more frequently than women (a ratio of about 3:1). However, attempted suicide is more common in young women than young men (a ratio of about 2:1). For emphasis, though, it can be noted that more young men commit suicide than do women. The tendency for attempted suicide to peak in younger years may reflect the relative powerlessness of the young, with a suicidal gesture being powerful.

- *Some, but not all, self-harming reflects suicidal behaviour* Many people who self-harm (for example, by cutting themselves) are very clear that they are *not* suicidal. Some self-harming activity is mainly directed at tension release or self-punishment – it does not signal a wish to die. Moreover, in some people, dramatic suicidal gestures are used as a communication to influence others (as in the actions of histrionic personalities when they are distressed). In the psychiatric literature, suicide (or 'completed' suicide) is usually distinguished from suicide attempts or 'parasuicide'. There are both empirical and cultural problems with this distinction. For example, a person who is found dying at their own hands may or may not be relieved if they are saved by others. An alternative example is that a person may not intend to commit suicide in a dramatic gesture that 'goes wrong'. In cultures where there is shame attached to suicide (or where it is illegal), parasuicide may be under-reported. For example, in India, suicidal behaviour is still a punishable legal offence. Suicide is also considered to be immoral according to some forms of strict religious observance. The moral and legal context can thus shape the norms of reporting about suicidal behaviour. A final empirical problem is that an open verdict is often recorded for people dying at their own hands – this makes precise estimates of suicide difficult and brings into question the validity of suicide data at times.

- *People with mental health problems are at greater risk of suicide* The reasons for this are contested and can be related back to the basic cultural assumption addressed at the outset (that suicidal action is always irrational). Empirically, the picture is by no means clear. For example, depressed behaviour seems to be linked to a tendency to commit suicide. However, not all depressed people commit suicide and some who show no obvious symptoms of depression can (shockingly) take their own life. Despite seasonal variations in mood (particularly in Northern Europe), suicide rates do not increase in the winter but are at their highest in the spring and summer. Women receive a psychiatric diagnosis more often than men but the latter commit suicide more often than the former. Having said all of this, some mental health problems are associated with an increased risk of suicide. Depressed patients who are older, male and abuse substances are at a significantly high risk. Those with a diagnosis of schizophrenia are also at a significantly high risk of suicide. Factors that might affect this correlation are loss of career or academic success, social exclusion and the impact of anti-psychotic medication, which includes distressing agitation (akathisia) and a drop in mood (acute dysphoria). Those with a diagnosis of schizophrenia are at a 14-fold rate of risk compared to the general population and, in the case of bipolar disorder, it is a 12-fold risk. However, despite these psychiatric correlations and the sociological trends noted above, no successful method has been found to accurately predict the risk of an *individual* committing suicide in either clinical or non-clinical populations.

Finally, we can note that a range of public health strategies to reduce rates of suicide have been introduced but to date their cost-effectiveness has not been proven. This may be because effectiveness is difficult to demonstrate unequivocally, given that suicide is a low frequency event and, as was noted above, the conditions of possibility for its emergence are varied and multi-factorial and not always readily understood from case to case. Sometimes, after the event, we know why a person committed suicide, sometimes we can make a fair estimate of motive and sometimes it remains a baffling mystery to those left behind.

See also: *biological interventions; physical health; risks to and from people with mental health problems.*

FURTHER READING

Alexander, M.J., Haugland, G., Ashenden, P. et al. (2009) 'Coping with thoughts of suicide: techniques used by consumers of mental health services', *Psychiatric Services*, 60 (9): 1214–21.

Bhui, K.S. and McKenzie, K. (2008) 'Rates and risk factors by ethnic group for suicides within a year of contact with mental health services in England and Wales', *Psychiatric Services*, 59 (4): 414–20.

Biddle, L., Brock, A., Brookes, S.T. et al. (2008) 'When things fall apart: gender and suicide across the life-course. Suicide rates in young men in England and Wales in the 21st century: time trend study', *British Medical Journal*, 336: 539–42.

Durkheim, E. (1951) *Suicide: A Study in Sociology*. Glencoe, IL: Free Press.

Gunnell, D., Middleton, N., Whitley, E., Dorling, D. and Frankel, S. (2003) 'Why are suicide rates rising in young men but falling in the elderly? A time-series analysis of trends in England and Wales 1950–1998', *Social Science & Medicine*, 57 (4): 595–611.

Hawton, K.E. and van Heeringen, K. (2000) *The International Handbook of Suicide and Attempted Suicide*. Chichester: Wiley.

Horne, J. and Wiggins, S. (2009) 'Doing being "on the edge": managing the dilemma of being authentically suicidal in an online forum', *Sociology of Health and Illness*, 31 (2): 170–84.

McDaid, D. (2016) 'Making an economic case for investing in suicide prevention: quo vadis?', in R.C. O'Connor and J. Pirkis (eds), *Handbook of Suicide Prevention: Research, Policy and Practice*. Chichester: Wiley Blackwell.

O'Connor, R.C. and Sheehy, N.P. (2001) 'Suicidal behaviour', *The Psychologist*, 14 (1): 20–4.

Scourfield, J. (2005) 'Suicidal masculinities', *Sociological Research Online*, 10: 2.

Social Class

DEFINITION

The term 'social class' has been used in a variety of ways in social science and remains contested. There is little doubt that all societies contain some people at the top who are rich and powerful and those at the bottom who are poor and powerless. The debates about social class, then, revolve around ways of defining and measuring differences in the strata that exist between these extremes.

KEY POINTS

- Problems in defining social class are outlined.
- The relationship between social class and mental health problems is discussed, along with difficulties in interpreting the meaning of the relationship.

Overall, the relationship between social class and mental health is straightforward. The lower a person's social class position, the higher the probability of them being diagnosed with a mental health problem. However, this broad generalisation contains contradictions and uncertainties, which are discussed below. Before that, it should be noted that social class remains contested within social science. Social stratification is defined within these debates by various combinations of labour market position, socio-economic status, prestige, educational level, rank and property.

A relevant shift in Western European societies in the past 50 years has been from a pyramid structure of class to one of a diamond. The peak for both remains the same (the minority who are very rich and powerful). However, there has been a reduction in blue-collar work, the traditional notion of manual working-class people working in manufacturing industries, and an enlargement of white-collar labour in service industries. The latter does not imply high levels of earning. Moreover, many in the service sector are in insecure employment. At the base of the new diamond is a group sometimes called the 'underclass', or what Marx and Engels called the 'lumpenproletariat'. These are people who are unemployed and often unemployable. They represent a social class which is reproduced, in a stable fashion, over several generations. They are chronically outside the labour market, poorly educated, living in poverty and susceptible to a range of social problems including substance abuse, mental health problems and criminality.

SOCIAL CLASS PREDICTS DIAGNOSIS

The overall correlation between social class and mental health – the class gradient of an inverse relationship between class position and prevalence of mental health problems – contains exceptions. Some diagnoses occur less frequently in lower class groups. These include eating disorders and obsessive-compulsive personality disorder. However, these are exceptions that prove the rule. The prevalence of those

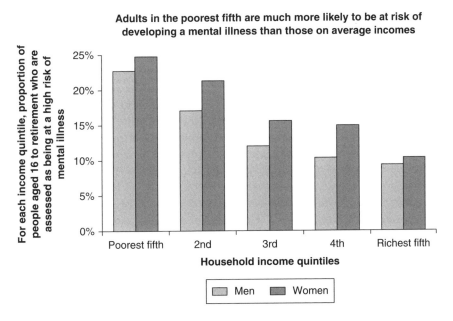

Figure 4.4   Data from England on social class and a diagnosis of mental illness

Note: It is notable that women in all social classes are more likely to receive a diagnosis of mental illness. This arises largely because of higher rates of diagnosed depression in primary care settings. (Men are over-represented by contrast in specialist secondary care facilities.)

diagnosed with anxiety states, depression, antisocial personality disorder and schizophrenia (between them the most common diagnoses made in specialist mental health services) is significantly higher in the poorest stratum of society. (The entry on Causes and Consequences of Mental Health Problems also points out that labour market disadvantage is important but not straightforward.) Data from England on social class and a diagnosis of mental illness are indicated in Figure 4.4.

The chronically unemployed are less distressed than those who are poorly employed (in stressful, poorly paid and insecure jobs). Single marital status is also a good predictor of mental health problems. As with class itself, the question then begged is whether the disadvantage of a single status is a product or cause of mental health problems, which leads to the next point.

THE DIRECTION OF CAUSALITY REMAINS UNCERTAIN

A problem for psychiatric epidemiology is that it only maps cases not causes. This is because, for the functional diagnoses, causes are unknown or in dispute. Consequently, two antagonistic hypotheses have arisen, when a correlation is found between the prevalence of a diagnosis and a social variable. The first assumes that social stress causes mental health problems. The second assumes that inherited or acquired causes of mental health problems lead to the patient being socially disadvantaged. In the first case, high prevalence rates in the lower classes are taken to indicate the particular stressors associated with poverty. In the second case, it is assumed that the patient's illness leads to a downward 'social drift'. Usually, the term 'social selection' hypothesis is used to connote this idea about social drift. A common intermediate position is the 'stress–vulnerability' hypothesis, which contends that patients susceptible to developing mental health problems may be buffered from this outcome by protective benign social conditions or precipitated into a mental health problem by adverse conditions. It is certainly the case that, in all social classes, people have a mixture of stressful events and buffering or protective experiences. However, the richer and more powerful a person is, the more likely it is that the ratio of the two favours the protective experiences. A further complication here is that each of the three hypotheses may be more likely for some problems than others. For example, post-traumatic stress disorder is fairly well predicted by external stressors. Emergency service workers and battered wives have high prevalence rates of PTSD. In the case of the 'common cold' of psychiatry, 'depression', higher rates are found in the unemployed. However, not all acutely stressed people develop PTSD and not all unemployed people are depressed. This point suggests that individual differences exist about vulnerability within the same social circumstances.

At the same time, diagnoses favoured for the social selection hypotheses, such as 'schizophrenia', do not follow neat genetic rules. Here, the converse argument applies: why is it that some people, but not others, become psychotic in those with a genetic loading? It is probable that the peculiar stressors affecting vulnerable individuals trigger a mental health problem. These cautions, about the interpretation of the interaction between social stress and individual vulnerability, indicate that any particular diagnostic outcome is likely to have multi-factorial antecedents or aetiological pathways.

THE RELEVANCE OF THE UNCERTAIN DIRECTION OF CAUSALITY

Much of the argument about direction of causality is linked to the ideological investment of the protagonists. It matters to those on the political left that there is an evidence base for the health-sapping effects of poverty and social disadvantage. Evidence for the social stress hypothesis is also evidence for the need for social justice. Equally, it matters to those on the political right that poverty and social disadvantage can be accounted for by the behaviour or biology of their inhabitants. Genetic faults or fecklessness in the poor can be used to justify a natural order of inequality. Leaving aside these ideological preferences, the personal consequences of having a mental health problem become an overriding consideration of patients rather than the causes. (This point is further discussed in the entries on Causes and Consequences of Mental Health Problems and on Stigma and Social Exclusion.) If the direction of primary causes remains in question, this is not the case for the relapse and maintenance of problems. In other words, a consequence of being stigmatised, socially excluded and living in poor conditions is that people with pre-existing mental health problems are made vulnerable to relapse and find recovery extra difficult, compared to those who are better off and more powerful.

See also: *causes and consequences of mental health problems; race; social exclusion; stigma.*

FURTHER READING

Dohrenwend, B.P. (1990) 'Socioeconomic status (SES) and psychiatric disorders: are the issues still compelling?', *Social Psychiatry and Psychiatric Epidemiology*, 25: 4–47.

Eaton, W.W. and Muntaner, C. (1999) 'Socioeconomic stratification and mental disorder', in A.V. Horwitz and T.L. Scheid (eds), *A Handbook for the Study of Mental Health*. Cambridge: Cambridge University Press.

Rogers, A. and Pilgrim, D. (2003) *Mental Health and Inequality*. Basingstoke: Palgrave.

Savage, M. et al. (2013) 'A new model of social class: findings from the BBC's Great British Class Survey Experiment', *Sociology*, (online) 2 April. doi: 10.1177/0038038513481128.

race

Race

DEFINITION

Race is controversial to define. Genetic distinctions between groups of humans (other than those based on sex) have little empirical basis. Racial distinctions arose from anthropological investigations carried out by colonial powers and reflected the social categorisations of colonised indigenous people. However, because of colonisation, the social identity of these people became real to them and others.

KEY POINTS

- Case studies of Afro-Caribbean and Irish people are provided to illustrate the relationship between race and mental health in a British post-colonial context.
- Implications for understanding racial differences in mental health are discussed.

As the above definition indicates, race is scientifically dubious but socially real. For example, people of African origin dispersed by the slave trade throughout the Americas and economic migration later in Europe now willingly call themselves 'black'. The relevance of this general sociopolitical point is that the health, including mental health, of previously colonised or enslaved people can be studied. When this happens, we find that it is the shared post-colonial context which predicts differences in mental health status, not particular physical characteristics such as skin colour. This is illustrated in the British post-colonial context by examining the mental health of Afro-Caribbean and Irish people.

THE MENTAL HEALTH OF AFRO-CARIBBEAN PEOPLE

The term Afro-Caribbean (increasingly shifting to 'African-Caribbean') refers to black people who either still live in the Caribbean or have moved to Britain. The term is now also used to describe their British-born children and grandchildren ('British-born blacks'). Britain is an ex-colonial power, which enslaved and forcibly transported African people. African-Caribbean people have higher rates of diagnosis for schizophrenia but lower rates for depression and suicide than indigenous whites (Cochrane, 1977). Young males are particularly likely to be diagnosed as psychotic. Higher rates of cannabis use in this group and their style of public behaviour, which is out of sync with the indigenous white culture, have been mooted as contributory factors in this picture. The cultural gap, in norms of behaviour and the problems of intelligibility that this creates, is discussed by Littlewood and Lipsedge (1997). Young male African-Caribbeans are particularly over-represented in secure provision and on locked wards (Mohan et al., 1997; Fernando et al., 1998). An unresolved debate about over-representation is whether it is actual (black and Irish people are mad more often) or whether it is a function of misdiagnosis (Sashidharan, 1993). The hypotheses are, of course, not mutually exclusive. Reviewing the competing hypotheses of raised prevalence rates of diagnosed schizophrenia in African-Caribbeans, Jablensky (1999) concluded that 'the causes of the Afro-Caribbean phenomenon remain obscure'.

THE MENTAL HEALTH OF IRISH PEOPLE

The data on Irish people highlight why the stresses of racism, based purely on skin colour, are not an adequate explanation for the differences in mental health status. Comparisons between Irish and other whites in Great Britain show the former to have twice the incidence of depression and psychosis and three times the rate of alcohol-related problems (Bracken et al., 1998). Only African-Caribbeans have higher rates of psychosis (Sproston and Nazroo, 2002). A variety of hypotheses about the over-representation of the Irish in psychiatric statistics addressing child-rearing practices, alienation from an imposed English ruling-class culture, poverty, the overbearing and sexually repressive nature of the Catholic Church and the confusions of a post-colonial identity can be found in the literature (Scheper-Hughes, 1979; Kenny, 1985; O'Mahony and Delanty, 1998). Also, the proximity of Great Britain to Eire and the ease of migration have enabled the Irish to leave home in less planned ways than other ethnic minorities. Unplanned migration increases the probability of depressive symptoms (Ryan et al., 2006).

IMPLICATIONS

What are the implications of comparing and contrasting these two ex-colonised groups for our understanding of the relationship between race and mental health?

The first point to emphasise is that, given the white skin of the Irish, racism based on skin colour may be a stressor but is not one that accounts for racial differences in mental health. A confirmation of this is that young Asian men are not over-represented in psychiatric populations but young African-Caribbean men are (Cochrane and Bal, 1989).

A second point is that, while both groups are post-colonial remnants of forced migration, the circumstances for each were different. The Irish were not enslaved but starved and dispossessed by British landlords. Africans lost or adapted their languages when they encountered English. In Ireland, Gaelic was suppressed – a trend of the English colonisers on the Celtic fringe throughout the British Isles.

Third, the circumstances of migration to Great Britain were similar in some ways but not others. Employment opportunities governed population movement in each. However, it was a continuous flow from the proximate Ireland over two centuries but only for prescribed limited periods for those from the Caribbean. During the 1950s and 1960s, they both encountered hateful notices in rental housing, such as 'No blacks. No Irish. No dogs.' Both were poor groups in unskilled or semi-skilled work. While the West Indian immigrants came to a perceived 'motherland', the island of Ireland was under continued British occupation and fought an unresolved war of independence with its colonising neighbour. Migrants criss-crossing the Irish Sea embodied this tension. These histories of slavery and starvation, and the alienation they created in both, culturally resonated down the generations of each group.

Fourth, as ex-colonised people, African-Caribbeans and the Irish have been recurrently stigmatised and rejected. For those born in Britain, they have nowhere to 'return to'. As a consequence, the mental health system, as an extension of the apparatus of coercive control of the state, is a repository for internal banishment. It is a place of segregation for those whose 'origin, sentiment or citizenship assigns them elsewhere' (Gilroy, 1987). A confirmation of this point is that these groups are also over-represented in the prison population, not just in involuntary specialist mental health services.

Fifth, and following on from the previous point, whatever the causal explanations for over-representation, the racial bias means that these groups are disproportionately dealt with by specialist mental health services. As the latter are dominated by coercion, this outcome can be thought of as a form of structural disadvantage for these groups, which leads to higher rates of social control for some black and ethnic groups compared to others.

See also: *eugenics; segregation; temporo-spatial aspects of mental abnormality.*

FURTHER READING

Nazroo, J. and Iley, K. (2011) 'Ethnicity, race and mental disorder in the UK', in D. Pilgrim, A. Rogers and B. Pescosolido (eds), *SAGE Handbook of Mental Health and Illness*. London: Sage.

Sproston, K. and Nazroo, J. (eds) (2002) *Ethnic Minority Psychiatric Illness Rates in the Community (EMPIRIC)*. London: Stationery Office.

REFERENCES

Bracken, P.J., Greenslade, L., Griffen, B. and Smyth, M. (1998) 'Mental health and ethnicity: an Irish dimension', *British Journal of Psychiatry*, 172: 103–5.

Cochrane, R. (1977) 'Mental illness in immigrants to England and Wales: an analysis of mental hospital admissions, 1971', *Social Psychiatry*, 12: 2–35.

Cochrane, R. and Bal, S. (1989) 'Mental hospital admission rates of immigrants to England: a comparison of 1971 and 1981', *Social Psychiatry*, 24: 2–11.

Fernando, S., Ndegwa, D. and Wilson, M. (1998) *Forensic Psychiatry, Race and Culture*. London: Routledge.

Gilroy, P. (1987) *There Ain't No Black in the Union Jack*. London: Hutchinson.

Jablensky, A. (1999) 'Schizophrenia: epidemiology', *Current Opinion in Psychiatry*, 12: 19–28.

Kenny, V. (1985) 'The post-colonial personality', *Crane Bag*, 9: 70–8.

Littlewood, R. and Lipsedge, M. (1997) *Aliens and Alienists: Ethnic Minorities and Psychiatry*. Harmondsworth: Penguin.

Mohan, D., Murray, K., Taylor, P. and Stead, P. (1997) 'Developments in the use of regional secure unit beds over a 12-year period', *Journal of Forensic Psychiatry*, 2: 321–35.

O'Mahony, P. and Delanty, G. (1998) *Rethinking Irish History: Nationalism, Identity and Ideology*. Basingstoke: Macmillan.

Ryan, L., Leavey, G., Golden, A., Blizard, R. and King, M. (2006) 'Depression in Irish migrants living in London: case control study', *British Journal of Psychiatry*, 18 (8): 560–6.

Sashidharan, S.P. (1993) 'Afro-Caribbeans and schizophrenia: the ethnic vulnerability hypothesis re-examined', *International Review of Psychiatry*, 5: 129–44.

Scheper-Hughes, N. (1979) *Saints, Scholars and Schizophrenics*. Berkeley, CA: University of California Press.

Sproston, K. and Nazroo, J. (eds) (2002) *Ethnic Minority Psychiatric Illness Rates in the Community (EMPIRIC)*. London: Stationery Office.

key concepts in mental health

Gender/Sex

> ## DEFINITION
>
> *Gender refers to descriptions of the role division of girls and boys and men and women in society. Sex refers to descriptions of a division based on biological features of the internal and external genitalia. Gender is a social description and sex is a biological one. In practice, often the two terms are used interchangeably in the professional literature.*

KEY POINTS

- The complex relationship between gender, sex and mental health is outlined.
- Factors accounting for the relationship are discussed.

SOME PRELIMINARY COMMENTS ON TERMINOLOGY

In social science, the term 'gender' is contested. Sometimes it is conflated with biological sex (see some of the references given below that demonstrate this point). However, sometimes 'gender' only signals the psychosocial features of conforming to, or being at variance with, normative expectations of a boy/man or a girl/woman. What is at issue here is whether sex, *not just gender*, is socially constructed. Researchers and political campaigners, trans-activists and radical feminists take opposing views on this matter.

The distinction between biological sex, on the one hand, and variance in social role and forms of conduct linked to current notions of masculinity or femininity in a society, on the other hand, has been complicated further by the recent heated controversy about trans identities. Gender critical feminists deny that transwomen are women and transmen are men, reversing the assertions of trans-activists. Accordingly, the long-term goal of gender critical feminists is to abolish the notion of gender, which for research purposes would take us back to a simpler time when we only made a distinction between the sexes. Some trans-activists favour a medicalised approach to gender alteration, but others reject this. For a longer discussion of this current debate, see Pilgrim (2018).

Whether or not trans phenomena represent forms of mental disorder or are merely variations on personal identity, requiring no medicalisation, merely self-identification, is then a matter of debate within and between these ideologically opposed groups. This ambiguity and current discursive confusion are mentioned here as a prelude to the reporting of the themes in the literature summarised below. However, some points are clear for now. For example, transwomen cannot develop puerpal psychosis or post-natal depression for the simple reason that they cannot give birth. However, some trans-activists point to an expanded medicalised future in which transwomen might receive a womb transplant.

SEX DIFFERENCES AND MENTAL HEALTH

The relationship between natal sex and mental health is complex and it contains a core contradiction. On the one hand, generally, women are more likely to receive a psychiatric diagnosis, although, as will be noted later, this claim is sometimes contested. On the other hand (and this claim is certain), men are more likely to be treated coercively within specialist mental health services. The key phrase here is 'more likely'. With the inevitable exception of diagnoses linked to female physiology, such as 'premenstrual tension' and 'premenstrual syndrome', men and women may receive any diagnosis. And, although secure mental health services are overwhelmingly populated by male patients, women can be found in them. While they are in a minority in secure services, women tend to be more vulnerable to abuse in them than are men.

Most of the over-representation calculated for women is accounted for by particular diagnoses (especially depression, panic disorder, agoraphobia, borderline personality disorder and eating disorders) (Lepine and Lellouch, 1995; Gelder et al., 2001). Most of the male over-representation in secure services is reflected in, and arises from, the higher prevalence of antisocial personality disorder and the management of some sex offenders within mental health facilities. The great majority of sex offenders are men. Sex differences are not apparent across the life span in relation to the diagnosis of the main functional psychoses of schizophrenia and bi-polar disorder but the dementias are more prevalent in women (because on average they live longer). The peri-natal period can affect the mental health of both women and men. Women giving birth can develop puerpal psychosis, and depressive and anxiety symptoms increase in both mothers and fathers (Gavin et al., 2005; Epifanio et al., 2015; Leach et al., 2016; Nath et al., 2016).

The inclusion or exclusion of certain diagnoses, when comparing men and women, can make the difference in representation between the two groups appear to be significant or non-existent. Moreover, claims about female over-representation have only appeared since the Second World War – there is little evidence from before then that sex differences in diagnosis were present. Arguments prevail, then, about whether levels of representation are real or whether they reflect methodological artefacts (Gove and Geerken, 1977; Busfield, 1982; Nazroo, 1995).

A number of points can be developed about this complex picture:

- *Professional decision-making may be gendered* Some feminists have argued that, from its inception, the profession of psychiatry has targeted female deviance (e.g. Chesler, 1972). Showalter (1987) argued that women were over-represented in the Victorian asylums. However, Busfield (1996) notes that a more careful look at the evidence for this claim reveals that

Showalter's case is unfounded. Women lived longer in the asylums so their numbers were greater. Busfield argues that female over-representation in the asylum system was thus an artefact of the life span and was not, as Showalter claims, evidence of a patriarchal psychiatric focus on female madness. There is some evidence that in primary care, GPs are more likely to identify mental health problems in women than men (Barrett and Roberts, 1978; Goldberg and Huxley, 1980). This is not merely a matter of more frequent contact (see the next point), but it also seems to reflect sex stereotyping by medical practitioners.

- *Gender representation may reflect type of service contact* There is a strong case for arguing that much of the gender difference can be accounted for by service contact differences and the style of help seeking. Women consult GPs more frequently than men (Rickwood and Braithwaite, 1994). Also, when men do consult, they are less disclosing about distress than women (Blaxter, 1990). As a consequence, diagnoses made in a voluntary context will be applied less often to men. Moreover, the high contact with primary care services has led to the excessive prescription of psychotropic drugs to women for neurotic distress (Gabe and Lipshitsz-Phillips, 1982). For this reason, iatrogenic addiction to prescribed medication is greater in women than men.

- *Academic and journalistic accounts may be gendered* There has been a tendency for the social scientific academic discourse to conflate gender with women (Cameron and Bernades, 1998). This has had the effect, at times, of skewing research interest in mental health, with the consequence that we know more about women's mental health than men's. A good example of this is the seminal study by Brown and Harris (1978) of women and depression. This began as a study of *social class* and depression in the community, with the original intention of studying male as well as female respondents. However, this gender-balanced aspiration was dropped because the researchers predicted that women were more likely to be at home to be interviewed than men. Another example of skewed interest is in relation to the consequences of higher levels of prescribed medication for women noted in the previous point. This has been associated with a portrayal in the mass media of women being weaker and more dependent than men because of their higher rate of addiction to prescribed drugs (Bury and Gabe, 1990).

- *Changes over the life span in gender differences in common mental health problems might implicate sex role differences* Prepubescent boys have more mental health problems than girls but this balance goes into reverse at puberty (Angold et al., 1998) and then later equalises in relation to the diagnosis of depression (Bebbington et al., 1998).

- *Social stress may generate real sex differences in mental health* Gove (1984) argues that the differences in rates of diagnosis are mainly a function of differences in social stress. This is most evident in relation to eating disorders and sexual victimisation. In the former case, social pressures about body image affect females more than males. In the latter case, women are more frequently victims of sex attacks than men. However, men are more frequently victims of physical assault from strangers. Domestic violence is often discussed in terms of singular female victimisation. However, the evidence suggests that sex differences are actually small or even non-existent (in terms of reported rates of assaults) (Rogers and Pilgrim, 2003). But women are more seriously injured in violent incidents and are more likely to remain traumatised (Nazroo, 1995). Trauma leads to a range of post-traumatic symptoms, including anxiety, depression and panic disorder. If trauma is gendered in society, then this will translate into gendered mental health problems.

- *Mental health services are an extension of the state apparatus of social control* This point is fairly unambiguous in relation to male dangerousness. Men are over-represented in both prisons and secure mental health facilities. Generally, men are violent more often than women. As a consequence, men with mental health problems are violent more often than women with mental health problems and they are treated more restrictively within the mental health system, as they are elsewhere.

To summarise, when we try to account for gender differences in diagnosis, treatment and service contact, a number of factors may be operating. Some of these are competing hypotheses. Some are not mutually exclusive. Also, the topic of gender exemplifies a tension between one explanatory approach, which focuses on constructs or the social negotiation of gendered mental health (for example, the potential bias in professional decision-making and the skewed academic focus on women), and another based on causal empirical claims of real differences. For example, because women suffer peculiar social stresses, live longer and contact health services more than men and in a different way, these real differences produce direct effects on the recorded incidence and prevalence of mental health problems. Gender differences probably represent the outcome of a mixture of real and socially-constructed processes. For now, though, the list provided above is not a formula for a strong consensus about this concluding point. It is more an arena of dispute.

See also: *causes and consequences of mental health problems; fear; forensic mental health services; primary care; sadness; temporo-spatial aspects of mental abnormality.*

FURTHER READING

Busfield, J. (1996) *Men, Women and Madness: Understanding Gender and Mental Disorder.* London: Macmillan.
Cameron, E. and Bernades, J. (1998) 'Gender and disadvantage in health: men's health for a change', *Sociology of Health and Illness*, 20 (5): 673–93.

REFERENCES

Angold, A., Costello, E.J. and Worthman, C.M. (1998) 'Puberty and depression: the roles of age, pubertal status and pubertal timing', *Psychological Medicine*, 28 (1): 1275–88.

key concepts in
mental health

Barrett, M. and Roberts, H. (1978) 'Doctors and their patients', in H. Smart and B. Smart (eds), *Women, Sexuality and Social Control*. London: Routledge and Kegan Paul.

Bebbington, P.E., Dunn, G., Jenkins, R., Lewis, G., Brugha, T., Farrell, M. and Meltzer, H. (1998) 'The influence of age and sex on the prevalence of depression conditions: report from the National Survey of Psychiatric Morbidity', *Psychological Medicine, 28* (1): 9–19.

Blaxter, M. (1990) *Health and Lifestyles*. London: Routledge.

Brown, G. and Harris, T. (1978) *The Social Origins of Depression*. London: Tavistock.

Bury, M. and Gabe, J. (1990) 'Hooked? Media responses to tranquilizer dependence', in P. Abbott and G. Payne (eds), *New Directions in the Sociology of Health*. London: Falmer Press.

Busfield, J. (1982) 'Gender and mental illness', *International Journal of Mental Health, 11* (12): 46–66.

Busfield, J. (1996) *Men, Women and Madness: Understanding Gender and Mental Disorder*. London: Macmillan.

Cameron, E. and Bernades, J. (1998) 'Gender and disadvantage in health: men's health for a change', *Sociology of Health and Illness, 20* (5): 673–93.

Chesler, P. (1972) *Women and Madness*. New York: Doubleday.

Epifanio, M.S., Genna, V., DeLuca, C., Roccella, M. and La Grutta, S. (2015) 'Paternal and maternal transition to parenthood: the risk of postpartum depression and parenting stress', *Pediatric Reports*, 7: 58–72.

Gabe, J. and Lipshitsz-Phillips, S. (1982) 'Evil necessity? The meaning of benzodiazepine use for women patients from one general practice', *Sociology of Health and Illness, 4* (2): 201–11.

Gavin, N.I., Gaynes, B.N., Lohr, K.N., Meltzer-Brody, S., Gartlehner, G. and Swinson, T. (2005) 'Perinatal depression: a systematic review of prevalence and incidence', *Obstetrics & Gynaecology, 106*: 1071–83.

Gelder, M., Mayou, R. and Cowen, P. (2001) *Shorter Oxford Textbook of Psychiatry*. Oxford: Oxford University Press.

Goldberg, D. and Huxley, P. (1980) *Mental Illness in the Community*. London: Tavistock.

Gove, W. (1984) 'Gender differences in mental and physical illness: the effects of fixed and nurturant roles', *Social Science and Medicine, 19* (2): 77–91.

Gove, W. and Geerken, M. (1977) 'Response bias in surveys of mental health: an empirical investigation', *American Journal of Sociology, 82*: 1289–317.

Leach, L.S., Poyser, C., Cooklin, A.R. and Giallo, R. (2016) 'Prevalence and course of anxiety disorders (and symptom levels) in men across the perinatal period: a systematic review', *Journal of Affective Disorders, 190*: 675–86.

Lepine, J.P. and Lellouch, J. (1995) 'Diagnosis and epidemiology of agoraphobia and social phobia', *Clinical Neuropharmacology, 18* (2): 15–26.

Nath, S., Psychogiou, L., Kuyken, W., Ford, T., Ryan, E. and Russell, G. (2016) 'The prevalence of depressive symptoms among fathers and associated risk factors during the first seven years of their child's life: findings from the Millennium Cohort Study', *BMC Public Health, 16*: 509.

Nazroo, J.Y. (1995) 'Uncovering gender differences in the use of marital violence: the effect of methodology', *Sociology, 29* (3): 475–9.

Pilgrim, D. (2018) 'Reclaiming reality and redefining realism: the challenging case of transgenderism', *Journal of Critical Realism, 17* (3): 1–17.

Rickwood, D.J. and Braithwaite, V.A. (1994) 'Social psychological factors affecting help seeking for emotional problems', *Social Science and Medicine, 39* (4): 563–72.

Rogers, A. and Pilgrim, D. (2003) *Mental Health and Inequality*. Basingstoke: Palgrave.

Showalter, E. (1987) *The Female Malady*. London: Virago.

gender/sex

Age

DEFINITION

This entry refers to the relationship across the life span between chronological age and mental health status.

KEY POINTS

- Childhood has been the focus of competing theories about the development of mental health problems.
- Childhood and older adulthood are times of particular vulnerability to mental health problems.

The relationship between age and mental health has been considered important broadly for two reasons. First, the idea that childhood is a phase of life when mental abnormality is primarily generated has held the attention of many researchers and theorists. Second, a longitudinal map of the relationship between age and mental health status reveals sociopolitical features about the life span. This section will address both of these points.

THE ROLE OF CHILDHOOD IN THE GENESIS OF MENTAL HEALTH PROBLEMS

In the entry on Causes and Consequences of Mental Health Problems, it was noted that explanations for mental health problems remain varied. Biodeterminism, especially if it focuses on genetic explanations, minimises the role of the post-natal environment. However, although many psychiatrists are biodeterminists, it is common for them to emphasise the interaction of biological vulnerability and environmental stressors. The latter are distributed unevenly across populations and across the life span.

Psychological theories place more of an emphasis upon the location of these uneven stressors in childhood. This can be seen in both psychoanalysis, with its emphasis on the dynamics of family life being internalised into psychodynamics in the child, and behaviourism, with its emphasis on the conditioning of anxiety responses. A further ambiguity is that some psychological theories, such as Kleinian psychoanalysis, conceded that individual differences in the inheritance of aggression can alter the proneness of the developing child to develop forms of psychopathology. By contrast, other psychoanalytical writers, such as Winnicott (1958) and Bowlby (1951), emphasise the direct impact in infancy of environmental insults. This branch of psychoanalysis is much closer to the view advanced by behaviourists. Social theories of mental abnormality also emphasise the role of vulnerability in childhood, although multi-factorial models, such as that offered by

Brown and Harris (1978), suggest that contemporary contextual factors, and not just historical ones, are important.

DIFFERENCES IN MENTAL HEALTH ACROSS THE LIFE SPAN

Whatever the competing theories say about childhood, one thing that is not in doubt is that general measures of mental health seem to indicate that it is a difficult phase of life. Community studies suggest that between 11 and 26 per cent of children manifest distress or dysfunction, although only 3 to 6 per cent of under-16s receive the attention of specialist mental health services (Bird et al., 1988; Costello et al., 1988). According to these studies, the prevalence of mental health problems in children has increased in recent times. Dysfunctional children then go on to experience educational disadvantage. In turn, this leads to labour market disadvantage in later life and an increased probability of criminal activity. Another consequence of increased identification or labelling of children with mental health problems has been the contention about the increase in psychotropic medication imposed on children (they cannot give adult informed consent) (Bentall and Morrison, 2002; Olfson et al., 2002; Timimi, 2002; McLeod et al., 2004; Sparks and Duncan, 2004).

When the family environment of distressed or dysfunctional children is studied, it is evident that they are subjected to high levels of neglect and abuse, with estimates ranging from 20 to 65 per cent (Quinn and Epstein, 1998). These pathogenic families are also disproportionately poor, although because of the range of mental health problems in childhood and variations in the mediating role of family life, it is important not to see the link between poverty and distress as being direct and simple. Not only do many poor families produce psychologically robust children, but also many richer families do not. What is at issue here are statistical tendencies. Poverty increases the risk of mental health problems (throughout the life span) but does not singularly determine those problems.

One of the main stressors in childhood with good predictive value is sexual abuse. The main version of this is intra-familial abuse, with step-fathers being more likely to be the abuser than biological fathers. Sexual abuse occurs in all social classes. Girls are more at risk of intra-familial abuse, but boys are more likely to be abused by paedophiles from outside the family (Rogers and Pilgrim, 2003).

Childhood problems transfer into adulthood. Longitudinal studies looking at cohorts of children from birth to adulthood (for example, the 1970 British Cohort Study and the 1958 National Child Development Study) demonstrate this abiding impact of early childhood difficulties. The interaction of social class position and existence of mental health problems becomes particularly relevant. These studies demonstrate that:

- The existence of psychological problems and lower paternal class in adolescence predicts enduring mental health problems in adulthood.
- Achieved social class in adulthood is also predicted by paternal class and the existence of psychological problems in adolescence.

- The continuation of psychological difficulties is greater for men than women.
- Women demonstrate more inter-generational social mobility than men.

The highest rates of mental health problems occur in children and in the very old (Wade and Cairney, 1997), and so we need to adopt a life-course approach to understanding both physical and mental health (Mheen et al., 1998). In old age, the biopsychosocial model finds its greatest fit. Older people encounter a number of interacting challenges to their mental health:

- The incidence and prevalence of dementia increase with age.
- However, twice as many people over 70 are depressed than are dementing.
- Depression in old age is a function of psychological factors, such as cumulative bereavement reactions, as peers die around survivors (Clayton, 1998).
- Depression is also a function of somato-psychological reactions to multiple illnesses. Ageing increases the chances of co-morbidity and the latter brings with it disability and pain. These experiences in turn are depressing. Only 3 per cent of men and 20 per cent of women referred to specialist mental health services in old age are physically well (Dover and McWilliam, 1992). Only one in five older medical inpatients recovers from a depressed mood before they die (Cole and Bellevance, 1997).
- There are gender differences in ageing. Women live slightly longer than men and so the prevalence of dementia is greater in females. When men are widowed, they cope less well than women with losing their spouse (Clayton, 1998). For this reason, the risk of suicidal behaviour increases in older men. So, too, does the risk of substance misuse. Alcohol abuse in older men increases the chances both of depressive episodes and of premature death from cirrhosis of the liver (Helsing et al., 1982).
- Social factors are also relevant to predicting mental health problems in older people. The direct impact of poverty is one factor. Another is the restricted access to close confiding relationships in older people as they lose intimacy when spouses and friends die. Also, social networks are restricted by changes in mobility. Housebound older people can less readily access their friends and relatives compared to younger days. Social contact is a protective factor against depression in all age groups and so limitations on such contact increase the risk of depression (Murphy, 1982). The chances of depression also increase with residential care (Blazer, 1994). A final social factor to consider is that of elder abuse. Older people are subjected to abuse sometimes by their informal or paid carers, with estimates or prevalence rates of abuse ranging from 8 to 15 per cent (Hydle, 1993). Paveza and colleagues (1992) found that 5.4 per cent of relatives of people with dementia were violent to patients within one year of the diagnosis. However, the same study found that 15.8 per cent of dementing patients were also violent, suggesting the possibility of an aggressive spiral in the carer–cared for relationship.
- Recent investigations of dementia have noted a cohort effect (Matthews et al., 2013). Basically, later-born older people have lower incidence rates of

dementia than those born earlier in the 20th century. This may be because of factors such as diet, exercise levels and medical care (for example, changes in the prescription of anti-hypertensive medication affect the incidence of vascular dementia).

See also: *causes and consequences of mental health problems; childhood adversity; physical health; social class*.

FURTHER READING

Matthews, F., Arthur, A., Barnes, L., Bond, J., Jagger, C., Robinson, L. and Brayne, C. (2013) 'A two-decade comparison of prevalence of dementia in individuals aged 65 years and older from three geographical areas of England: results of the Cognitive Function and Ageing Study I and II', *The Lancet*, 382 (9902): 1405–12. Online first 17 July, doi: 10.1016/S0140-6736(13)61570–6.

Timimi, S. (2002) *Pathological Child Psychiatry and the Medicalization of Childhood*. Hove: Brunner-Routledge.

REFERENCES

Bentall, R.P. and Morrison, A.P. (2002) 'More harm than good: the case against neuroleptics to prevent psychosis', *Journal of Mental Health*, 11: 351–6.

Bird, H., Canino, G., Rubio-Stipec, M. et al. (1988) 'Estimates of the prevalence of childhood maladjustment in a community survey in Puerto Rico', *Archives of General Psychiatry*, 43: 1120–6.

Blazer, D.G. (1994) 'Epidemiology of late-life depression', in I.S. Schneider, C.F. Reynolds, B.D. Lebowitz and A.J. Friedhoff (eds), *Diagnosis and Treatment of Depression in Late Life*. Washington, DC: American Psychiatric Press.

Bowlby, J. (1951) *Maternal Care and Mental Health*. Geneva: World Health Organization.

Brown, G. and Harris, T. (1978) *Social Origins of Depression*. London: Tavistock.

Clayton, P.J. (1998) 'The model of distress: the bereavement reaction', in B.P. Dohrenwend (ed.), *Adversity, Stress and Psychopathology*. Oxford: Oxford University Press.

Cole, M.G. and Bellevance, F. (1997) 'Depression in elderly medical inpatients: a meta-analysis of outcomes', *Canadian Medical Association Journal*, 157: 1055–60.

Costello, E.J., Edeibrook, C.S., Costello, A.J., Dulcan, M.K., Burns, B. and Brent, D. (1988) 'Psychiatric disorders in primary care: the new hidden morbidity', *Paediatrics*, 82: 415–23.

Dover, S. and McWilliam, C. (1992) 'Physical illness associated with depression in the elderly in community-based and hospital patients', *Psychiatric Bulletin*, 16: 612–13.

Helsing, K.J., Comstock, G.W. and Szklo, M. (1982) 'Causes of death in widowed populations', *American Journal of Epidemiology*, 116: 524–32.

Hydle, I. (1993) 'Abuse and neglect in the elderly – a Nordic perspective', *Scandinavian Journal of Social Science*, 21 (2): 126–8.

Matthews, F., Arthur, A., Barnes, L., Bond, J., Jagger, C., Robinson, L. and Brayne, C. (2013) 'A two-decade comparison of prevalence of dementia in individuals aged 65 years and older from three geographical areas of England: results of the Cognitive Function and Ageing Study I and II', *The Lancet*, 382 (9902): 1405–12. Online first 17 July, doi: 10.1016/S0140-6736(13)61570–6.

McLeod, J.D., Pescosolido, B.A., Takeuchi, D.T. and Falkenberg White, T. (2004) 'Public attitudes toward the use of psychiatric medications for children', *Journal of Health and Social Behavior*, 45 (1): 53–67.

Mheen, H., Stronks, K. and Mackenbach, J. (1998) 'A life course perspective on socioeconomic inequalities in health', *Sociology of Health and Illness*, *20* (5): 754–77.

Murphy, E. (1982) 'Social origins of depression in old age', *British Journal of Psychiatry*, *141*: 135–42.

Olfson, M., Marcus, S.C., Weissman, M.M. and Jensen, P.S. (2002) 'National trends in the use of psychotropic medications by children', *Journal of the American Academy of Child & Adolescent Psychiatry*, *41* (5): 514–21.

Paveza, G.J., Cohen, J.G. and Esdorfer, C. (1992) 'Severe family violence and Alzheimer's disease: prevalence and risk factors', *Gerontologist*, *32* (4): 493–7.

Quinn, K.P. and Epstein, M.H. (1998) 'Characteristics of children, youth and families served by local interagency systems of care', in M.H. Epstein, K. Kutash and A. Duchnowski (eds), *Outcomes for Children and Youth with Behavioural and Emotional Disorders*. Austin, TX: Pro-Ed.

Rogers, A. and Pilgrim, D. (2003) *Mental Health and Inequality*. Basingstoke: Palgrave.

Sparks, J.A. and Duncan, B.L. (2004) 'The ethics and science of medicating children', *Ethical Human Psychology and Psychiatry*, *6* (1): 25–40.

Timimi, S. (2002) *Pathological Child Psychiatry and the Medicalization of Childhood*. Hove: Brunner-Routledge.

Wade, T.J. and Cairney, J. (1997) 'Age and depression in a nationally representative sample of Canadians', *Canadian Journal of Public Health*, *88*: 297–302.

Winnicott, D.W. (1958) *Collected Works*. London: Hogarth Press.

The Pharmaceutical Industry

DEFINITION

The pharmaceutical industry is the generic term used to describe the activity of the drug companies, which research and market medication. Given the central role of the latter in psychiatric practice, the industry plays a central role in mental health work.

KEY POINTS

- Shifts in the salience of drug treatments are outlined.
- The role of the drug companies in maintaining the dominance of a biomedical approach to treatment is discussed.

The success of the pharmaceutical industry over the past 50 years has been intimately entwined with both changes, and custom and practice, in the medical profession. This point has been particularly applicable to the treatment of mental health problems for two reasons. First, although psychiatrists have certainly been eclectic (with some specialising in psychotherapy and a small number flirting with psychosurgery), the profession's treatment response has been overwhelmingly medicinal. Second, most mental health problems have been treated in primary care. GPs in the main have used drugs to treat 'mild to moderate' conditions, dominated by diagnoses of anxiety states and depression. For this reason, it is hardly surprising that the pharmaceutical industry has frequently targeted GPs when marketing psychotropic medication.

The symbiotic relationship between the medical profession and the drug companies can be thought of in three historical phases.

BEFORE THE 1950S – THE PRE-REVOLUTIONARY PHASE

It would be wrong to accuse the drug companies of being the primary determinant of the biomedical emphasis in psychiatry. From the beginning, in the Victorian period, the psychiatric profession emphasised biological causation. The shell-shock problem of the First World War momentarily diverted attention from this trajectory, allowing psychological theory and practice into the mental health service arena, but other than during periods of warfare it was a question of 'business as usual' in asylum psychiatry. Prior to the 1950s, psychiatrists had only a few biological options to calm patients: bromides, barbiturates, paraldehyde, opiates and a small number of synthesised tranquillisers, such as scopolamine. As a result, a medicinal response to madness was augmented by psychosurgery, seclusion, shocks (electrically or chemically induced), wet packs and baths. During this phase, the psychiatric profession tended to view drugs as one of a few options to combine to manage madness. They were not ascribed special curative powers. However, this was about to change.

THE 1950S – THE 'PHARMACOLOGICAL REVOLUTION'

After the Second World War, a number of drugs were introduced to treat mental health problems. For this reason, this period has been characterised as the 'pharmacological revolution'. This discourse of revolution was reflected in the aspirations claimed for drug treatments. It is at this point that terms like 'antipsychotic' and 'antidepressant' were coined. During the 1950s, the pharmaceutical industry began to compete vigorously to synthesise and market a few types of drug in response to specific mental disorders. Lithium salts were introduced for mood disorders. The first anti-psychotic was introduced (chlorpromazine), as well as the first anxiolytic (minor tranquillizer) to treat anxiety states – the benzodiazepine, Librium. Two types of antidepressants also appeared: the tricyclic drugs and the monoamine oxidase inhibitors.

AFTER THE 1950S – THE REVOLUTION POSTPONED?

Once the pattern of pharmacological optimism had been established, drugs began to dominate psychiatric practice. Some in the profession demonstrated that ward activity and psychosocial interventions were important components of treatment and rehabilitation. Others were to show that anti-psychotic and antidepressant medication had their best impact if complemented by psychological interventions. All too often, however, patients, whatever their diagnosis, were to find themselves being treated singularly with pills or injections. The reputation (but not the use) of drug treatments was to decline for a number of reasons.

Average dose levels of anti-psychotics began to rise, with the consequence that an international pandemic of iatrogenic movement disorders became evident. After the 1960s, psychotic patients were made obvious by their shuffling gait, twitching limbs and grimacing faces. In primary care, a different iatrogenic problem emerged. The widespread use of the benzodiazepines as minor tranquillisers and sleeping pills meant that many patients had become addicted to drugs that no longer had any therapeutic value for them. (The benefits of benzodiazepines wane after a couple of weeks.)

More iatrogenic problems were to follow. Because of high dose levels ('mega-dosing') and drug cocktails ('polypharmacy'), the anti-psychotics began to cause acute cardio-toxicity and sudden death in some patients. An irony here is that chlorpromazine was originally sold over the counter in oral form to prevent nausea and sickness. It only became a danger to life when it was administered by mental health professionals in injected form. Death rates also rose because of poor control of the adverse movement disorder effects of anti-psychotics.

One particular minor tranquilliser was to create a widely reported iatrogenic tragedy. In the early 1960s, Contergan (thalidomide) was marketed widely to GPs. It soon became evident that its administration during pregnancy was to create congenital deformities. Before the drug was withdrawn, over 6,000 babies had been born with severe physical abnormalities.

During the 1980s, newer forms of anti-psychotic and antidepressant agents were introduced, with claims to greater efficacy and fewer movement disorder effects than the older drugs, which had constituted the 'pharmacological revolution'. Yet, these were also not without their problems. Some caused blood abnormalities and had to be monitored closely (clozaril). Others were deemed unsafe in clinical practice and were withdrawn because of their cardio-toxic effects (sertindole). The new antidepressants proved particularly controversial as it became evident that they were associated with raised suicide rates and aggression in some patients.

Defenders of the continued central use of drugs for mental health problems point out that the risks that they create to patients have to be set against the benefits that accrue. For example, the newer antidepressants may raise the chances of suicide, but the older ones were more toxic and so created more accidental deaths. Also, untreated depression itself increases the risk of suicide. Moreover, drugs are cost-effective because they are much cheaper to deploy than labour-intensive alternatives (such as counselling or family therapy).

Probably the biggest credibility problem that the medical profession has in relation to drug treatments is the dominant role of the latter. User groups largely complain not of drug treatments *per se*, but of their unimaginative use. Typically, if a drug is not working, the prescriber will raise the dose level, try another version of the same class or add another drug. Patients (and their relatives) will ask for talking treatments instead of, or as well as, drug treatments. These demands reflect poor supply in mental health service routines. Ironically, these reasonable expectations are consistent with the evidence that maximum therapeutic effects occur when treatment packages combine drugs and talking treatments.

Doctors are over-reliant on drug company information to guide their practice and their professional training emphasises the prescription pad. Investment in psychological treatments is a low priority. Finally, the drug companies are highly enmeshed in the continued professional development of psychiatrists and GPs. They typically fund training events and use these as opportunities to promote new drugs and maintain a continued focus on a medicinal approach to mental health problems.

See also: *biological interventions; psychological interventions; segregation.*

FURTHER READING

Breggin, P. (1993) *Toxic Psychiatry*. London: Fontana.

Breggin, P. and Breggin, G. (1994) *Talking Back to Prozac*. New York: St. Martin's Press.

Brown, P. and Funk, S.C. (1986) 'Tardive dyskinesia: barriers to the professional recognition of iatrogenic disease', *Journal of Health and Social Behavior*, 27: 116–32.

Cosgrove, L., Bursztajn, H.J., Krimsky, S., Anaya, M. and Walker, J. (2009) 'Conflicts of interest and disclosure in the American Psychiatric Association's clinical practice guidelines', *Psychotherapy & Psychosomatics*, 78: 228–32.

Fisher, S. and Greenberg, R.P. (eds) (1997) *From Placebo to Panacea: Putting Psychiatric Drugs to the Test*. New York: Wiley.

Harris, G. and Carey, B. (2008) 'Researchers fail to reveal full drug pay', *The New York Times*, 8 June. Available at www.nytimes.com/2008/06/08/us/08conflict.html?pagewanted=all

Healy, D. (1997) *The Anti-depressant Era*. London: Harvester.

Healy, D. (2004) 'Psychopathology at the interface between the market and the new biology', in D. Rees and S. Rose (eds), *The New Brain Sciences: Perils and Prospects*. Cambridge: Cambridge University Press.

Klass, A. (1975) *There's Gold in Them Thar Pills*. Harmondsworth: Penguin.

Moncrieff, J. (2008) *The Myth of the Chemical Cure*. Basingstoke: Palgrave Macmillan.

Tyrer, P., Harrison-Read, P. and van Horn, E. (1997) *Drug Treatment in Psychiatry: A Guide for the Community Mental Health Worker*. Oxford: Butterworth/Heinemann.

Warfare

DEFINITION

'State of war, campaigning, being engaged in war …' (Concise English Dictionary).

- The impact of war on mental health policy and on psychiatric theory and practice is described.
- The governmental preoccupation with the dangerousness of patients is placed in the context of the scale of violence associated with modern warfare.
- The mental health impact on non-combatants in war conditions is summarised.

This entry appears in a book on mental health for two main reasons. First, warfare has been an important determinant of shifts in mental health policy and professional theory and practice. Second, it provides a global backdrop of violence against which to judge patient dangerousness.

THE IMPACT OF WAR ON POLICY, THEORY AND PRACTICE

By the end of the 19th century, the system of large asylums was defining the stable present and likely future of psychiatry. This institutional containment of madness, on behalf of civil society, was at the centre of this policy emphasis. All of this was to change with the First World War.

The eugenic emphasis in the asylums transferred poorly to these new conditions. Working-class volunteers and officers and gentlemen ('England's finest blood') broke down with predictable regularity in the war of attrition between 1914 and 1918 (Stone, 1985). 'Shell shock' (since variously dubbed 'war neurosis', 'battle fatigue' or 'post-traumatic stress disorder') simply could not be accounted for within the eugenic framework preferred by the medical superintendents of the civilian asylums. This view was tantamount to treason, if applied to soldier patients who were not conscripts. An alternative view, offered by the 'shell-shock' doctors, was that some form of interaction, between extreme external stress and inner psychological vulnerability, accounted for the symptoms evident in the casualties of the trenches (Salmon, 1917). These patients were not the assumed degenerates of the asylum system but decent, ordinary and, in civilian life, apparently mentally stable people, who had broken down under conditions of extreme adversity (Keane, 1998).

A psychosocial approach to mental disorder was thus made possible by the conditions of warfare. Moreover, the jurisdiction of psychiatry consequently shifted and expanded. Neurosis had been of little concern to the alienists and mad-doctors of the Victorian period. Conditions of warfare obliged all parties – psychiatrists, politicians, civil servants and the relatives of returning soldiers – to take another version of mental disorder seriously.

This wider view of the role of psychiatry in society influenced the first major British reform of mental health legislation since the 1890 Lunacy Act. The 1930 Mental Treatment Act introduced a voluntary status for some boarders in mental hospitals and indicated the beginnings of community care. By the time that a second period of hostility with Germany was becoming evident in the late 1930s, the government did not call upon asylum doctors for advice. Instead, the legacy of the shell-shock doctors was rewarded by a psychoanalyst, J.R. Rees, being appointed as head of the Army Psychiatric Services in 1938.

The Second World War was to have two major impacts in subsequent decades. First, the inability of the military medical services to deal individually with a new generation of traumatised combatants between 1939 and 1945 led to experiments in group work. Both group psychotherapy and therapeutic communities were created in this wartime period in military hospitals. Their legacy was to shape post-war NHS psychotherapy.

Another major impact of the Second World War was the invention of the term 'institutional neurosis', which was also called 'institutionalism' or 'institutionalisation'. (The last of these terms has proved to be confusing. In the literature, it also describes the policy of mass segregation in the asylums.) The germ of the concept of institutional neurosis came from the visit of a medical student with the Red Cross to observe the opening of the concentration camps. Russell Barton (1958) watched as skeletal inmates in unsanitary conditions paced around with arms folded. When asked to move to fresher and cleaner conditions by the liberating forces, the inmates refused. After the war, Barton noticed that psychiatric patients in the large asylums manifested similar stereotypical behaviour and an irrational dependency on the institution.

A final example of the impact of the Second World War occurred during the 1960s and 1970s in Italy. The shame of fascism and the sensitivities of warehousing devalued people out of sight and mind, given the post-war evidence of the labour and death camps, led to a strong movement for desegregation. In 1978, Law 180 was passed to close all large mental hospitals in Italy. A resonance about the camps probably influenced (but did not solely determine) the hospital run-down and closure throughout Western Europe.

WARFARE AS INSTITUTIONAL VIOLENCE

An irony of the governmental preoccupation with people with mental health problems as a source of violence is one of scale. If all of the acts of violence committed by individuals, globally, in the last 100 years (whether or not they were considered to be mentally disordered) were added together, the total would pale into insignificance in the context of warfare. The latter has been responsible for the recurrent mass killing of swathes of the civilian population by the military wing of the state in many countries during the same period. As Žižek (2008) has noted, by individualising the topic, we easily lose sight of systemic violence and the scale of its destruction.

The problem with the use of terms such as 'First World War' and 'Second World War' is that they understate the unending nature of global warfare. For example, between 1945 and 1990 there were 150 wars, leading to the deaths of 22 million people (Goldson, 1993). Since 1990, we have seen wars in the Balkans, the Middle East and Africa, all of which have continued this trend of state-sponsored mass killing. The pattern of modern warfare has been less and less about military casualties and more and more about the annihilation, persecution and traumatisation of millions of unarmed civilians. The psychological consequences for survivors are now immeasurable, as they extend into subsequent generations (Solkoff, 1992).

Unlike the patients they are concerned to control, for fear of violence towards others, politicians are unconstrained in their decision-making about embarking on or prolonging warfare. Far from being distrusted or socially controlled for their dangerous actions, politicians in this context are often the beneficiaries of violence. They stand to gain (and occasionally lose) votes. The loss of their liberty is rarely an outcome for them.

THE IMPACT OF WARFARE ON CIVILIAN MENTAL HEALTH

In 2005 the World Health Organization reported that for those living in areas of armed conflict, around 10 per cent will develop a serious mental disorder and another 10 per cent will have degrees of functional impairment. As well as PTSD, other common symptoms identified were depression, anxiety and insomnia, as well as back problems and gastro-intestinal disturbances (World Health Organization, 2005).

Although the shell shock problem has led to a focus on the mental health of combatants, in war zones they now tend to be in a minority. Miller and Rasmussen (2010) note that the trauma focus inherited from the combatant literature now needs to be placed in a wider social context for those civilian populations affected. For residents in war zones, all aspects of their daily life, which usually provide routines and the psychological stability or 'ontological security' they ensure, are disrupted.

If work is reduced or rendered impossible, then this affects earnings and access to basic necessities; the already poor will be made poorer. Supplies of water, fuel and electricity are constantly disrupted. Schooling may be rendered impossible and entering public spaces is fraught with danger. Homes may be lost or badly damaged. The uncertainty created by episodic violence is constantly distressing. A shortage of food supplies may soon lead to starvation and malnutrition. Together, these discontinuities to ordinary life and basic need satisfaction create open-ended and so chronic stressors on the population and all the likely symptoms of distress in their wake. The latter are added to the outcome we now associate more stereotypically with PTSD.

See also: *eugenics; mental health policy; risks to and from people with mental health problems; secondary prevention.*

FURTHER READING

Devakumar, D., Birch, M., Osrin, D. et al. (2014) 'The intergenerational effects of war on the health of children', *BMC Medicine*, 12: 57.

Murthy, R.S. and Lakshminarayana, R. (2006) 'Mental health consequences of war: a brief review of research findings', *World Psychiatry*, 5 (1): 25–30.

Shephard, B. (2002) *A War of Nerves: Soldiers and Psychiatrists 1914–1994*. London: Pimlico.

REFERENCES

Barton, W.R. (1958) *Institutional Neurosis*. Bristol: Wright and Sons.

Goldson, E. (1993) 'War is not good for children', in L.A. Leavitt and N.A. Fox (eds), *The Psychological Effects of War and Violence on Children*. Hillsdale, NJ: Erlbaum.

Keane, T.M. (1998) 'Psychological effects of human combat', in B.P. Dohrenwend (ed.), *Adversity, Stress and Psychopathology*. Oxford: Oxford University Press.

Miller, K.E. and Rasmussen, A. (2010) 'War exposure, daily stressors, and mental health in conflict and post-conflict settings: bridging the divide between trauma-focused and psychosocial frameworks', *Social Science & Medicine*, 70 (1): 7–16.

Salmon, T.W. (1917) 'The care and treatment of diseases and war neuroses: "shellshock" in the British Army', *Mental Hygiene*, 1: 509–75.

Solkoff, N. (1992) 'Children of survivors of the Holocaust: a critical review of the literature', *American Journal of Orthopsychiatry*, 62: 342–58.

Stone, M. (1985) 'Shellshock and the psychologists', in W.F. Bynum, R. Porter and M. Shepherd (eds), *The Anatomy of Madness*, Vol. 2. London: Tavistock.

World Health Organization (2005) *Resolution on Health Action in Crises and Disasters*. Geneva: World Health Organization.

Žižek, S. (2008) *Violence*. London: Profile.

Index

index

273